The authors of this book provide an entirely new perspective on how emotions influence mental and physical health. They present recent thinking about the development and regulation of emotions and argue that several common but difficult to treat psychiatric illnesses, including drug addictions, eating disorders, panic disorder, and post-traumatic stress disorders, are a consequence of an inability to regulate distressing emotions through mental processes. The book also advances a model in which dysregulated emotions may alter other bodily systems and thereby contribute to the development of physical illnesses and diseases. This book offers a valuable and stimulating reference for clinicians and researchers alike.

**DISORDERS OF AFFECT REGULATION**
Alexithymia in medical and psychiatric illness

# Disorders of affect regulation
## Alexithymia in medical and psychiatric illness

Graeme J. Taylor
*University of Toronto*

R. Michael Bagby
*University of Toronto*

James D.A. Parker
*Trent University, Peterborough, Ontario*

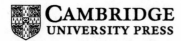

CAMBRIDGE
UNIVERSITY PRESS

PUBLISHED BY THE PRESS SYNDICATE OF THE UNIVERSITY OF CAMBRIDGE
The Pitt Building, Trumpington Street, Cambridge, United Kingdom

CAMBRIDGE UNIVERSITY PRESS
The Edinburgh Building, Cambridge CB2 2RU, UK www.cup.cam.ac.uk
40 West 20th Street, New York, NY 10011-4211, USA www.cup.org
10 Stamford Road, Oakleigh, Melbourne 3166, Australia
Ruiz do Alarcón 13, 28014 Madrid, Spain

First published 1997
First paperback edition 1999

*Typeface* Bembo 10.5/12pt. *System* Linotron 202

*A catalogue record for this book is available from the British Library*

*Library of Congress Cataloguing in Publication data*

Taylor, Graeme J.
    Disorders of affect regulation: alexithymia in medical and
psychiatric illness/Graeme J. Taylor, R. Michael Bagby, James D.A.
Parker
        p.   cm.
    Includes bibliographical references and index.
    ISBN 0 521 45610 X (hardback)
    1. Alexithymia.   2. Emotions – Health aspects.   3. Personality and
emotion.   I. Bagby, R. Michael.   II. Parker, James D.A. (James
Donald Alexander), 1959–   .   III. Title.
    [DNLM: 1. Affective Symptoms.   2. Mental Disorders.   3. Substance
Use Disorders.   WM 171 T241D   1996]
    RC540.T39   1996
    616.89–dc20   96–8520 CIP
    DNLM/DLC
for Library of Congress

ISBN 0 521 45610 X hardback
ISBN 0 521 77850 6 paperback

Transferred to digital printing 2003

To the memory of my friend and colleague Arthur H. Sohn   GJT

To the memory of my uncle James W. Bagby III      RMB

For Anne and Dorothy               JDAP

# Contents

# Foreword
# Alexithymia: the exception that proves the rule – of the unusual significance of affects

by James S. Grotstein, MD
University of California, Los Angeles

THE HEART HAS ITS REASONS THAT
REASON KNOWS NOT OF.

Pensées: *Pascal*

The work of these authors represents a signal contribution to the study of affects, emotions, and feelings, whether from the perspective of empirical research or for its clinical application to psychoanalysis and psychotherapy. Alexithymia, the construct they have nominated to represent a cluster of deficits in the capacity to process emotions from the cognitive perspective, reveals by its cognitive processing failure its healthy, intact counterpart in the normal individual and thereby helps illuminate the unusual significance of emotional life for all of us. Advances in developmental psychology, neurobiology, infant development research, trauma research, new concepts of personality development, and newer concepts in psychoanalysis have all contributed to the evolution of a new and distinct entity, that of *self-regulation* in general and of *affect regulation* in particular. In regard to the latter it should be understood that one's ability to regulate one's affects is paired in turn with the need to allow these affects to regulate one's thinking and behaviour.

The role of affects in psychoanalytic theory has evolved over time from Freud's early discharge model and, as such, as a step-child to the instinctual drives, to its presently emerging status as subordinating the drives within the broad sweep of its new found relevance. In this new conceptual model, dysregulated emotions escape from the individual's self-regulating, self-organizing reciprocal feed-back loop and may instead pathologically alter biopsychosocial systems at random. Implicit in this new conception is the sense of an intimate, almost indivisible, connection between affects and their contribution to the cognitive processing of them as the valid data of one's own personal experience. What had become lost sight of in Freud's original formulation of libido theory has now re-emerged in the more suitable garb of affects – as the more all-inclusive entity. If we were to re-read Freud today, I think a good case could be made for our being able to substitute affect for libido – or, for that matter, the whole ensemble of associated ideas subsumed under his concept of the pleasure principle. The very concept of 'sexualization of trauma', for instance, or the 'libidinization of experience' are but other ways of talking about *personalizing* one's relationship to the event so as to claim a *personal subjective sense of agency* in terms of one's response to it. At the extreme alexithymic individuals are virtually organismic automatons functioning in a one- to two-dimensional world, one that is deprived of the fullness of feeling.

Affect theory is, in other words, the study of *how we were personally 'affected' by the event* as well as being able to gauge the importance, significance, and meaning for us in terms of cognitive evaluation, planning, adaptation, etc. Affects, like the drives which they now are understood to include, constitute the 'adjectives', the definers, of human experience as well as the on-going reformulators of the *meaning* and *significance* of that experience. Consequently, affects, though rooted in biology, now include a cognitive/experiencing dimension as well as a behavioural one. As a result, affects cognitively extend to such functions as attention, appraisal, amplification, imagination, mental representation, defense mechanisms, dreams, and verbal communication. Affects allow us to value, validate, and appreciate the objects we depend on and allow them, when internalized within us, to grow in value. This mutuality is predicated upon the idea of the sociability of feelings. That is fundamentally how we develop and mature – from the basis of our identifications with ever-valued and ever-valuing internal objects – who also can be mourned – with value. The fate of the alexithymic individual is more starkly different.

The authors proffer the concept of alexithymia as a personality construct that reflects a significant disorder in affect regulation, one that constitutes an important risk factor for psychological and physical disease, and they implicate it in somatoform disorders, eating disorders, substance abuse, panic disorder, and other illnesses. Drs Taylor, Bagby, and Parker conceive of alexithymia as an affect processing disorder that interrupts or seriously interferes with the organism's self-organizing and re-organizing processes, all part of a hitherto mysterious third area of involvement, one that is situated between the physiology of the soma and the cerebral processes of the mind.

Alexithymia, as a disorder of affect regulation and mediation, finds its cognitive analogue in the thought disorders of schizophrenics. Psychoanalysis and psychotherapy deal fundamentally with the emotional life of the individual, but we have begun to realize that the tools they have traditionally employed were borrowed from cognitive thinking *about* emotions. Analysts and therapists have long known that their patients were generally afraid of their feelings, both in experiencing them and in knowing about them. The construct of alexithymia offers a partial rationale for this fear. If feelings cannot be processed, then the feeling, as *signifier* of internal states automatically becomes the *signified* horror that it would normally signal. Thus, becoming aware of one's feelings runs the risk in these cases of unleashing raw proto-affect avalanches. As a consequence, affect-unprepared individuals (those with alexithymia) must instigate a coarctation of the affect cascade that otherwise would inundate them. When we consider some of the symptoms associated with alexithymia, such as anhedonia, paucity of phantasy, imagination, and dream life, etc., might it be that alexithymia represents a defect of primary process, one that I have already postulated occurs in schizophrenia?

The significance of alexithymia is that it is the exception that proves the rule; that is, from its perspective a whole panorama of failed emotional processing becomes apparent, and we get a vaster perspective of the importance of emotional life in a holistic sense. We know what we have hitherto only intuited; that affects are the '*silent service*' of our self-organizing and self-maintenance processes which interface both with soma and with mind *particulately* and comprises them *holistically* at the same time.

The authors present alexithymia in the context of a broad nosology. It not only constitutes an inherent personality aberration in its own right, but it also constitutes a secondary accompaniment of trauma, and also emerges secondarily as a consequence of attachment and bonding failures. The authors go further, however, and suggest that alexithymia may be a universal feature to one degree or another in all human beings. Fairbairn (1952) similarly conceived of schizoid nosology as comprising a unique personality type *and* at the same a virtually universal factor in every individual. Kohut (1971, 1977) likewise applied this double theory to narcissism. Perhaps the overall significance that the alexithymia construct offers us is as a model in those affected for the failure of affects to be regarded as valid signals for mental processing.

Now that emotions, affects, and feelings are worthy, enfranchised partners to cognitive mental life, we can evaluate how they interact with one another – from the point of view of their separate but equal status, but we must also consider that they are so intricately intertwined that they are functionally indivisible (holistic). Yet if we were to separate them for a moment and compare abstract thought with pure feeling, an interesting feature quickly comes to light. Thoughts occupy the third to fourth dimensions of space and time in terms of length, width, breadth, and linear succession. They belong, as Bion (1962, 1963) advises us, to the sensuous domain of perception. Proto-affects, on the other hand, are non-sensuous and may be time-less, chaotic, dimensionless, unbounded, infinite. Whereas anxiety may adaptively help prepare us for anticipated dangers in the future, panic, by contrast, is dramatic in its terrifying immediacy, is direction-less in its vector, and is experienced as unbounded, infinite, and eternal, i.e. there *is* no past or future, and there *is* no space. Whereas Freud reminded us, from the hegemony of the instinctual drive perspective, that psychic trauma represented the irruption of the drives into the ego, we now see that the feared content of the unconscious is not so much the drives as it is the chaos, infinite sets, unmodified inherent pre-conceptions, and 'beta elements' (Bion's [1962] term for the unmentalized data of human experience [Mitrani, 1995]), all of which are under the proto-affective umbrella, that constitutes the potentially threatening agent.

In-between the experience of mild and severe emotions there exists the capacity in all of us to be both logical as well as illogical. We are born with the propensity for illogical thinking, according to the infant developmentalist, Eugene Subbotsky (1993), and that propensity is probably what Freud meant by primary process and what Klein assumed to be the basis for unconscious phantasy. Matte-Blanco (1988) refers to this dual capacity as *bi-logic*, which includes the *asymmetrical logic* of Freud's secondary process and the *symmetrical logic* of his primary process. Together, they comprise what he terms the *heterogenic mode* of thinking. Emotions veer toward *symmetry*, thus their propensity to be personal, exaggerated, and seemingly irrational. Matte-Blanco (1988) states:

> We know . . . that thinking is the purest expression of the hetero-genic mode: the abyss of the incompatibility between the ways in which both modes of being live in the world. . . . Feeling is not normal logical thinking but also contains or expresses some type of bi-logical thinking. When Pascal said that the heart has its reasons which Reason does not understand, it seems to me that . . . he was, unawares, referring to the fundamental antinomy of human beings and world (p. 76).

Later he states:

> If the whole world becomes one and indivisible, to our limited intel-lect this amounts to the complete disappearance of the heterogenic

mode; like a ferocious beast, the symmetrical or indivisible mode had 'eaten up' all that there was to eat! (p. 81).

Finally:

In the end nothing is found which leads to a clear and neat psychological distinction between emotion and the unconscious (p. 84).

In other words, Matte Blanco seems to equate the symmetry and the infinite sets of the unconscious with the existence of emotional life, the latter of which then gradually becomes modified as it interacts with the asymmetry of bivalent logic.

The matter of boundlessness or infinity, to which I alluded above, has been addressed recently by a number of different but converging contributions, which include Bion's (1965, 1972, 1992) concept of 'transformations in "O"' and his 'beta element's', Lacan's (1966) concept of the 'Register of the Real', and Kauffman's (1993, 1995) ideas about chaos and complexity theory. One must also cite the seminal ideas of Kant (1787), especially his concept of 'the thing-in-itself', the 'noumenon'. What Freud (1923) called the 'seething cauldron' was meant to be representative of the peremptory irruption of the instinctual drives into the ego. Freud was not yet aware of the probability that what 'seething' force was more apposite for the affects than the drives. Kant's, Bion's, Lacan's, Matte-Blanco's, and Kauffman's contributions help us to reinterpret the id as being characterized by symmetry (boundlessness), infinity, chaos, complexity, and ineffability. Bion's concept of 'O' and Lacan's concept of the Real each deal with the domain of the ineffable, which is Absolute Reality, Ultimate Truth, the domain that can never be embraced by imagination and symbolization. When one is unprepared to experience it, it approximates the specular catastrophe of Sodom and Gomorrah. When one is ready, it can become spiritually transcendent (Grotstein, 1996). Klein (1940), working with Freud's original model of drives and affects, made a signal contribution by formulating an epigenesis of the processing of affects. She conceived that the early infant wishes to preserve the pleasure ego by evacuating its painful feelings of persecutory anxiety into the object through splitting and projective identification in the paranoid-schizoid position. As the infant developmentally progresses, it becomes more able with the object's help to tolerate and to own its own feelings. This accomplishment is a feature of the attainment of the depressive position. One can say that the earlier infant is developmentally 'alexithymic' but, with normal maturational epigenesis, achieves lexithymia. Bion (1959, 1962), following in Klein's footsteps, conceived of the *container and contained* model in which mother's emotional/cognitive processing ('alpha function', 'reverie') of her infant's raw projected feelings of distress transformed them into gentle, defused interpretations for the infant to learn about its feeling repertoire.

Silvan Tomkins (1962, 1963), amongst others, has helped to launch this new conception of the superordinating role of affects that allows for a distinction between positive and negative affects and for their being innate preconceptions that included the drives as subordinated within them. Lichtenberg (1989) completed the task by re-examining the drives in terms of complex motivational systems. In addition, we now have reason to believe that affect regulation is of critical importance for infant brain development. Recently, Schore (1994) summarized a vast array of neuro-developmental research and concluded that the mother's skill in the proper affective attunement (containment) of her infant has a direct effect on the quantity and quality of her infant's brain development, especially up to and including the practising subphase of separation–individuation, particularly involving the orbito-frontal cortex.

Alexithymia, the disorder of affect regulation, expression, and experience, reveals its normal counterpart in its very dysfunction, a hitherto hidden order that orchestrates affects and which unites them in some kind of synthesis with cognition, adaption, and *inter*personal as well as *intra*-personal relationships. I should like to proffer two models to embrace the new concept of affects that the authors are proposing, each of which is virtually interchangeable with the other and which together belong to the dual-track principle. One is the image of the virtual or abstract '*Siamese-twin*', and the other is the concept of *holography*. In the former, one can conceive of affects and cognition as both separate and yet at the same time paradoxically connected. The putative 'appearance' of their separateness in the twinship is for experiential discriminatory convenience. Actually, they can never really be separated.

Holography offers yet another point of view. A hologram is created when two laser beams are directed in such a way that one beam is aimed directly at the ultimate target while the other beam is directed toward an object that is so arranged that the laser beam penetrates it and is then refracted toward the target. The resulting shimmering image represents a visual paradox insofar as it is, on one hand, holistic but, on the other, represents a virtually infinite number of minute simulacra of the holistic entity. These models are my attempts to help comprehend the complexity of this new model of affect ↔ cognition ↔ perception ↔ sensation ↔ behaviour, which can be expressed both *with* the reversible arrows and simultaneously *without* them – as if they were a holistically one.

Cartesian dualism was a product of the Enlightenment and, in its proverbial linearity, constrained the concept of the psyche and soma into two polarized twins which had been arbitarily separated from one another with the former being assigned the role of dominance. This model is implicit in Newtonian physics. In our current century the emergence of such new ideas as the *law of relativity* (Einstein) and *the principle of uncertainty* (Heisenberg) superimposed another cohering order atop the Newtonian. From a more practical standpoint we can understand the application of this principle in our clinical work as the emergence of such ideas as intersubjectivity, the two-person model, contextualization theory, information theory, cybernetic reciprocal feed-back loops, and organismic self-organizing directedness toward self-regulation – and self-information – instead of the earlier notion of the prime aim of instinctual drives and affects being to discharge in order to reduce unpleasurable tension.

Alexithymia, as a construct about a defect in emotional processing in relationship to cognition, throws a new light on the role of emotions, affects, and feelings. Perhaps we can analogize the role that affects play with thoughts with that of prosody and language, in which prosody adds a critical and ineffable dimension to the overall meaning of the narrative. Prosody in addition to timber are what allows one to recognize the distinctive, unique features of the other's identity on the telephone. Another analogue for the relationship between affect and cognition is one borrowed from neurophysiology. We now know that the ascending and descending tracts of the reticular activating system are situated astride the distributions of the peripheral and subcortical nervous systems and constitute a self-instigating module for its self-organizing and self-regulating functions.

Thanks to this seminal work and the numerous other contributions that are summarized in it, we can now see cognition and emotions as two sides of the same coin – fundamentally indivisible but yet *appearing* to be divisible for perceptual and conceptual simplicity and convenience. The same 'Siamese-twinship' unity seems to be true for the relationship between affects and the instinctual drives, whose new-found unity is best expressed in the all but forgotten word *passion*.

There were many contributions that prefigured this great paradigm shift in psychoanalysis and psychiatry. Freud's original discharge model for affects and drives gradually revealed its limitations. Hartmann's (1939) conception of adaptation represented a significant attempt to portray the notion of the importance of the interrelationship between the infant and mother. Erikson (1959) carried this idea even farther in terms of the epigenesis of modes and modalities in the infant and child for interaction with a reciprocally evolving cultural environment. Bowlby 1969, 1973, 1980, 1988a) codified this idea with his pivotal concepts of attachment and bonding. Ferenczi (1951, 1988), Fairbairn (1952) and Winnicott (1952) anticipated Bowlby's contributions. Bion (1959, 1962), as mentioned earlier, simultaneously developed the conception of the container and contained in terms of the mother's capacity to absorb, contain, process, and interpret her infant's affect states. His contribution is especially apposite to the construct of alexithymia insofar as he specified the task of the containing mother – and the analyst by implication – to be, unlike Winnicott's 'holding environment', a processing, that is, an interpretive *naming of feelings* function.

The authors also proffer some helpful suggestions for treatment. Analogous to Bion's (1959, 1962) concept of maternal containment, they advocate that analysts and therapists who have primary or secondary alexithymic patients in their case load would do well to spend more time in educating them about their feelings and be able to show them the importance of appreciating the messenger service they impart, for which they ultimately would be grateful.

# Acknowledgments

The idea for this book grew out of a program of research on the alexithymia construct that we have conducted over the past 12 years. During that time, our thinking was stimulated by discussions with many clinicians and researchers in the fields of psychoanalysis, psychiatry, personality psychology, developmental psychology, and psychosomatic medicine, but we would particularly like to thank Drs Jack Brandes, Morris Eagle, John Elliott, John Flannery, Ray Freebury, Renata Gaddini, James Grotstein, Henry Krystal, Richard Lane, Mark Haviland, Joyce McDougall, John Nemiah, William Rickles, John Salvendy, Peter Sifneos, Herbert Weiner, Thomas Wise, and the late Dr Arthur Sohn.

We are grateful also for the encouragement and support of our colleagues in the Departments of Psychiatry at the Clarke Institute of Psychiatry, Mount Sinai Hospital, and University of Toronto, and in the Departments of Psychology at Trent University and York University. We especially thank Dr Mary Seeman for her enthusiasm for our work, and for ensuring the survival of our research program during her tenure as Psychiatrist-in-Chief at Mount Sinai Hospital. We also thank Dr Joel Sadavoy, current Psychiatrist-in-Chief at Mount Sinai Hospital, and Dr Paul Garfinkel, Chairman of the Department of Psychiatry at the University of Toronto, for their ongoing support. Though our work has been largely a labour of love, we could not have proceeded without the funds generously provided by the Laidlaw Foundation, the Samuel Lunenfeld Research Institute, the Mount Sinai Hospital Department of Psychiatry, and two private donors. Dr Michael Bagby received funding also from the Social Sciences and Humanities Research Council of Canada, the Clarke Institute of Psychiatry Research Fund, and the York University Part-time Faculty Research Fund. Dr James Parker received Post-Doctoral Fellowships from the Social Sciences and Humanities Research Council of Canada and the Ontario Mental Health Foundation. Interest in alexithymia and disorders of affect regulation has increased considerably over the past decade and there are now numerous investigators in many different countries who are conducting research studies on this topic. We have had the privilege of being able to exchange ideas and/or work collaboratively with several investigators in different parts of the world, and express our appreciation to Drs Marvin Acklin, Michael Bach, António Barbosa, Margarita Beresnevaité, Michael Bourke, Cinzia Bressi, Rui Mota Cardoso, Roberto Delle Chiaie, Karen Cohen, Isao Fukunishi, Giordano Invernizzi, Juhani Julkunen, Jussi Kauhanen, John Krystal, Wolfgang Linden, Carmen Loiselle, Mark Lumley, Manas Mandal, Franco Orsucci, Piero Porcelli, Michael von Rad, Hyo-Deog Rim, David Ryan, Peter Shoenberg, Jouko Salminen, Paul Schmitz, Luigi Solano, Orlando Todarello, Willem Trijsburg, Ad Vingerhoets, Colin Wastell, Paul Yelsma, Sotiris Zalidis, Sharon Zeitlin, and Michael Ziegler.

Special thanks go to Dr Jocelyn Foster, Editor of Medical Sciences at Cambridge University Press, for her endless patience and understanding over the delays in completing the manuscript, and for guiding us through the many production stages. We are indebted also to Helen Taylor for invaluable library research and literature reviews she provided during the writing of the manuscript, and to her and Susan Dickens and Kirstin Bindseil for their assistance in organizing the extensive bibliography for the book. Difficulties in locating resource materials were surmounted with the help of Salma Mirshak through her knowledge of complex cataloguing principles.

Finally, and most important, we would like to express appreciation to the many patients and university students who participated in the investigations reported in this book and to those other patients who shared personal experiences that have been an invaluable source of ideas for us.

# Acknowledgment of permission for use of material

Some of our theoretical ideas and most of our empirical research were originally reported at conferences and in scientific articles. We are grateful to the following publishers for granting us permission to use their material. Parts of Chapters 1 and 10 were published in G.J. Taylor, Psychosomatics and self-regulation. In J.W. Barron, M.N. Eagle, and D.L. Wolitzky (Eds.), *Interface of Psychoanalysis and Psychology*, pp. 464–88, Washington DC: American Psychological Association; copyright 1992, American Psychological Association, adapted with permission. Parts of Chapters 2 and 11 were published in G.J. Taylor, R.M. Bagby, and J.D.A. Parker (1991). The alexithymia construct: a potential paradigm for psychosomatic medicine. *Psychosomatics*, **32**, 153–64, used by permission of the American Psychiatric Press. Parts of Chapters 1, 2, 3, 4, and 11 were published in G.J. Taylor (1994). The alexithymia construct: conceptualization, validation, and relationship with basic dimensions of personality. *New Trends in Experimental and Clinical Psychiatry*, **10**, 61–74, Copyright 1994, CIC Edizioni Internazionali, used with permission. Parts of Chapters 3 and 4 are reprinted from R.M. Bagby, J.D.A. Parker, and G.J. Taylor (1994). The Twenty-Item Toronto Alexithymia Scale – I. Item selection and cross-validation of the factor structure. *Journal of Psychosomatic Research*, **38**, 23–31, and R.M. Bagby, G.J. Taylor, and J.D.A. Parker (1994). The Twenty-Item Toronto Alexithymia Scale – II. Convergent, discriminant, and concurrent validity. *Journal of Psychosomatic Research*, **38**, 33–40, with kind permission from Elsevier Science Ltd, Kidlington, UK. Parts of Chapters 6, 7, and 8 were published in J.D.A. Parker, G.J. Taylor, R.M. Bagby, and M. Acklin (1993). Alexithymia in panic disorder and simple phobia: a preliminary investigation. *American Journal of Psychiatry*, **150**, 1105–7, Copyright 1993, American Psychiatric Association; and in G.J. Taylor, J.D.A. Parker, and

R.M. Bagby (1990). A preliminary investigation of alexithymia in
men with psychoactive substance abuse. *American Journal of Psychiatry*,
**147**, 1228–30, Copyright 1990, American Psychiatric Association;
reprinted by permission. Part of Chapter 9 was published in M.P.
Bourke, G.J. Taylor, J.D.A. Parker, and R.M. Bagby (1992).
Alexithymia in women with anorexia nervosa: a preliminary investigation. *British Journal of Psychiatry*, **161**, 240–3, used by permission of
the Royal College of Psychiatrists.

The NEO PI and NEO PI-R profile forms in Chapter 4 are repro-
duced by special permission of the publisher, Psychological Assessment Resources Inc., 16204 North Florida Avenue, Lutz, Florida
33549, from the NEO Personality Inventory-Revised, by Paul Costa
and Robert McCrae, Copyright 1978, 1985, 1989, 1992 by PAR, Inc.
Further reproduction is prohibited without permission of PAR, Inc.

The modified version of the Beth Israel Hospital Psychosomatic
Questionnaire in the Appendix is adapted from P. Sifneos (1973). The
prevalence of 'alexithymic' characteristics in psychosomatic patients.
*Psychotherapy and Psychosomatics*, **22**, 255–62, with permission of the
publisher S. Karger AG, Basel.

# Introduction

A DEEP CONCERN WITH EITHER MIND OR
BODY OR BOTH APPEARS HISTORICALLY TO
LEAD TO CONCERN WITH AFFECT.

*Silvan Tomkins, 1981*

Over the past two decades, there has been an expanding scientific interest both in the development and regulation of affects, and in the impact of dysregulated affects on mental and physical health. This interest in affects has been prompted by the development of new technologies and experimental methods for investigating brain functions, and by fascinating findings from observational studies of the infant–caregiver relationship. While the former have advanced our understanding of the brain mechanisms involved in emotions, the latter have led to reformulations of the nature, functions, and early development of affects that have important clinical implications. At the same time, the development of new measurement instruments has enabled researcher–clinicians to investigate temperamental or dispositional differences in affectivity, and to conduct empirical studies to explore the role of dysregulated affects in a variety of medical and psychiatric illnesses. Indeed, the study of affects has become an exciting interdisciplinary activity involving developmental psychology, personality psychology, neurobiology, psychoanalysis, biological psychiatry, psychophysiology, psychosomatic medicine, and the communication sciences.

The aim of this book is to show how some of the theoretical models and research resulting from this interdisciplinary activity provide a new clinical perspective from which certain medical and psychiatric illnesses can be reconceptualized as disorders of affect regulation. We will focus predominantly on recent work on the personality construct known as *alexithymia*, which reflects difficulties in affective self-regulation and is thought to be one of several possible risk factors for a variety of medical and psychiatric disorders.

The idea that affects, in particular excessive and unmodulated levels of affect, can influence adversely mental and bodily health has been expressed by physicians and philosophers since ancient times, although the emphasis placed on affects has ebbed and flowed through different eras. In the Greco-Roman era, for example, Ascelepiades attributed mental disorders to emotional disturbances; Galen classified the passions as the sixth of the non-natural causes of disease; Plato associated 'erotic madness' with human love; and Cicero described four main 'perturbations' or passions (sorrow, fear, joy, and libido), which could be moderated by reason, but could cause diseases of the soul if they became excessive. Addressing the treatment of mental disorders, Aristotle advocated the use of catharsis, including music, wine, and aphrodisiacs, to release disturbing emotions or passions (Mora, 1967).

Following the Greco-Roman era, and throughout the Middle Ages, more primitive concepts were invoked as causal explanations of disturbing human behaviour, such as the influence of evil spirits, witches, or demons; these explanations led to exorcisms, torture, and other cruelties to the mentally ill. Interest in the emotions began to return during the sixteenth century with Johann Weyer's rejection of the belief in witchcraft, and the humane approach of Paracelsus, who gave the passions a role in the pathogenesis of both mental and physical diseases (Mora, 1967; Weiner, in press).

At the onset of the seventeenth century, Wright (1601) published his book *Passions of the Minde in Generalle* in which he asserted that the passions engender humors that can alter bodily function and structure, and that humors can also breed passions. Wright believed that the seat of the passions was in the heart; while moderate joy was seen as promoting health, excessive joy was thought to dilate the heart and to possibly cause sudden death. The negative passions of fear, sadness, and despair were considered more dangerous to the body as they were thought to constrict the heart.

Wright's linking of the passions with temperament and the corporeal humors extended Hippocrates' (fourth century BC) description of four basic temperaments or emotional orientations (sanguine, choleric, melancholic, and phlegmatic), which had been attributed to the preponderance of different bodily fluids (blood, phlegm, and various forms of bile), with an excess of black bile being the most frequently mentioned cause of mental illness. The typology of four temperaments, and the explanatory humoral theory, anticipated the modern notion that individuals are characterized by certain fundamental personality traits, which are believed to be determined largely by constitutional factors.

Robert Burton's (1621) famous essay on melancholia, which was published two decades after Wright's book appeared, re-emphasized emotional factors in the causation of mental illness, but identified the brain, rather than the heart, as the affected body part. The work of several illustrious seventeenth century physicians, including Thomas Willis, Thomas Sydenham, and William Harvey, focused attention on the influence of the emotions on bodily function and structure, and also causally linked distressing and uncontrolled emotions with hysteria and hypochondriasis (Weiner, in press).

The idea that emotions sometimes induce physical disease was explored further during the eighteenth century by several eminent physicians including William Falconer (1796), who wrote a book entitled *The influence of the passions upon disorders of the body*, and Jerome Gaub, who was professor of medicine and chemistry at the University of Leiden. In a major essay (translated in Rather, 1965), Gaub described the harmful effects on the body of disturbing emotions, in particular excessive anger, unexpressed grief, fear and terror, unrestrained joy, and unrequited love; he also discussed the beneficial effects of hope, joy, love, and tranquillity, as well as the therapeutic value of releasing suppressed emotions and the modulating effect of correct reasoning (as Cicero had postulated during the second century BC). Indeed, Gaub anticipated the modern notion that certain cognitive capacities, through the regulation of emotions, have a regulatory influence also on the functioning of the body: 'The first instance from which one can see that a tranquil mind making use of right reason aids the health in many ways is that it adjusts and regulates both its own functions and those attributable to the body. . . .' (Gaub, 1763, in Rather, 1965, p. 156).

Although there were major reforms affecting the care of the mentally ill during the late eighteenth century and throughout the nineteenth century, advances in biology diverted attention from the emotions to single-factor linear conceptions that mental disorders could be explained only by organic changes in the central nervous system (Kraepelin, 1909–1915) and that bodily disease had its origin in disease of the cell (Virchow, 1858). The adoption of germ theory in the latter part of the nineteenth century, and the development of new biomedical technologies at the beginning of the twentieth century, led to a greater separation of the organic elements of disease from emotional malfunctioning, thereby reinforcing a reductionistic biomedical model of disease, which has prevailed throughout the present century (Engel, 1977).

The work of Pierre Janet, and the emergence of psychoanalysis at the turn of the century, led to the rediscovery of the role of emotions in the pathogenesis of mental disorders, and eventually also to the formalization of psychosomatic medicine as a discipline concerned with the

influence of emotions on bodily processes (Dunbar, 1935). Although
Freud (1905) focused primarily on the role of unconscious conflict and
associated affects in the formation of psychoneurotic symptoms, and
avoided any psychoanalytic investigation of physical disease, he
echoed Gaub's view that depressive affects could bring about bodily
disease in predisposed individuals, and that feelings of joy and happiness could have a rejuvenating effect on the body.

It is evident from this brief historical overview that the relations
between emotions and mental and bodily health have, for the most
part, been conceptualized in terms of the balance between negative and
positive emotions and how well emotions are regulated. In accounting
for changes in health, however, most writers have advanced a interactional dualistic theory in which emotions are given a linear–causal
role in altering mental or bodily functions. The principle of dualistic
interactionism (Wallace, 1988a), which was formulated most strongly
by the seventeenth century French philosopher Rene Descartes, has
profoundly influenced modern thinking about mind–body relations
and generated much controversy and confusion even within the relatively small field of psychosomatic medicine. In our view, Cartesian
dualism and interactionist theory have also limited progress in understanding the role of emotions in health and illness. 'Emotions', as
Weiner (in press) has emphasized, 'do not cause anything. They are
part and parcel of adaptive and maladaptive organismic responses.'

The principle of self-regulation, however, can certainly be applied to
emotions; it is a biological principle that is basic for all living systems
(Emde, 1988a). Though the principle of self-regulation emerged from
the work of Claude Bernard and Walter Cannon on the homeostatic
mechanisms that regulate and maintain constant conditions in an
organism's *milieu intérieur*, it extends beyond physiological systems to
include self-regulation in behavioural systems, as recognized by general systems theory (Taylor, 1987a). It is now established that the seat
of the emotions is in the brain, rather than in the viscera, and that
neuromodulator projection systems regulate the physiological arousal
and motor/expressive activity in emotional behaviour; failures in these
neuromodulator systems produce affect dysregulation and certain
types of psychopathology.

Affects, however, though rooted in biology, are generally viewed as
composite states, which include a cognitive/experiential component as
well as physiological and behavioural/expressive components (Dodge
& Garber, 1991). Thus, cognitive processes such as attention, appraisal, amplification, mental representation, imagination, defense
mechanisms, dreams, and verbal communication are also involved
in the processing and regulation of affects (Izard & Kobak, 1991;

Rachman, 1980; Salovey, Hsee & Mayer, 1993). And while affects are subject to regulatory action, it has become increasingly evident that affects themselves play an important role in organizing mental functioning and behaviour (Ciompi, 1991; Emde, 1988b; Frijda, 1986). The focus of this book will be on the cognitive/experiential component of affects, in particular on deficits in the subjective awareness and cognitive processing of affects, which comprise the alexithymia construct. The notion that certain medical and psychiatric illnesses are essentially disorders of affect regulation will be conceptually elaborated, and supporting evidence from empirical research will be reviewed and critically evaluated.

Before discussing clinical disorders involving disturbances in affective self-regulation, it is necessary to provide an historical and conceptual framework for understanding the normal development and regulation of affects and the function of affects in everyday human life. The first chapter therefore will present an overview of contemporary theories of emotion and of normal affect development and affect regulation, and also review findings from recent infant and child observational studies that link the development and regulation of affects with early relationships. The important role of imaginative processes in affect regulation will be outlined, and attention directed to the influence of neurobiological and cultural factors.

Chapter 2 defines and describes the salient features of the alexithymia construct and relates this construct to disturbances in the self-regulation of affects. The historical background of the construct is reviewed, and attention given to types of early childhood experiences that might affect adversely the development of affects and a capacity for imagination, and thereby limit the ability to modulate states of emotional arousal.

Chapter 3 outlines evidence supporting the validity of the alexithymia construct, and also critically reviews the various instruments that have been developed to measure the construct.

Chapter 4 provides an overview of some contemporary models of personality structure, and then reviews a body of empirical research examining the relations between alexithymia, positive and negative affects, and basic dimensions of personality. Recent empirical research on alexithymia and psychological defense style is also reviewed.

Chapter 5 presents an overview of the neurobiology of emotion, with an emphasis on the role of the two cerebral hemispheres in the experience, expression, and regulation of affects. The chapter then reviews research exploring possible neural mechanisms underlying alexithymia.

Chapters 6 through 9 provide the theoretical rationale for reconceptualizing certain psychiatric disorders as disorders of affect regulation, and also review a substantial body of recent empirical research examining the associations of the selected disorders with alexithymia. Chapter 10 reviews the associations between alexithymia and certain medical illnesses and diseases, and shows how the concept of affect dysregulation can be integrated into a new and sophisticated medical model that avoids dualistic interactionism and is based on the view that living organisms are self-organizing systems involving complex cybernetic feedback loops.

It is well recognized that patients suffering from the illnesses that we conceptualize as disorders of affect regulation are difficult to treat and make extensive use of health care facilities. Chapter 11 addresses the issue of treatment with an emphasis on modified psychotherapeutic approaches, and a discussion of several other modalities that may be used separately or integrated with individual psychotherapy.

Chapter 12 concludes the book with a short discussion of future directions that might be taken to extend further or refine the alexithymia construct and the concept of disorders of affect regulation.

# The development and regulation of affects

Although affects have long been considered a basic and essential feature of human experience, there has never been any clear agreement on a definition and theory of affects; and only recently have psychologists and psychiatrists shown a serious interest in how affects develop and come to be regulated. Some psychologists distinguish between emotions and affects, but their definitions of these constructs are inconsistent; others use these terms synonymously but distinguish them from the word feelings. In this chapter, we will review contemporary theories and recent research on affect development and affect regulation. First, however, we will summarize several major theories and conceptualizations of emotion, and also discuss the relations between emotion and cognition and the role of affects in the organization of the personality.

## Emotions, affects, and feelings

In the modern era, controversy about the definition of the construct of emotion has existed since the publication over 100 years ago of William James's now famous essay entitled 'What is an emotion?' While James (1884) and Lange (1885) believed that emotions result from the afferent feedback to the brain of different patterns of peripheral autonomic nervous system activity and other bodily states (i.e. emotions were construed as nothing but the awareness of different physiological changes in response to arousing stimuli – the 'James–Lange theory'), Cannon (1927) argued that emotions arise from the subcortical regions of the brain and that the autonomic responses are merely an output component of the brain processes that define the experience of emotion

(Porges, 1991). Darwin also viewed physiological changes as integral parts of emotional states (McNaughton, 1989); however, he focused on the expressive aspects of emotions and their communicative functions.

In his monumental work *The expression of the emotions in man and animals*, Darwin (1872) reported his detailed observational findings that the facial and bodily display of certain emotions is similar in human infants and adults and across different cultures, and also remarkably similar to the non-vocal emotional expressions of phylogenetically lower animal species, especially non-human primates. Darwin proposed that there are certain innate discrete emotions that manifest themselves via distinct patterns of facial expression and postural muscle activity, which occur in a reflex-like manner and result from the direct action of the central nervous system. He regarded these expressions as part of larger action patterns in lower species that had 'evolved into an independent signalling or communicative function which was important for social adaptation' (Basch, 1976, p. 760). Darwin recognized that emotional expressions, through their signal function, promote bonding between mothers and infants and the forging of relationships between individuals within a social group. From Darwin's point of view, emotions are basically adaptive and help to organize behaviour in ways that increase the chances of survival.

Several contemporary emotion theorists also emphasize the expressive aspects and/or adaptive functions of emotions or affects. For example, Plutchik (1980, 1993) defines emotions as communication and survival mechanisms based on evolutionary adaptations; Tomkins (1962) regards affects as innate biological motivating mechanisms; Izard (1977) and Ekman (1993) highlight the role of facial emotional expressions as sources of affective feedback to the self as well as communications to other people; and Watson and Clark (1994) view an emotion as 'an organized, highly structured reaction to an event that is relevant to the needs, goals, or survival of the organism' (p. 89).

Though there is no consensus about the definition of emotion, there is general agreement that emotional responding in humans involves three interrelated systems or sets of processes: (1) *neurophysiological processes* (largely autonomic nervous system and neuroendocrine activation); (2) *motor or behavioural-expressive processes* (e.g. facial expressions, crying, changes in posture and tone of voice); and (3) a *cognitive-experiential system* (subjective awareness and verbal reporting of feeling states) (Dodge & Garber, 1991; Frijda, 1986; Izard & Kobak, 1991; Watson & Clark, 1994). From an evolutionary perspective, emotions are solely biological phenomena in animals that do not have the neocortical development necessary for the development of cognition, but they acquire a psychological component in humans that permits reflective awareness and intentional activity (Frijda, 1986).

While the word *feeling* refers to the subjective, cognitive–experiential domain of emotion response systems, and the word *emotion* refers to the neurophysiological and motor-expressive domains, *affects* are composite states encompassing all three domains (as was outlined in the Introduction to this book), as well as mental representations of feeling states intertwined with memories of experiences that give personal meaning to current feeling states (Schwartz, 1987; Sifneos, 1988). As noted earlier, however, there is an inconsistent use of these terms among psychologists and psychiatrists. Basch (1976) and Nathanson (1992), for example, use the word affect to describe the biological portion of emotion and the word emotion to refer to a level of affective maturation that captures the biography of an individual. In contrast, Sandler (1972) and Sifneos (1988) reserve the term emotion for the physiological processes and subsume both subjective feeling states and the bodily changes occurring in emotion under the heading of affect. Most authors use the terms emotion and affect interchangeably (e.g. Emde, 1991; Jones, 1995; Krystal, 1988; Osofsky, 1992; Watson & Clark, 1994), and some even fail to distinguish these terms from the term feeling (e.g. Rapaport, 1953; Schaffer, 1964). Given that there is no agreed upon differentiation between emotions and affects in the literature, and to avoid confusing the reader, we have adopted the style of most authors and use the terms emotion and affect interchangeably throughout this book.

## Modern theories of emotion

As noted earlier, the ideas of Darwin are clearly discernible in many modern theories of emotion. During the 1960s, Silvan Tomkins (1962, 1963) proposed that affects constitute a primary innate biological motivating system. He identified eight innate affects, each characterized by a specific facial expression, and gave them two-word group names to describe the nature of the affect and the range over which it may be experienced. The positive innate affects are *interest–excitement* and *enjoyment–joy*; the negative affects are *distress–anguish*, *anger–rage, fear–terror, shame–humiliation*, and *contempt–disgust; surprise–startle* functions as a neutral affect. Tomkins (1984) later separated contempt–disgust into two separate affects, thus making nine innate affects.

Contrary to Freud, who related all behaviour to the instinctual drives, Tomkins (1984) maintained that affects are the primary factors in motivation; indeed, Tomkins argued that drives derive their power from affects, which function as amplifiers. Tomkins viewed cognition also as separate from the affect system. Employing general systems theory, he proposed that 'emotions can control cognitions or be controlled by them or be integrally interconnected with them' (Magai & McFadden, 1995, p. 230). During childhood development, individuals form 'ideo-affective' structures, which are organizations of affect and cognition that become prominent features of personality and influence a broad range of behaviours, including information processing and strategies of affect regulation (Magai & Hunziker, 1993; Magai & McFadden, 1995). Although Tomkins identified a small number of basic emotions, he regarded them as very conditionable, which allows for the development of a large variety of ideo-affective organizations.

Plutchik (1980, 1993), also drawing theoretical inspiration from Darwin, conceptualizes emotions as adaptive mechanisms related to survival that have developed over the evolutionary history of the species. He proposes that emotions have a genetic basis, and he shares with Tomkins the belief that there is a small number of basic or primary emotions (although his list is slightly different from that of Tomkins). In an attempt to link emotions with personality traits, Plutchik identifies a large number of secondary emotions that are derived from mixtures or blends of the primary emotions. In his view, it is habitual styles in the likelihood of experiencing particular primary or secondary emotions that form the basis of personality structure.

Izard (1971, 1977), who was influenced by both Tomkins' work and the writings of Darwin, proposed a *differential emotions theory* that attempts to relate emotion processes with other subsystems of personality, including cognition, and also with findings from neurophysiological research. Like Tomkins and Plutchik, Izard identifies a set of basic emotions (he adds *guilt* to Tomkins' list of nine innate affects, and replaces distress–anguish by the affect of *sadness*). He labels these 'fundamental' emotions because each emotion has a specific innately determined neural substrate, a characteristic facial expression and sometimes bodily response, and a unique subjective or phenomenological quality. The theory holds that the 'fundamental emotions are motivators and organizers of behaviour, not merely responses to an appraisal process' (Izard & Buechler, 1980, p. 168).

Izard (1977) conceptualizes the personality as a network of six subsystems: the homeostatic, drive, emotion, perceptual, cognitive, and motor subsystems. These subsystems can function relatively autonomously but are also complexly interrelated. Of particular importance are the interactions that occur between cognitive processes and affects:

Such interactions are innumerable and they vary with the particular person–environment transaction. Affective–cognitive structures are psychological organizations of affect and cognition – traitlike phenomena that result from repeated interactions between a particular affect or pattern of affects and a particular set or configuration of cognitions (p. 45).

As with Tomkins' concept of ideo-affective organizations, Izard (1977) links personality traits with combinations of affective-cognitive structures. Structures that involve the fundamental emotion of *interest* are thought to have the most dramatic consequences for personality organization. 'Interest is the most frequently experienced positive emotion. It is an extremely important motivation in the development of skills, competencies, and intelligence' (p. 212). Not surprisingly, Izard links interest–cognitive structures with individual differences in creative and artistic abilities, as well as with the ability to form and maintain close interpersonal relationships. In our view, the affect of interest underlies the dimension of personality referred to as *openness to experience* (McCrae & Costa, 1985), which has an important role in self- and affect regulation and will be described in detail in Chapter 4.

Although Freud was strongly influenced by Darwin's evolutionary theory and emphasis on the importance of the instincts for survival and reproduction (Sulloway, 1979), he conceptualized affects as derivatives of the instinctual drives rather than as primary motivating factors. Anxiety, for example, in Freud's (1895a) early writings, was regarded as transformed libido. Being secondary to drives, affects were essentially discharge processes occurring only when the drive was not fully gratified. Freud came close to divorcing affects from drives in 1926, as Sandler (1972) and Jones (1995) have noted, when he pointed out that anxiety could function also as a signal affect in response either to the perception of dangers in the real world or to the threatening nature of drive-related impulses. However, Freud never systematized his thinking about the difference between affects and drives.

Over several decades after Freud's death, a few eminent psychoanalytic theorists made attempts to modify Freud's conception of affects; however, they never succeeded in fully separating affects from the framework of drive theory. The emergence of attachment theory (Bowlby, 1969, 1973), self psychology (Kohut & Wolf, 1978), and Sullivan's (1953) interpersonal theory provided alternative ways of conceptualizing affects, but these ideas were not integrated into mainstream psychoanalysis. Consequently, for most of the present century, psychoanalysis has been without a satisfactory theory of affects.

In recent years, however, and prompted partly by Tomkins' affect theory and findings from human infant research, a number of psychoanalysts and psychoanalytic psychotherapists have made vigorous efforts to revise the psychoanalytic theory of affects and to view affects, rather than drives, as the primary motivators in human life (Basch, 1976; Emde, 1988a,b; Jones, 1995; Karush, 1989; Kissen, 1995; Krystal, 1988; Nathanson, 1992; Schwartz, 1987; Spezzano, 1993). A lucid and comprehensive discussion of this new psychoanalytic theory of affect is provided by Jones (1995), who conceptualizes affects as 'the experiential representation of a non-symbolic information-processing system that can serve as the central control mechanism for all aspects of human behavior' (p. xxi).

Though Darwin clearly established the biological basis of emotions, some emotion theorists argue that emotions are primarily psychological phenomena and that cognitive activity causally precedes emotions (e.g., Lazarus, 1991; Ortony, Clore, & Collins, 1988). The cognitive approach to emotion was stimulated by the work of Schachter and Singer (1962) and their attempts to surmount inadequacies in the James–Lange theory of emotion. According to Schachter (1964), certain environmental stimuli have the potential to generate a general state of autonomic arousal. This general state is subsequently modified into different emotional experiences by the emotional meanings that the aroused person gives to different situational stimuli. There is no emotional experience when there is no autonomic arousal; nor when the arousal is attributed to non-emotional sources (Frijda, 1986). By demonstrating in experimental studies that emotional experiences can be determined by the way people interpret their arousal, Schachter and Singer (1962) initiated an enormous amount of theorizing and empirical research on the link between cognition and emotion.

One of the strongest proponents of a cognitive theory of emotion is Lazarus (1991), who argues that *cognitive appraisal* of the significance of the person–environment relationship is both sufficient and necessary for emotional experience; 'without a personal appraisal (i.e. of harm or benefit) there will be no emotion; when such an appraisal is made, an emotion of some kind is inevitable' (p. 177). According to this theory, each emotion is guided and generated by its own particular pattern of appraisal.

Much of the controversy over the relations between emotion and cognition stems from different ways in which theorists define the term cognition. As Zajonc (1984) has noted, Lazarus's argument is unassailable because he includes cognition (as a necessary precondition) in his definition of emotion. Plutchik (1980) also regards cognitive appraisals as precursors of all emotional states, but his definition of cognition includes perception. Davidson & Ekman (1994) point out that 'if "cognitive" is taken to include basic sensory information processing, then most, if not all, emotions will have some cognitive contribution' (p. 232). However, if one restricts the definition of cognition to processes based in the hippocampus or neocortex of the brain, there is evidence that affects can arise independent of cognitions (Davidson & Ekman, 1994; LeDoux, 1994). Moreover, both phylogenetically and ontogenetically, affects precede the development of cognition (Zajonc, 1984). Jones (1995) notes that, by making cognitive appraisal a precursor of emotional reactions, the cognitive theory of emotion resembles Freud's early drive-discharge model, which did not allow affects to be thought of 'as nonsymbolic signals that, in and of themselves, conveyed information' (p. 22).

While we subscribe to a primacy of affect theory, we concur with Zajonc (1984) that this does not mean that affects are always primary. Cognition becomes linked inseparably with affects early in development, and also functions as one of several types of emotion-activating systems (Izard, 1994). Indeed, as Jones (1995) points out, if affects are primary processes, 'the experience of any affect is itself cognitive because it adds to our knowledge about our body or our world' (p. 23). Moreover, as we will elaborate in the next section and in subsequent chapters, cognitive processes play a vital role in the regulation of affects.

### The concept of affect regulation

As biologically based phenomena, emotions involve a readiness to action, a notion that is implicit in the Latin verb *emovere* (meaning 'to move out' or 'expel') from which the word emotion is derived. Consequently, as Frijda (1986) has pointed out, people not only have emotions, they also manage or handle them. The actions taken to influence what emotion we have and how these emotions are experienced and expressed are encompassed in the concept of affect (or emotion) regulation (Gross & Muñoz, 1995; Kopp, 1989; Schore, 1994). This concept is part of the broader construct of self-regulation, which refers to the autonomous functioning of the organism, a universal and general mechanism found in both biological and cognitive behaviours (Emde, 1988a; Taylor, 1987a, 1992b; Wilson, Passik & Faude, 1990).

Although the concept of affect regulation is currently a growing area of interest for researchers and clinicians in both the developmental area

(Campos, Campos & Barrett, 1989; Garber & Dodge, 1991; Kopp, 1989; Schore, 1994) and the field of adult mental health (Gross & Muñoz, 1995), regulation has been a part of emotion theories throughout history, as we noted in the Introduction to this book. In reviewing the historical background to the concept, Dodge and Garber (1991) point out that Freud's theory of psychosexual development was one that essentially dealt with 'the struggle between internal emotional impulses and attempts by the individual to control or regulate their expression' (p. 3). Darwin similarly observed regulatory aspects of emotions in his studies on behavioural expressions of emotion.

Notwithstanding these early predecessors of affect regulation, many contemporary theorists conceptualize the regulation of emotions as an integrative interactional process among the three domains of emotion response systems and with the environment. The model proposed by Freud (1923, 1926) is essentially one in which an individual's instinctual drives and emotional desires are regulated by ego defense mechanisms (i.e. cognitive processes), the failure of which results in psycho-pathology (Dodge & Garber, 1991). As outlined in the previous section, recent theories proposed by cognitive psychologists view both the elicitation and regulation of emotion as secondary to some form of cognitive processing.

Adopting the broader conceptualizations of Dodge and Garber (1991), Izard and Kobak (1991), and Gross and Muñoz (1995), we regard affect regulation as a process involving reciprocal interactions between the neurophysiological, motor–expressive, and cognitive–experiential domains of emotion response systems. As activation in any one response domain alters or modulates activation in the other two domains, all three domains are involved in the regulation of emotion. Also, one aspect of responding in a particular domain may modulate another aspect of responding in the same domain. In addition to the *interdomain* and *intradomain* regulation of emotion, an individual's interaction within social relationships and other aspects of the environment provide *interpersonal* regulation that may be supportive (e.g. soothing) or disruptive (e.g. arguing) (Campos *et al.*, 1989; Dodge & Garber, 1991). Clearly, social bonds, language, dreams, fantasy, play, crying, smiling, and defense mechanisms all play a role in emotion regulation, as does afferent feedback from peripheral autonomic activity and the musculoskeletal system. Affects them-selves may also regulate other affects; for example, activation of the positive affect of interest may attenuate fear and sadness and thereby alleviate a tendency to depression; and shame may attenuate joy (Izard & Kobak, 1991).

It is important to emphasize that the regulation of emotion does not necessarily mean controlling emotions. Affects have important organizing, motivating, and adaptive functions, and are not meant to be tightly controlled (Ciompi, 1991; Izard & Kobak, 1991). These functions occur more successfully when the activity in one or more component of affect response systems is used as information about the state of the self within its environment, thereby providing feedback that helps the affect system to regulate itself. As Izard and Kobak (1991) emphasize, it is the reciprocal influences among the component systems that provide inherent regulatory mechanisms; as a prime example, one affect may be influencing the perception and cognitive appraisal of an event while these processes are, in turn, activating another emotion. Similarly, play or other imaginative activity enhance the positive emotions of interest and enjoyment; these have regulatory feedback effects serving not only to minimize negative emotions, as we just indicated, but also to motivate further playful activity that intensifies the interest (Tomkins, 1962; Izard & Kobak, 1991).

The cognitive skills required to effectively monitor and self-regulate emotions are encompassed in a recently introduced construct known as *emotional intelligence* (Goleman, 1995; Salovey, Hsee & Mayer, 1993). Such skills include an ability to accurately appraise one's emotions and use them in adaptive ways, and an ability to comprehend the feelings of other people and make empathic responses (Salovey & Mayer, 1989/90). As we will elaborate in the next chapter and throughout the book, people who have difficulty regulating their emotions typically manifest deficits in this set of cognitive skills.

### Affect development

Although there is evidence that the basic innate emotions are present in the neonate and are fundamentally the same in infants across cultures, these initially are experienced and expressed behaviourally and physiologically. The subjective–experiential aspect of the basic emotions, and also other more complex emotions (such as love, pride, happiness and envy), develop during early childhood, with cognition and socialization playing important roles in this development.

Most developmental psychologists and psychoanalytic theorists postulate an epigenetic sequence for affect development. During infancy, the behavioural–expressive manifestations of affects are the infants' language – their means of communicating their needs, desires, and satisfactions to the caregiver; the subjective–experiential component of affects consists of undifferentiated precursor states of *contentment* and *distress* (Hesse & Cicchetti, 1982; Krystal, 1988; Osofsky, 1992). In the course of maturation, affects evolve from these two precursor states into a range of specific emotions (Krystal, 1988). As outlined first by Schur (1955), and later by Krystal (1974), this involves a progressive desomatization and differentiation of the affect precursors and, as language develops, the gradual construction of symbolic representations of emotions (also referred to as cognitive schemata), which thereafter can be communicated verbally.

Although Piaget (1967, 1981) did not address the topic of affect development very extensively, he proposed that affect development follows a course that is parallel and complementary to cognitive development. Lane and Schwartz (1987) subsequently integrated Piaget's theory of cognitive development with Werner and Kaplan's (1963) ideas about symbolization and language development, and thereby conceptualized a cognitive–developmental model for understanding the organization of emotional experience. In this model, as Lane and his colleagues (1990) explain, 'the experience of emotion is hypothesized to undergo structural transformation in a hierarchical developmental sequence of progressive differentiation and integration' (p. 125).

There are five levels of emotion organization and awareness in the model: (i) *sensorimotor reflexive* (emotion is experienced only as bodily sensations, but may be evident to others in the individual's facial expression); (ii) *sensorimotor enactive* (emotion is experienced as both a body sensation and an action tendency); (iii) *preoperational* (emotions are experienced psychologically as well as somatically, but they are unidimensional and verbal descriptions of emotion are often stereotyped); (iv) *concrete operational* (there is an awareness of blends of feelings and the individual can describe complex and differentiated emotional states that are part of his or her subjective experience; and (v) *formal operational* (there is an awareness of blends of blends of feelings, as well as a capacity to make subtle distinctions between nuances of emotion, and an ability to comprehend the multidimensional emotional experience of other people).

Lane and Schwartz's cognitive–developmental model not only provides an extremely useful framework for conceptualizing the development of affects during early childhood, but it also helps explain individual differences in the experience, expression, and ability to regulate affects, and in the capacity to empathize. As a dimensional model of affect development independent of other aspects of cognitive development, it can be applied also to the construct of emotional intelligence, which 'may or may not correlate with other types of intelligence' (Salovey & Mayer, 1989/90, p. 187). As Lane and

Schwartz (1987) indicate, some 'highly intelligent individuals may be quite unsophisticated in their awareness of their own emotional reactions or those of others' (p. 136).

Although seemingly unaware of Lane and Schwartz's important contribution, Frosch (1995) has recently proposed a similar approach to conceptualizing the organization of emotions. Influenced also by Piaget's theory of cognitive development, Frosch makes an important distinction between emotions that are organized at a *preconceptual* level (i.e. early in, or prior to, the preoperational stage) and emotions that are organized on a more *abstract, logical, and reality-oriented* level (i.e. in the concrete or formal operational stages). At the preconceptual level of organization, affects are experienced as sensations, perceptions, or impulses to action, and there is an associated inability to move freely into the world of imagination and fantasy. Normal affect development involves a move away from a perceptually bound affectomotor existence to a conceptual world of abstraction.

There is an obvious parallel between Frosch's distinction between preconceptual and conceptual levels of organization and Melanie Klein's (1935) formulation of paranoid–schizoid and depressive positions. As elaborated by Segal (1957, 1964), Brown (1985), and Stein (1990), these two mental positions designate different ways of regulating intense affects, especially love and hate, with primitive defenses and a concrete type of mentation characterizing the paranoid–schizoid position, and mature defenses and a capacity for symbolization and abstract thinking emerging in the depressive position.

### The role of early relationships

Clearly, affect development and the development of cognitive skills for regulating affects are intimately related to the infant and young child's relationships with parents. Through her attunement to the behavioural emotional expressions of her infant, the primary caregiver (who is usually the mother) is guided to respond with appropriate caregiving and facial and other emotional expressions that, in turn, help organize and regulate the emotional life of the infant (Stern, 1984). As Emde (1988a) indicates: 'Mother hears a cry and acts to relieve the cause of distress; she sees a smile and hears cooing and cannot resist maintaining a playful interaction' (p. 31).

Developmental research has shown that during this phase in the infant–mother relationship, and especially as the infant develops more capacities, infant and mother display periodic runs of affective synchrony as they regulate and adapt to each other's behaviours and changing needs (Emde, 1988a; Stern, 1984). According to Osofsky (1992), 'it is possible to observe a matching of mental states between the infant and the parent as well as both parties' abilities to share feelings' (p. 236). She emphasizes that 'Being able to share emotions is extremely important for affective development because it is the sharing of emotions with the infant that indicates that a feeling state is understood' (p. 236). The sharing and 'mirroring' of positive emotions in particular, and the experience of safety in the early family environment, have an important influence on the affective development of the child and on his or her emerging self- and object representations (Beebe & Lachmann, 1988; Emde, 1988a, 1991; Osofsky, 1992; Stern, 1985).

Normal affect development does not occur when the parents are unable to read the emotional cues of the infant, and fail to function as external regulators of the infant's emotional states. This regulatory function of the caregiver was appreciated by the psychoanalyst Bion (1962, 1965), who conceptualized the infant–mother relationship as one in which the mother functions as a *container* for receiving and sharing the infant's primitive sensations and emotions; once in the containing space, these *beta elements* (as Bion referred to them) are transformed through the mother's cognitive processes into meaningful affects and other aspects of experience (*alpha elements*) that can be conveyed back to the infant (i.e. the mother functions as a thinking apparatus for the infant).

With the emergence of symbolization and language during the second year of life, the child's level of subjective emotional awareness gradually increases as the parents teach words and meanings for their child's somatic emotional expressions and other bodily experiences (Edgcumbe, 1984; Emde, 1984; Furman, 1992). The acquisition of language has a dramatic impact on the child's developing capacity to regulate affects, both at the intrapersonal level and through relationships with others. 'With language', as Kopp (1989) points out, 'children can state their feelings to others, obtain verbal feedback about the appropriateness of their emotions, and hear and think about ways to manage them' (p. 349). Talking about feelings with an attuned parent extends the sense of 'being felt with' (Furman, 1992), and enables the child to directly enlist aid in alleviating distressing feelings. Moreover, the verbalization of affects leads to new experiences and a growing awareness of more complex and differentiated emotional states (Stern, 1985). This will occur only if the child is reared in a family environment where feelings are verbally labeled and validated.

In an early observational study of nursery school children, Katan

(1961) noted that teaching a child to name feelings and express them in words not only enhances affect regulation by channelling motor behaviour into verbal expressiveness, but also has a favourable effect on the developing functions of thinking, integration, and distinguishing fantasies and wishes from reality. Indeed, several developmental psychologists strongly emphasize that the ability to form verbal representations helps the child to organize and integrate affective experiences, and to reflect on his or her subjective states and plan affect regulating strategies (Bretherton et al., 1986; Dunn & Brown, 1991; Greenberg, Kusche & Speltz, 1990; Kopp, 1989; Stern, 1985).

The capacity verbally to represent and think about subjective experiences also allows the child to begin to contain and tolerate the tensions generated by feelings and needs without always having to rely on parents. In addition to developing affect tolerance (Krystal, 1975, 1988), the child learns to use feelings of anxiety, depression, and other affects as *signals* that can be evaluated and used to guide behaviour that might eliminate or change stressful situations. The emergence of these capacities, in particular the ability to represent the idea of an affect and other subjective experiences, and the awareness that one can be aware of one's own mental state and that of others, imply that the child has acquired an understanding of the concept of mind, an understanding that burgeons in the third year of life (Bretherton & Beeghly, 1982; Fonagy, 1991; Hobson, 1994).

Research studies on attachment styles in infancy and childhood have confirmed that the sensitivity and responsiveness of the primary caregiver to the child's emotional states is a major determinant of the way the child learns to regulate distressing affects and to relate to other people (Bretherton, 1985; Goldberg, MacKay-Soroka, & Rochester, 1994). Children who become securely attached have experienced optimal and consistent responsiveness and learned that modulated emotional expression has positive outcomes. They are able to sustain higher levels of symbolic play than insecurely attached children, and display more positive affect, as well as a greater adaptability and competence in their subsequent relationships (Malatesta, 1990; Slade & Aber, 1992).

Deficient caregiving results in insecure patterns of attachment behaviour and impedes the development of effective affect regulating skills. Attachment researchers originally classified insecurely attached infants and young children into two types – 'avoidant' and 'ambivalent/resistant' – but later added a third type, which they call 'disorganized/disoriented' (Main, 1991; Main, Kaplan & Cassidy, 1985). Studies have found that the insecure–avoidant pattern is associated with maternal insensitivity to infant cues, especially rejection of proximity-seeking behaviour; the insecure–ambivalent pattern is associated with unpredictability of maternal responsiveness; the parental behaviour associated with the disorganized/ disoriented pattern is not yet known, but researchers speculate that the parents at times may appear frightened and/or frightening to the child as a result of their own unresolved psychic trauma (Main, 1991).

Like secure attachment behaviour, the three insecure patterns reflect different strategies used by the child to regulate affective arousal during interactions with, and separations from, the parents. Whereas securely attached children are able to seek and receive comfort from the parents when emotionally distressed, avoidant children have learned to keep their distance and to suppress outward displays of emotion; though affects are hidden, the avoidant attachment style revolves around an axis of fear and anger (Magai & Hunziker, 1993), which, in later childhood, may lead to inappropriate expressions of hostility in social relationships (Kobak & Sceery, 1988). In contrast, children with an ambivalent attachment style display escalating amounts of affective distress, either anxiety, sadness, and helplessness that might elicit a nurturant response, or anger that is sometimes self-defeating. Children with a disorganized/disoriented attachment style display a diverse array of unusual and inexplicable behaviours such as sudden immobility and a dazed expression, or approaching the parent with the head averted; such behaviours suggest that dissociation is being used to regulate affect (Liotti, 1992).

Following the lead of Bowlby (1969, 1973, 1988b) and other psychoanalytic theorists, who emphasize the influence of the inner representational world on both subjective experience and outward behaviour, attachment researchers have moved from a behavioural approach to a representational approach. They now describe the influence of early attachment experiences on the evolving internal representations of the self and others, and have begun to investigate how the 'internal working model' of attachment influences future relationships as well as affect regulating strategies in adolescence and adulthood (Goldberg, 1991; Main et al., 1985; Slade & Aber, 1992). What is internalized, as West and Sheldon-Keller (1994) explain, 'is the child-in-relation-to-the-attachment-figure, rather than the attachment figure per se, creating a cognitive/affective schema of this first attachment relationship' (p. 45). Subsequent attachment events either reinforce or modify this initial schema.

Similar conceptions of the inner representational world have been proposed by many contemporary psychoanalytic object relations theorists, including Kernberg (1984), who acknowledges that affects are the primary motivational system, and links them intimately with internalized object relations. Self psychology, in its conception of 'self–selfobject relationships', stresses the importance of empathic attunement and the regulatory functions provided by relationships throughout life; but it also conceptualizes an internalization in childhood of affective experiences with 'mirroring' and 'idealized' parental selfobjects, which have a major impact on the child's developing sense of self, capacity to experience and regulate affects, and interpersonal relationships (Kohut, 1977, 1984).

Though some investigators use different labels to describe insecure attachment patterns in older children and adults, there is strong suggestive evidence that the attachment styles developed in childhood remain relatively stable across the life span and may even be transmitted between generations (Goldberg, 1991; Slade & Aber, 1992). Furthermore, studies of adolescents and adults have found that those with secure attachment styles report low levels of negative affect, and form strong relationships with others to whom they turn for support when emotionally distressed (Kobak & Sceery, 1988; Mikulincer & Orbach, 1995; Priel & Shamai, 1995; Schaffer, 1993; Shaver & Brennan, 1992). Individuals with insecure styles of attachment were found to experience less positive affect than those with secure attachments, and also manifested deficits in the ability to self-regulate anxiety, depression, and other negative affects.

## Imagination and the self-regulation of affects

Although initially the infant's precursor emotional states of contentment and distress are regulated primarily by the responses of an empathically attuned caregiver, even babies who become securely attached display some independent affect regulating behaviours such as sucking on their fingers and thumbs, rubbing their genitals, rocking their bodies, and fingering parts of the caregiver's body or clothing (Kopp, 1989). These elemental forms of affect regulation have been studied by Winnicott (1953) and Gaddini (1978), and also by Tustin (1981), who refers to the objects or body parts used by the infant as *sensation-objects*. Such objects, through the motoric rhythms and tactile sensuous experiences they provide, are thought to help preserve in the infant an illusion of 'oneness' with the mother. All three psychoanalytic theorists regard the infant's use of sensation-objects, during the first month's of life, a precondition for the later development of *transitional objects* and *transitional phenomena*.

Defined by Winnicott (1953) as the child's 'first creation' or imaginative act, the transitional object emerges at around four to six months of life and reaches its peak at about eighteen months. It is a special object such as a soft toy, a small blanket, or a piece of wool, which the child selects and repeatedly seeks out during states of distress, especially anxious states evoked by separations from the mother. Used by the child for self-soothing and comforting, the transitional object functions as an important regulator of affect. While this function is related initially to the textural and olfactory properties of the object (softness, and odours it collects from milk and mother's pheromones), the child gradually endows the transitional object with meaning so that it becomes a symbol for the mother and bridges the space created by her temporary absence. Although Winnicott believed that the use of transitional objects was virtually universal, findings from several studies suggest that transitional objects are a more necessary creation in infants who are weaned early or otherwise have less close contact with their mothers (Taylor, 1987a). However, most studies do not take account of transitional phenomena, such as babblings, humming tunes, and creating imaginary companions, which many infants and children use to induce pleasurable affects or to modulate distressing states.

Winnicott and several more recent theorists (e.g. Deri, 1984; Mayes & Cohen, 1992) regard the relatedness between the infant and an empathically attuned mother as the necessary matrix for the gradual development of the child's imagination and creative capacities. From its roots in the sensation-objects and transitional object of the infant, and aided by the maturation of neocortical structures and functions (Schore, 1994), the child's imaginal capacity evolves into forming a mental image of the mother in her absence, and eventually to creating fantasies, dreams, interests, and play that go beyond images derived directly from external objects. These capacities play an important role in personality development and in the self-regulation of affects throughout life. As Mayes and Cohen (1992) indicate:

> Imagination . . . encompasses a number of interrelated functions and concepts, including the capacity to create a fantasy, the ability to use such a fantasy in the service of affect regulation and/or defense, the synthesis of memories and percepts into the mental image of a person or thing which is not present, and the inner world of mental representations, as opposed to the external world of sensory perceptions (pp. 24–25).

The role of fantasy in affect regulation, especially the induction of positive affective experiences, is very evident in children's play, an activity that usually first occurs in interactions with parents. Singer (1979) regards play in early childhood as an adaptive resource by which children can organize complex experiences into manageable forms, and thereby avoid extreme negative affects and maximize the occurrence of the positive affects of interest and joy. Izard and Kobak (1991) similarly view play as one of the most important developmental processes through which children learn to integrate affect, cognition, and action. 'It is through play that children have repeated opportunities to rehearse verbal and motoric responses to their emotion-feeling states. In their various types of play, children make connections among their feelings, thoughts, and activities' (p. 317). Children who are unable to engage in imaginative play show degrees of failure in integrating cognitions with emotions, as well as a disturbance in the symbolic function of fantasy and an inability to identify with the feelings of others (Galenson, 1984; Tustin, 1988).

Another important way in which imaginal activity regulates affects, as well as instinctual wishes, is through the creation of symbolic wish-fulfilling types of dreams. In addition to modulating affects through the mechanisms of displacement, condensation, and symbolization, dreams are thought to help organize and store affect-laden recent events in long-term memory (Taylor, 1987a). Individuals with an inadequate ability to symbolize are unable to transform affective experiences into creative stories; consequently, their dreams are either banal or highly disturbing, the latter type appearing to attempt to regulate intense emotions through 'evacuation' (Segal, 1981; Taylor, 1987a).

Though children eventually relinquish their transitional objects, individuals generally acquire interests and engage in activities that provide similar solacing functions (Horton, 1981). These include religion, reading, music, and artistic creativity, as well as meditation, daydreaming, and the pursuit of hobbies. As Eagle (1984) points out, however, the development of interests may reflect the unfolding of an innate predisposition; they secondarily come to serve some of the affect regulating functions initially provided by the primary attachment figures. And, as was noted earlier, interests generate the positive affects of interest and enjoyment, and thereby strengthen social relationships, which provide further affect regulating functions. Individuals who have constricted imaginations and fail to develop interests, and who also lack supportive social relationships, may rely on less effective methods to regulate affects such as excessive eating or consumption of alcohol, issues that will be taken up in later chapters.

## Toward an integrated model

In this chapter, we have emphasized the role of early relationships in affect development and in the acquisition of affect regulating capacities. These are complex developmental processes, however, that are influenced by other factors as well, including temperament and neurobiological structures and functions, and the reciprocal interactions between these endowments and the early social environment (Schore, 1994). For example, some innate neurological defect in an infant may affect the way it attempts to engage with an appropriately attuned mother; alternatively, a mother with an endogenous depressive disorder is likely to be emotionally unavailable and insensitive to her infant's emotional signals (Cicchetti, Ganiban & Barnett, 1991). There is accumulating evidence also that early social relationships can affect the organization and homeostatic setting of neurobiological systems, including the physiological component of emotion response systems (Field, 1985; Hofer, 1987). As Schore (1994) has elaborated, the degree to which the mother stimulates and modulates the infant's affect–arousal states and maintains them within a moderate range may influence the ongoing balance between the sympathetic and parasympathetic components of the autonomic nervous system. Whereas secure-infants are protected from extreme high and low arousal states and develop an optimal balance between these two autonomic systems, it is thought that insecure–avoidant infants develop an ongoing parasympathetic bias, and that insecure–ambivalent infants develop a bias toward a predominance of the sympathetic system over the parasympathetic system.

Cultural factors also may exert an influence on affect development and affect regulation. Child-rearing practices, for example, may be different in some cultures, and emotional expressions (non-verbal and through language) may have different meanings across cultural groups. Cultural differences may exist also in the way different groups appraise emotionally relevant situations, and sociocultural norms influence how people think about and express various emotions (Mesquita & Frijda, 1992).

Though a great deal of progress has yet to be made, emotion theorists and researchers are now taking an integrated approach toward understanding the development and regulation of affects. This includes attempts to conceptualize the complex interactions between cognition, affect, and attachment behaviour. Crittenden (1994), for example, relates successful affect development and regulation to the experience of secure attachment; it provides predictable positive outcomes to affective communications, and thereby facilitates a satisfactory integration of affective information with cognition information. Consequently, the child is able to 'use cognition to moderate affect and affect to inform cognition' (p. 134). Crittenden goes on to suggest that insecurely attached children show various degrees of failure in integrating cognition with affect: insecure–avoidant children come to distrust affectively based information and learn to rely on cognition to organize behaviour and control affect; insecure–ambivalent children, who are unable to predict the outcome of affective communications, come to distrust cognitively-generated information, and function on the basis of unregulated affect.

Though modified to some extent by socialization experiences throughout childhood and adolescence, the way in which affect, cognition and attachment behaviour are integrated and mentally represented during the formative years has a major influence on the organization of the personality and accounts for important individual differences in adult life (Bowlby, 1988b; Kissen, 1995; Magai & Hunziker, 1993; Magai & McFadden, 1995; Malatesta, 1990). In the following chapters we will describe how continuing splits between affect and cognition in insecurely attached individuals appear to be a risk factor for a variety of medical and psychiatric disorders.

# [2] Affect dysregulation and alexithymia

Because the capacities for experiencing and regulating affects cognitively are acquired during the developmental years, opportunities easily arise for failure (Dodge & Garber, 1991; Taylor, 1992b). Such failures result in a proneness to affect dysregulation that is evident in personality traits or psychopathology and poor physical health. The major psychopathologies and physical pathologies are conceptualized in this book as disorders of affect regulation and are linked to failures at, or regressions to, lower levels within the model of an epigenetic sequence of affect development proposed by Lane and Schwartz (1987).

As was noted in the previous chapter, the self-regulation of affect has been linked also with the recently introduced construct of emotional intelligence (Goleman, 1995; Salovey et al., 1993). Individuals who are described as low in emotional intelligence manifest difficulties in the accurate appraisal and expression of emotion, in the effective regulation of emotion, and in the ability to use feelings to guide behaviour (Salovey & Mayer, 1989/90). As a continuum construct, emotional intelligence at its lower end corresponds to the preconceptual levels of emotion organization and regulation within Lane and Schwartz's hierarchical model. Lane and Schwartz, and also Salovey and his colleagues, acknowledge that individuals functioning at the lower levels of these conceptual frameworks have been described previously in the literature as *alexithymic*. Although this personality trait has generated interest only recently among emotion theorists and researchers, the construct of alexithymia emerged more than 20 years ago and has its origins in clinical observations that were made even earlier on both medical and psychiatric patients.

In this chapter we will review the historical background and clinical features of the alexithymia construct, and then discuss several criticisms of the construct and some similarities and differences between alexithymia and related constructs. We will consider also some factors that might contribute to failures in affect development and in the cognitive processing and regulation of emotion that are reflected in the alexithymic personality trait.

## Historical background

The alexithymia construct evolved from clinical observations that were made initially on patients suffering from one or more of the so-called classical psychosomatic diseases. For many years the psychic disturbance in these patients was conceptualized according to Freud's model of psychoneurotic pathology and psychosomaticists attempted to relieve somatic symptoms by identifying and interpreting conflicts over unconscious drive-related wishes.[1]

However, some of the early leaders in psychosomatic medicine believed that psychosomatic diseases could not be explained by analogy with the psychoneuroses; they reported observations which suggested that it is a disturbance in the cognitive processing of emotions, rather than intrapsychic conflict, that predisposes people to psychosomatic illnesses. For example, MacLean (1949) noted that many psychosomatic patients show an apparent inability to verbalize feelings. Using his model of a 'triune brain' (which will be described in Chapter 5), MacLean speculated that, instead of being relayed to the neocortex (which he referred to as the 'word brain') and finding expression in the symbolic use of words, distressing emotions find immediate expression through autonomic pathways and thereby result in physiological changes that may lead to physical disease.

Ruesch (1948) observed a similar disturbance of verbal and symbolic expression among psychosomatic patients and patients with post-traumatic syndromes; he attributed this to the continuation of an 'immature' or 'infantile personality' into adult life. In addition to dependency and a childlike way of thinking, Ruesch's patients were unimaginative, used direct physical action or bodily channels for emotional expression, failed to use affects as signals, and showed an excessive degree of social conformity.

In the early 1950s, Horney (1952) and Kelman (1952) described similar characteristics in certain psychiatric patients who were respond-

---

1. The classical psychosomatic diseases and early psychosomatic theories and treatment approaches will be reviewed in Chapter 10.

ing poorly to psychoanalytic treatment because of a lack of emotional awareness, paucity of inner experiences, minimal interest in dreams, concreteness of thinking, and an externalized style of living. These psychiatric patients were prone to developing 'psychosomatic' symptoms and often engaged in binge eating, alcohol abuse, or other compulsive behaviours, seemingly to avoid experiencing feelings of inner emptiness. Although Horney and Kelman recognized that these characteristics were not restricted to any specific type of neurosis, they attributed them to strong defenses against unconscious conflicts.

A decade later, however, the French psychoanalysts Marty and de M'Uzan (1963) described a similar utilitarian thinking style and conspicuous absence of fantasy in physically ill patients, which they attributed to deficits in personality organization rather than to neurotic defenses. They referred to this cognitive style as *pensée opératoire* and later introduced the term *vie opératoire* to describe the associated externalized mode of existence (Marty & DeBray, 1989).

The significance of these early observations was not fully appreciated until the early 1970s after Sifneos (1967) and Nemiah and Sifneos (1970) had begun to investigate systematically the cognitive and affective style of patients suffering from classical psychosomatic diseases. The results of their studies, and those of subsequent investigators (Shands, 1975; Vogt *et al.*, 1977; von Rad, Lalucat & Lolas, 1977), confirmed that many patients with classical psychosomatic diseases have a marked difficulty describing subjective feelings and a communicative style characterized by a preoccupation with minute details of external events and by a paucity or absence of drive-related fantasies. Sifneos (1973) coined the word *alexithymia* (from the Greek: *a* = lack, *lexis* = word, *thymos* = emotion) to denote this cluster of cognitive and affective characteristics. Like the French psychoanalysts, Nemiah and Sifneos (1970) and Nemiah (1977) proposed a deficit model for understanding alexithymia and the psychosomatic process.

Around this time, and unaware of the studies on medically ill patients, Krystal (1968) and Krystal and Raskin (1970) were observing similar characteristics among patients with severe posttraumatic states and patients with drug dependence; Wurmser (1974) described deficits in the verbal affective expression and imaginal capacity of drug addicts; and Bruch (1973) reported a comparable set of personality traits in patients with eating disorders.

In recognition of the growing interest in the construct, alexithymia was selected as the main theme of the 11th European Conference on Psychosomatic Research held in Heidelberg, Germany, in 1976 (Bräutigam & von Rad, 1977). At that conference a consensus was reached that a precise definition of the alexithymia construct was needed, as well as validational research and development of reliable and valid instruments for measuring the construct.

## The alexithymia construct

Since the Heidelberg Conference the alexithymia construct has been refined theoretically, largely through a program of research that sought to validate the construct in the process of developing a reliable and valid instrument for measuring it (Taylor *et al.*, 1990*a*). As it is presently defined, the alexithymia construct is composed of the following salient features: (i) difficulty identifying feelings and distinguishing between feelings and the bodily sensations of emotional arousal; (ii) difficulty describing feelings to other people; (iii) constricted imaginal processes, as evidenced by a paucity of fantasies; and (iv) a stimulus-bound, externally orientated cognitive style (Nemiah, Freyberger & Sifneos, 1976; Taylor, 1994; Taylor, Bagby & Parker, 1991).

At first glance, some individuals who are labelled alexithymic appear to contradict this definition of the construct because they experience chronic dysphoria or manifest outbursts of weeping, anger, or rage. Intensive questioning, however, reveals that they know very little about their own feelings and, in most instances, are unable to link them with memories, fantasies, higher level affects, or specific situations (Nemiah *et al.*, 1976; Robbins, 1989; Taylor, 1987*b*). Indeed, in a report of his preliminary clinical observations, Sifneos (1967) noted that these patients commonly mentioned anxiety or complained of depression; but, when questioned further about their anxiety, they talked 'only about nervousness, agitation, restlessness, irritability and tension'; when asked about depression, they talked about 'sensations of emptiness, void, boredom, and pain' (pp. 3–4).

On the basis of some other early clinical observations, several additional characteristics have been associated with the alexithymia construct, including a tendency toward social conformity, a tendency toward action to express emotion or to avoid conflicts, an infrequent recollection of dreams, a somewhat stiff wooden posture, and a paucity of facial emotional expressions (Krystal, 1979; Nemiah *et al.*, 1976; Ruesch, 1948; Sifneos, Apfel-Savitz & Frankel, 1977). However, while these characteristics often are associated with alexithymia, they are not part of the theoretical core of the construct. Indeed, as we will describe in Chapter 3, social conformity, a tendency toward action, and the ability to recall dreams did not emerge as essential features of alexithymia in the process of validating the construct. Clinical experience suggests it is the quality of dreams more than the ability to recall them that best characterises alexithymia. When dreams are recalled they either contain explicit archaic mental content (e.g. scenes of violence or perverse sexuality) or they merely replay a daytime experience without the usual dream work of symbolization, condensation, and displacement (Levitan, 1989; Taylor, 1987a).

Even without these additional characteristics, alexithymia is conceptualized as a multifaceted construct. Although the salient features of the construct can be distinguished conceptually, they are related logically: the ability to identify and communicate feelings to others is obviously contingent on an ability to distinguish one's feelings from the bodily sensations that accompany emotional states; and an externally orientated cognitive style reflects an absence of inner thoughts and fantasies, as well as a low range of emotional expressiveness. It should be emphasized also that alexithymia is conceptualized not as a categorical (all-or-none) phenomenon, but as a dimensional construct (or personality trait) that is distributed normally in the general population.

**Alexithymia and failures in affect regulation**

Though the alexithymia construct is defined in terms of identifiable cognitive characteristics, these characteristics reflect deficits both in the cognitive–experiential domain of emotion response systems and at the level of interpersonal regulation of emotion. Unable to identify accurately their own subjective feelings, alexithymic individuals verbally communicate emotional distress to other people very poorly, thereby failing to enlist others as sources of aid or comfort. As noted earlier, their limited ability to identify and describe subjective feelings has been linked to a failure to elevate emotions from a preconceptual level of organization to the conceptual level of mental representations in Lane and Schwartz's (1987) model of affect development.

The associated restricted imaginal capacities also limit the extent to which alexithymic individuals can modulate anxiety and other emotions by fantasy, dreams, interest, and play (Krystal, 1988; Mayes & Cohen, 1992). Lacking knowledge of their own emotional experiences, alexithymic individuals cannot readily imagine themselves in another person's situation and are consequently unempathic and ineffective in modulating the emotional states of others (Goleman, 1995; Krystal, 1979; Lane & Schwartz, 1987). Clinical reports of restricted gestures and near expressionless faces in some alexithymic individuals

(Nemiah *et al.*, 1976), together with preliminary evidence of a reduced ability to recognize posed facial expressions of emotion (which will be reviewed in later chapters), suggest that alexithymia may involve deficits in the behavioural-expressive domain of emotion response systems as well.

Given the impaired emotion-processing and emotion-regulating capacities thought to underly alexithymia, it is not surprising that alexithymia has been conceptualized as one of several possible personality risk factors for a variety of medical and psychiatric disorders involving problems in affect regulation. For example, hypochondriasis and somatization disorder might be viewed as resulting, at least in part, from the alexithymic individual's limited subjective awareness and cognitive processing of emotions, which leads both to a focusing on, and amplification and misinterpretation of, the somatic sensations that accompany emotional arousal; this corresponds to the sensorimotor reflexive level in Lane and Schwartz's model. An inability to modulate emotions through cognitive processing might explain also the tendency of alexithymic individuals to discharge tension arising from unpleasant emotional states through impulsive acts (Keltikangas-Järvinen, 1982) or compulsive behaviours such as binge eating, substance abuse, perverse sexual behaviour, or the self-starvation of anorexia nervosa; this corresponds to the sensorimotor enactive level in the model. Further, as suggested originally by MacLean (1949), the failure cognitively to regulate distressing emotions might result in exacerbated responses in the autonomic nervous system and neuro-endocrine systems, thereby producing conditions conducive to the development of somatic diseases. Dysregulation or heightened activation of the autonomic nervous system would be expected to produce a proneness to dysphoric as well as somatic symptoms, a disposition that would overlap the trait of neuroticism (or negative affectivity), which will be discussed further in Chapter 4, and which Eysenck (1963; Eysenck & Eysenck, 1985) views in terms of a lability of the autonomic nervous system.

In addition to a proneness to undifferentiated negative affective states, alexithymic individuals show a limited capacity to experience positive emotions such as joy, happiness and love. Indeed, Krystal (1988) and Sifneos (1987) have described many of these individuals as being anhedonic. Although schizophrenic and depressed patients also tend to exhibit anhedonia, not all schizophrenic and depressed patients are alexithymic (Sifneos, 1987; Stanghellini & Ricca, 1995). And, while many schizophrenic individuals show minimal outward display of emotion, recent research suggests that they actually experience as much positive and negative emotion as normal individuals (Kring *et al.*, 1993). Also, preliminary research with a non-psychiatric population has shown alexithymia to be associated with social anhedonia, but not with pleasant physical situations, even when controlling for depression and other negative affect (Prince & Berenbaum, 1993). None the less, there is evidence that an absence of pleasurable affect in both alexithymia and depression is related to the personality dimension of positive affectivity or extraversion (see Chapter 4), which is largely independent of negative affectivity and is thought to involve a separate functional brain system (Emde, 1991; Watson & Clark, 1992; Watson, Clark & Carey, 1988). In Krystal's (1988) view, the finding of anhedonia in an alexithymic individual indicates a traumatic origin to the problem.

### Clinical illustration

To give the reader some idea of the clinical features of alexithymia, we report some short excerpts from a videotaped interview with an alexithymic patient. The patient, a divorced physiotherapist in her late-forties, had been referred to a craniofacial pain clinic for multidisciplinary assessment of several puzzling and medically unexplained somatic symptoms including facial pain, a burning sensation on the top of her head, and episodes of weakness. The patient had experienced these symptoms for eight years following surgical drainage of an infected sinus. The initial phase of the interview focused on the history of the patient's illness and the various investigations and treatments she had received. The patient spoke fluently and provided a very detailed account of the course of the illness and the changes it had caused in her life. However, when the doctor inquired about her emotional response to the illness, the patient displayed a striking inability to describe inner feelings:

DR  Can you say more about your feelings as a result of all these medical problems.

PT  Uhm – I really can't pin things down. As I say, I have always – you know – uhm – life to me is what you make of it in spite of things, and I've never been one to get terribly emotional about what's going on – trying to be analytical about it, and, as I maintain, all the way along, I knew it started from that infection of the sinus. And I think the basis of the bottom line of what's behind what is going on is that I was never put on antibiotics.

The patient continued to talk about her symptoms without mentioning any associated affects, and displayed an operative mode of thinking (*pensée opératoire*) as she described both her symptoms and external events in excessive detail and without any reference to inner experiences. After she had described a typical episode of physical symptoms, the doctor inquired once more about her emotional response.

DR Do you feel anything emotionally at those times?
PT No.
DR Nothing at all?
PT No. I'm just so weak, I'm just drained. Uhm – the only comparison I can make to that is after I had surgery about 20 years ago, I went into shock, and it's the same thing. Like when the phone finally woke me up that day – uhm – I had been to the hospital in the morning and I could hardly function to get there. They did not know what to do, so they didn't do anything. This is what I'm infuriated about.
DR (grasping the opportunity) Can you tell me a bit about that fury?
PT Well, I just feel that I'm – uh – that it's an exercise in futility trying to get to the source of what's going on.
DR What's it like to be feeling furious?
PT Well, it's an expression I use, but really it's hard to put it in words.
DR Can you try and put it into words?
PT It's – its – it's relating what's happened and not getting any answers and I think in view of the fact that I had a culture done when this pressure built up . . .
DR (interrupting the patient as she was again about to provide more details of her illness) That's not really putting the fury into words is it?
PT No, it's not.
DR Can you try and explain the fury? What is it like for you to feel furious?
PT It's hard to put it in words. (silence)

It is important to note that, although the patient used the word 'infuriated' to label an emotional state, she was unable to elaborate on the subjective nature of this emotion. The patient's inarticulateness and inability to describe inner feelings is further illustrated in a later portion of the interview in which the doctor inquires about other specific emotions the patient might experience.

DR It's hard for you to describe the feeling of fury. Do you have trouble describing most of your emotions?
PT I've never really given any thought to it.
DR Do you ever get depressed?

PT   No. I'm not the depressive type, no. What's been happening to me is bound to – uhm – to tell in certain ways I suppose.

DR   Do you know what depression is like?

PT   Yes, I think so. I've certainly looked after a number of people who have been depressed.

DR   Have you felt it yourself?

PT   I don't think so.

DR   Never, ever?

PT   No, I don't really think I have.

DR   What about sadness?

PT   No, I don't think so.

DR   What sort of emotions do you usually experience?

PT   I find that hard to say.

DR   If somebody was to ask you what sort of moods you have, how would you answer that?

PT   Well, I'm not a moody person, and – uhm – I think, as I say, I know I've been in three comas, and after the first one I just didn't seem to have any expression to my face. The physiotherapists that I've worked with would ask if I was mad at them and I said, well, you know me, if I were mad, you know, you would know about it.

DR   How would they know about it?

PT   We've discussed it; I'm not a moody person. I don't go around getting mad at people.

DR   Do you ever get mad?

PT   Oh sure. I can blow my top. I don't hold things in, I get it out of my system.

DR   What about sad feelings; do you ever get sad?

PT   I suppose everybody does to a degree. But I don't think I ever have.

DR   Do you ever cry?

PT   I have been weepy here telling you about what's going on and that surprises me. I think it's just the total frustration, as I say.

DR   It surprises you to find yourself crying! What does it feel like when you cry?

PT   I really don't know, because I think it's just frustration that brings it on.

DR   (referring to an earlier interview during which the patient had become tearful) You were crying, or you were about to cry the other day when we were interviewing you. Do you know what you were feeling when you started to become tearful?

PT   I really don't. And that's what surprised me. I think it's relating this over and over, it's bad enough living it.

Despite the patient's claim that she understands the term depression, it is evident in this portion of the interview that she has difficulty identifying emotional states and has a limited vocabulary for describing feelings. She seems to experience the subjective component of emotions largely as an undifferentiated state that she labels 'frustration' and which is devoid of any associated fantasies. Unaware of the subjective feeling of sadness, the patient is surprised to find herself crying; also, it seems that physiotherapy colleagues could recognize the affect of anger in her facial expression when the patient herself was unaware of feeling angry. Rather than experiencing anger as a signal affect that could lead to reflection about external events and be used to guide behaviour, the patient implies that she becomes aware of her anger only when it is intense. But, instead of fantasizing angry actions, the patient experiences anger as an entity that should be discharged through explosive outbursts. In a later portion of the interview the doctor inquired about the patient's emotional response to other stressful events including the breakdown of her marriage and her inability to return to work.

DR This illness must have had quite an effect on you. It has altered the course of your life; your husband left you, and you are no longer able to work. How has all of that made you feel?

PT Well, I feel that I have got to get to the source of it. And I feel that it can't be put off. Having things diagnosed and not getting – but maybe I have been at fault because maybe I was thinking in terms of just things that have progressed from the sinus infection. As I say, . . .

DR (again interrupting the patient as she was about to give more mundane details of her illness) What effect has it all had on you emotionally? What effect on your nerves and on your emotions?

PT Well, all my friends, my family and my friends, are amazed at how calm I can be about it? I can't go to pieces – it's not going to help the situation. I did burst into tears once and – uhm – after I had my living room carpet replaced and I thought, well – that's lunacy, what on earth am I doing that for? But I just looked at it and I thought I should have spent the money on a trip; the way I felt, I thought I'm not getting any better, why am I spending money on the house?

DR Do you know why you burst into tears?

PT Uhm – I just think, at that time, I just had the weakness come on, and I just knew I was going to be going through one of these infectious bouts, and I thought why on earth did I waste my money on this for, I might as well have gone on a trip.

DR Was that because you felt disappointed or upset?

PT I just felt here we go again.

## Criticisms of the alexithymia construct

Although there is consensus about the clinical features and definition of the alexithymia construct, there has been controversy and debate as to whether it is a stable personality trait, a transient state secondary to psychological distress associated with acute illness or some other stressful situation, or a coping response to chronic illness (Ahrens & Deffner, 1986). Some critics have argued that alexithymia can be explained merely by cultural or social class differences in emotional expressiveness (Borens et al., 1977; Kirmayer, 1987; Prince, 1987) or by communication difficulties specific to the patient/physician relationship (Musaph, 1974). Others regard alexithymia as a defense against neurotic conflict (Hogan, 1995; Knapp, 1983; Wilson & Mintz, 1989), rather than a type of affect deficit as Sifneos (1994) and Nemiah (1977) have proposed. Some even claim not to 'agree with' or 'believe' in the concept of alexithymia, failing to realize that constructs do not exist in the sense that material things do, but represent hypotheses which behavioural scientists rely on to explore human thought and behaviour (Wallace, 1988b).

Given that a child's intelligence and social and family environment influence the development of language skills and verbal emotional expressiveness, one might expect alexithymia to show some association with intelligence, educational level, and socioeconomic status. Preliminary investigations of the relationships between alexithymia and these variables have demonstrated either no associations or weak positive associations with lower socioeconomic status, lower educational level, and lower intelligence (Kauhanen et al., 1993; Kirmayer & Robbins, 1993; Parker, Taylor & Bagby, 1989b).

There is no doubt that the verbal expression of emotion is influenced also by prevailing cultural attitudes and by constraints imposed by certain languages (Leff, 1977; Mesquita & Frijda, 1992). It seems unlikely, however, that the constricted imaginal processes facet of the alexithymia construct could be explained merely by cultural influences. Preliminary evidence that alexithymia is not a culture-bound construct is provided by reports of alexithymia in both clinical and non-clinical populations in diverse cultures, and by the successful cross-validation of a self-report measure of the construct in many different countries including Italy, India, Japan, and Korea; these data will be reviewed in later chapters.

With regard to the trait versus state controversy, Freyberger (1977) and others have observed a constriction of emotional expression and imaginal activity in some medically ill patients undergoing hemodialysis or organ transplantation and in others who are transitorily suffering from a life-threatening state and are in an intensive care unit. Freyberger called this alexithymia-like phenomenon *secondary alexithymia* and reported that it may become a permanent feature in patients whose disease takes a chronic course. Recent empirical studies of patients undergoing kidney transplantation or receiving hemodialysis therapy have confirmed that the development of alexithymic characteristics is a not infrequent response to these stressful procedures; it appears to be a protective strategy involving the defense of denial (Fukunishi, 1992; Fukunishi, Saito & Ozaki, 1992*b*).

Sifneos (1988, 1994) uses the term *secondary alexithymia* somewhat differently than Freyberger to refer to alexithymic characteristics resulting from developmental arrests, massive psychological trauma in childhood or later on in life, sociocultural factors, or psychodynamic factors. He contrasts this with *primary alexithymia*, which he attributes to neurobiological deficits. As we will discuss later, however, the etiology of alexithymia probably involves multiple factors, including constitutional–inherited variations in brain organization and deficiencies in the early family and social environment. Moreover, massive psychological trauma may not only overwhelm the ego and produce a regression in affective functioning but also evoke lasting changes in neuronal excitability that contribute to the clinical features of alexithymia. Also, arrests in the development of affects and affect regulating capacities during childhood generally become pervasive features of the personality that endure across time and situations. We find it less confusing therefore to simply distinguish between alexithymia as a stable personality *trait* that is independent of etiology and alexithymia that is *state-dependent* and disappears after the evoking stressful situation has changed; the latter corresponds to Freyberger's concept of secondary alexithymia. Strong empirical support for alexithymia being a stable personality trait, rather than just a consequence of psychological distress, has been provided by several prospective studies which will be reviewed in Chapters 4 and 8.

Because some alexithymic patients manifest psychoneurotic symptoms and show evidence of unconscious drive-related conflicts, some clinicians and researchers resort to a neurotic conflict model to explain alexithymia. They overlook Freud's (1898) description of patients with admixtures of deficit-related and conflict-related symptoms, and ignore findings from recent empirical studies that support an independence of alexithymia from psychoneurotic pathology (Taylor, Bagby & Parker, 1993). Other clinicians report the emergence of primitive emotions and fantasies during the course of intensive psychoanalytic psychotherapy and conclude also that alexithymia is entirely a result of defensive operations, particularly denial, repression, avoidance, reaction formation, and externalization (Hogan, 1995; Knapp, 1981, 1983). While empirical research (which will be reviewed in Chapter 4) has shown an association between alexithymia and the use of 'immature' or primitive defense mechanisms, these critics of the alexithymia construct forget that primitive defenses emerge (a) when there is an absence or failure of higher level defenses, and (b) for the purpose of regulating intense and disruptive emotions that are not fully represented mentally and remain organized on a preconceptual level (Dorpat, 1985; Fonagy, 1991; Frosch, 1995; Robbins, 1989; Stein, 1990). As with other types of psychic deficit, the presence of alexithymia is likely to both initiate and intensify ordinary developmental conflicts (Killingmo, 1989).

**Relationships between alexithymia and other constructs**

Two psychological constructs with which alexithymia is closely related are *psychological mindedness* and *emotional intelligence*. Whereas emotional intelligence is a recently formulated construct, the concept of psychological mindedness has been employed for several decades to refer to a set of skills that are thought to enhance the prospects of successful insight-orientated psychotherapies. In contrast to alexithymia, however, there is little empirical research evaluating the validity of these two other constructs. Furthermore, the construct of psychological mindedness has been defined in a variety of ways and is not always distinguished from other concepts such as insightfulness, self-awareness, and introspectiveness (Taylor, 1995).

In an attempt to establish a generally agreed upon definition of the construct, Appelbaum (1973) proposed that psychological mindedness is 'A person's ability to see relationships among thoughts, feelings, and actions, with the goal of learning the meanings and causes of his experience and behaviour' (p. 36). This broad definition places psychological mindedness within the 'openness to experience' dimension of the five-factor model of personality (McCrae & Costa, 1985, 1987), which will be described in Chapter 4. In developing an operational definition and measure of psychological mindedness, Conte et al. (1990, 1995) identified four facets to the construct: access to one's feelings, willingness to talk about one's intrapsychic and/or interpersonal problems, a capacity for behavioural change, and an interest in why people behave the way they do. Though alexithymia is a more narrowly defined construct, concerned exclusively with the processing and regulation of affect, there is clearly considerable overlap with the psychological mindedness construct. In later chapters we will report some empirical research showing that alexithymia is related strongly and negatively to both psychological mindedness and openness to experience. Such findings help explain the unfavourable response of alexithymic patients to traditional psychodynamic psychotherapy.

In their conceptualization of emotional intelligence as a dimensional construct encompassing a set of skills involved in the appraisal, expression, and regulation of emotion in oneself and others, as well as the use of feelings to guide one's thinking and actions, Salovey *et al.* (1993) appropriately place severe alexithymia at the extreme lower end of the construct. This relationship has not been tested empirically, as no measure of the emotional intelligence construct has yet been developed. Closely related to emotional intelligence, however, is the *affective orientation* construct for which there is a valid measure. Formulated by Booth-Butterfield and Booth-Butterfield (1990), affective orientation is defined as 'the degree to which individuals are aware of and use affect cues to guide communication' (p. 451). Given that alexithymic individuals have difficulty in recognizing and labeling their emotions and in using affects as signals that guide behaviour, one would expect them to score low on affective orientation. Empirical evidence of an inverse relationship between the two constructs will be presented in Chapter 3. Though the constructs of alexithymia, emotional intelligence, and affective orientation all involve cognitive skills that relate to an awareness of emotions, the alexithymia construct also encompasses a cognitive style (*pensée opératoire*) that reflects deficits in imaginal processing that further limit the ability to self-regulate emotions.

Some theorists have suggested that alexithymia may overlap with the construct of *inhibition* (King, Emmons & Woodley, 1992) or be part of the *repressive coping style*, which is identified by high scores on social desirability scales (indicating high defensiveness) and low scores on measures of anxiety despite high levels of physiological arousal (Bonanno & Singer, 1990). Though there is evidence that long-term inhibition of emotional expression results in heightened autonomic arousal that can have adverse effects on physical health (Berry & Pennebaker, 1993; Pennebaker, 1985), inhibition differs from alexithymia in being a conscious act of suppression rather than a failure to fully differentiate emotions and integrate them with increasingly developed cognitive structures. And, although the repressive coping style involves a decoupling of the subjective awareness of affect from the physiological arousal, and has been linked also with certain medical illnesses (Bonanno & Singer, 1990; Schwartz, 1990), repression is essentially an unconscious ego defense mechanism for keeping certain thoughts and feelings out of awareness (King et al., 1992). Recent empirical studies have shown that repressors score low on measures of alexithymia, and that alexithymia is most similar to the sensitizing style of high-anxious individuals who acknowledge negative emotional experiences but have difficulty regulating them (Myers, 1995; Newton & Contrada, 1994). As Newton & Contrada (1994) point out, however, alexithymic individuals are distinguished from high-anxious individuals by their diminished fantasy life and externally orientated cognitive style.

Closely related to repression is the concept of *dissociation* with which alexithymia may also be confused. Like alexithymia, dissociation occurs on a continuum and may be found in normal individuals but is more prevalent among persons with major psychiatric disorders (Bernstein & Putnam, 1986). Though Freud often used 'dissociation' synonymously with 'repression' (Erdelyi, 1990), dissociation is nowadays considered a separate mechanism in which there is 'a disruption of the normal integration of cognition, affect, behaviour, sensation and identity' (Atchison & McFarlane, 1994, p. 591).

Nemiah (1989) points out that Freud's conceptualization of dissociation also differed significantly from Janet's formulation of the phenomenon. Whereas Freud attributed dissociation to 'the *active* repression of undesirable and emotionally painful mental contents by an ego that was strong enough to banish them from conscious awareness', Janet viewed dissociation as resulting 'from a *passive* falling away of mental contents from an ego that was too weak to retain them in consciousness' (p. 1528). Using modern terminology, Nemiah indicates that Freud's formulation was based on a psychodynamic *conflict* model of symptom formation, while Janet employed an *ego-deficit* model of psychopathology. As outlined earlier, the latter model has also guided the conceptualization of the alexithymia construct. And although alexithymia and dissociation are distinguishable constructs, they are related positively and both may be associated with trauma (Berenbaum & James, 1994).

**Developmental factors in the etiology of alexithymia**

Although multiple factors are thought to play a role in the etiology of alexithymia (Nemiah, 1977), including sociocultural influences and neurobiological deficits or variations in brain organization (which will be described in Chapter 5), psychoanalytic theorists have mostly emphasized the contribution of early developmental deficiencies

(Krystal, 1988; McDougall, 1980a, 1982a; Taylor, 1987a). Their speculations are supported by observational studies of infants and children in interaction with their primary caregivers.

As we outlined in Chapter 1, the development of affects and affect regulating capacities is facilitated early in life by the experience of affect sharing and 'mirroring' of affective expressions with the primary caregiver, and subsequently by engaging in pleasurable playful interactions and being taught to name and talk about feelings. Numerous studies have demonstrated that when the primary caregiver is emotionally unavailable, or when the child is subjected repeatedly to inconsistent responses because of parental 'misattunements', the child is likely to manifest abnormalities in affect development and affect regulation, as well as an insecure attachment style (Emde, 1988a,b; Osofsky, 1992; Osofsky & Eberhart-Wright, 1988; Stern, 1985). If the infant's affective cues are consistently rejected, and especially if the caregiver's own affective responses also are misleading, the infant becomes behaviourally avoidant and less emotionally expressive of both positive and negative affects, and fails to learn the meaning and signal function of affects (Crittenden, 1994; Goldberg et al., 1994). The mothers of insecure–avoidant infants are often low in emotional expressiveness themselves (Bretherton, 1985). Infants who experience inconsistent responses to their affective communications develop an insecure–ambivalent attachment style, and have difficulty regulating emotional distress (Slade & Aber, 1992).

According to Crittenden (1994), insecure attachment styles (as we noted toward the end of Chapter 1) are associated with inner schemata or representational models that reflect failures in the integration of affective information and cognitive information. Whereas insecure-avoidant children develop problems with the recognition and expression of affect and learn to rely on cognition, insecure–ambivalent children fail to use cognition to regulate affect. Though Crittenden's proposals have yet to be validated, they provide an original and interesting conceptualization of the development of problems in affect regulation that should guide future studies aimed at exploring the role of parental behaviour and infant attachment styles in the etiology of alexithymia.

It has been observed also that some mothers interfere with their child's creation of a transitional object, either by prohibiting every attempt on the infant's part to use precursor objects, or by offering themselves to the infant as the only source of satisfaction (Gaddini, 1978; McDougall, 1974). Such intrusions inhibit the emergence of imaginal activities in the infant, including the ability to create fantasies and play, and thus block the development of important affect regulating capacities (Deri, 1984; Tustin, 1988). Without the experience of transitional relatedness, these children may continue to rely on sensation objects or autosensual activity to reduce tension, such as self-rocking, excessive thumbsucking, hair-twirling, and masturbation. These primitive modes of affect regulation reflect a preconceptual level of emotion organization, and may have their counterpart in adolescence and adulthood in the form of sensation-dominated activities such as excessive smoking or alcohol consumption (see Chapter 8), or rumination and bingeing and vomiting, as seen in patients with bulimia nervosa (see Chapter 9). Ogden (1989) encompasses this primitive level of emotion organization in his concept of the *autistic-contiguous* mode of generating experience, which is in dialectical relationship with the paranoid–schizoid and depressive modes of experience described by Kleinian psychoanalysts.

There is some evidence that insecure attachment styles in infancy, and the associated problems in affect development and affect regulation, are related sometimes to a depressive or anxiety disorder in the mother and/or to unresolved loss and trauma (Manassis *et al.*, 1994; Radke-Yarrow *et al.*, 1985). There is evidence also that maltreated children are at risk for developing affective and behavioural dysregulation (Shields, Cicchetti & Ryan, 1994); such children are most likely to manifest a disorganized/disoriented attachment style, which has been linked to parents who elicit fear in the child rather than a sense of security, and who may have been abused themselves (Cicchetti *et al.*, 1991). Research findings suggest that the affect regulating problems of maltreated children are, in part, a consequence of their parents' disapproval of the expression of affect and failure to teach them words to label emotions and other inner states (Cicchetti *et al.*, 1991).

A recent empirical study with groups of undergraduate university students similarly found that alexithymia was associated with retrospective reports of not feeling emotionally safe during childhood and of a family environment in which members were not permitted to express their feelings directly. Higher degrees of alexithymia were associated with low levels of positive communication in the family, such as expressions of sympathy or praise (Berenbaum & James, 1994).

The findings from the observational studies of maltreated children are consistent with the theoretical formulations of Krystal (1978b; 1988), who has written extensively on the relations between trauma and affects. In his view, alexithymia is a consequence of psychic trauma experienced by the infant before affects have been fully desomatized, differentiated, and represented verbally. Among the consequences of infantile psychic trauma, Krystal includes arrests in affect development and in the development of imagination, a lifelong anhedonia, and a fear of affects themselves; affects become overwhelming and traumatic to the child because of their inchoate nature and the immature state of the child's mind. Krystal (1978a) describes associated disturbances in the development of self- and object representations, and in the acquisition of a capacity for self-care. van der Kolk (1987) has described similar cognitive changes and disturbances in affect regulation in children who have suffered the psychological trauma of loss of an attachment figure at a very early age.

According to Krystal (1988), alexithymia can result also from psychic trauma at a later stage in childhood, or from catastrophic trauma during adolescence or adult life. Although affect development is more advanced, the ego of the older child or adult is overwhelmed by the traumatic event; this results in a rapid regression of affects to a preconceptual level of organization with dedifferentiation and resomatization. In formulating these ideas, Krystal was presumably influenced by his early observations of alexithymic characteristics among drug addicts and survivors of concentration camps or other massive traumas, which were noted earlier and will be detailed in Chapters 7 and 8.

In his discussion of the relations between alexithymia, affects, and trauma, Krystal (1988) makes the point that, before there is sufficient ego development, the infant is unable to mobilize such defenses as denial, repression, or depersonalization to moderate the impact of psychic trauma. Indeed, Freud (1915a) regarded repression as a defense mechanism that cannot arise until experiences have been represented psychically and there is a cleavage between conscious and unconscious mental activity. Whereas repression was considered a defense against instinctual wishes, Freud (1940) conceptualized denial as a defense against perceptions and thought it involved a 'splitting of the ego'. As Cohen and Kinston (1984) have elaborated, however, Freud (1915a) made an important distinction between *primal repression* and *repression proper*. Though repression proper is a defensive process that evolves out of primal repression, it involves a rejection from the conscious mind of already formed instinctual wishes and other representations. Primal repression, on the other hand, is akin to another idea of Freud's (1918), viz., his concept of *foreclosure* in which aspects of experience have been repudiated and never represented psychically.

Cohen and Kinston (1984) relate primal repression to the experience of traumatic events, especially parental failure to meet the infant's emotional needs during the preverbal period of development, that were never comprehended cognitively, but are encoded as 'prerepresentational experiential elements including sensory impressions, stereotyped actions, physiological reactions, and isolated images and affects' (p. 38). Even in adult life, severe trauma can overwhelm the ego and evoke primal repression and an associated regression in affective functioning. Dorpat (1985) considers primal repression (and also dissociation) a form of primitive denial and believes it involves an arrest in cognitive functions that ordinarily serve to represent, integrate, and regulate experience. We will elaborate on the relations between alexithymia and primitive defense mechanisms in Chapter 4.

### The interpersonal relationships and communicative mode of alexithymic individuals

Consistent with the view of attachment theorists, one would expect the faulty self- and object representations constructed by alexithymic individuals during childhood, as well as their deficits in affect regulation, to strongly influence the types of interpersonal relationships they establish in adult life. Clinicians report that alexithymic individuals tend to establish markedly dependent relationships, but that these relationships are highly interchangeable; alternatively, they prefer to be alone and to avoid people altogether (Krystal, 1988; McDougall, 1980a; Robbins, 1989; Taylor, 1987a). These clinical observations suggest the persistence from childhood of insecure–ambivalent and insecure–avoidant attachment styles.

A recent study in the field of adult attachment research (Schaffer, 1993) has provided empirical evidence that alexithymia is associated most strongly with a compulsive care-seeking style of insecure attachment, which is a subtype of ambivalent attachment, and secondarily with a compulsive self-reliant attachment style, which is a subtype of avoidant attachment.[1] Despite the type of attachment, however, the study showed that highly alexithymic individuals tend to employ oral and somatic styles of affect regulation such as bingeing on food or developing a somatic symptom; these styles of affect regulation were not experienced as being particularly efficacious. In contrast, securely attached individuals showed low levels of alexithymia, and employed interpersonal behaviour and fantasies of talking to a caring person to help regulate affect. Such styles of affect regulation were experienced as successful. Future studies might employ the Adult Attachment Interview to classify attachment styles, as this measure also detects the presence of unresolved trauma (West & Sheldon-Keller, 1994).

---

1. In this study the attachment styles were assessed with the Reciprocal Attachment Questionnaire developed by West and Sheldon-Keller (1994).

In addition to using attachment theory and psychoanalytic object relations theory to conceptualize the interpersonal relationships of alexithymic individuals, several clinicians have used aspects of psychoanalytic theory to try and understand the *pensée opératoire*, or externally orientated communicative style, that is especially problematic in the psychotherapeutic situation. McDougall (1978), for example, observed that alexithymic patients use speech as 'an *act* rather than a symbolic means of communication of ideas or affect' (p. 179). Like Krystal (1988), she assumed that this communicative style is a consequence of early psychic trauma.

In attempting to understand the countertransference reactions evoked by this non-symbolic communicative style, McDougall (1982*b*) and Taylor (1977, 1984*b*) have reported that some alexithymic patients make extensive use of projective identification to discharge unbearable mental states into others. Langs (1978/79) refers to this cognitive style as a type B communicative mode, which he contrasts with a symbolic and interpretable type A mode used by most psychoneurotic patients. However, patients who are more severely alexithymic seem to make little use of projective identification. Their non-symbolic communicative style corresponds to a type C communicative mode described by Langs, in which language is used to create impenetrable barriers that seal off access to any inner mental life and prevent the formation of meaningful emotional connections with other people. Both type B and type C communicative modes can evoke countertransference boredom, which is typically experienced during psychoanalytic therapy with alexithymic patients (Taylor, 1984*b*). Whereas the type A mode reflects cognitive functioning at the level of the depressive position in Kleinian theory, the type B communicative mode indicates functioning in the paranoid/schizoid position, which is characterized by concrete thinking and organization of emotions at a preconceptual level (Brown, 1985). The type C mode seems to be associated with a greater use of primal repression, suggesting a history of very early infantile trauma and reflects functioning in the sensory-dominated autistic–contiguous position. We will return to the communicative modes of alexithymic individuals in Chapter 11.

# [3] Measurement and validation of the alexithymia construct

In any field of scientific inquiry, it is necessary to demonstrate the validity of a new hypothetical construct and to show that it is not merely a new name for an already established construct. Until recently, however, the need to subject alexithymia to a rigorous evaluation of construct validity was ignored, perhaps because the construct was derived from psychoanalytic observations, a field in which empirical research has been relatively neglected. As Lesser and Lesser (1983) have pointed out, there was a risk that alexithymia would be reified as most of the early advocates of the construct took its validity for granted and directly embarked on investigations to compare levels of alexithymia in different clinical populations. Most of this research was conducted with rather hastily constructed measures of alexithymia whose psychometric properties had not been adequately evaluated. Subsequent research (which will be described in this chapter) has shown that many of these measures lack adequate reliability and validity, thus questioning the validity and generalizability of results from the various studies that used them.

The development of a reliable and valid instrument for measuring a construct is in fact a widely used method of construct validation in the field of personality research (Hogan & Nicholson, 1988). Indeed, Cronbach and Meehl (1955) have argued that the validity of a construct cannot be evaluated independently of the tests that purport to measure that construct. In the case of a multifaceted construct like alexithymia, validational research should be able to demonstrate that the subordinate concepts of the construct can be measured separately and that they are related empirically (Carver, 1989).

In this chapter, we review our own extensive program of research that was aimed at evaluating the validity of the alexithymia construct through the development of a self-report scale (the Toronto

Alexithymia Scale) for measuring it. First, however, we review other available instruments for measuring alexithymia, including observer-rated questionnaires, self-report scales, and projective techniques. To guide clinicians and researchers in selecting suitable measures, we describe not only the psychometric properties of the available measures, but also how the measures were developed and the extent to which they support the validity of the construct. Later in the chapter, we review some additional empirical support for the validity of the alexithymia construct, which has come from studies that have used an experimental approach to construct validation.

## Observer-rated questionnaires

### Beth Israel Hospital Psychosomatic Questionnaire

The Beth Israel Hospital Psychosomatic Questionnaire (BIQ) was developed by Sifneos (1973) to provide a systematic, standardized assessment of alexithymia. It is a 17-item, forced choice questionnaire completed by an interviewer. The method of interviewing involves an initial period of unstructured conversation followed by repeated exploration of the patient's ability to describe feelings and to report fantasies and dreams (Nemiah et al., 1976). The BIQ appears to have good face validity with eight 'key' items pertaining directly to the alexithymia construct (Apfel & Sifneos, 1979). Only these eight 'key' items are used in obtaining the alexithymia score. Although alexithymia is considered a dimensional construct, a cut-off score of 6 has been arbitrarily established, yielding a dichotomous classification of alexithymic and non-alexithymic subjects.

The eight 'key' items on the BIQ were developed by Sifneos (1973) on the basis of his clinical observations of differences in the cognitive-affective style between psychoneurotic patients and patients with 'classical' psychosomatic diseases (Nemiah & Sifneos, 1970). Consequently, initial support for the validity of the BIQ was based not on its ability to measure the alexithymia construct but on results of a comparison study in which a group of patients with 'psychosomatic' diseases scored much higher than a group of patients with neurotic complaints and a variety of psychiatric diagnoses (Sifneos, 1973).

Later studies adhered to the theoretical construct of alexithymia and examined the relationships between the BIQ and projective measures of the capacity for emotional expressiveness and capacity for fantasy. Lesser, Ford and Friedmann (1979), for example, administered the BIQ and the Rotter Sentence Completion Test to a group of patients attending either a psychosomatic or a psychiatric outpatient clinic. The BIQ correlated significantly with the number of words per sentence (an index of the capacity to fantasize) and with the number of sentence completions containing a reference to an affective state (an index of the capacity for emotional expressiveness). Sriram *et al.* (1987*a*) administered the BIQ and the Thematic Apperception Test (TAT) to a group of patients with psychogenic pain disorder. Separate indices were calculated from the responses to the TAT cards – total word count, as a measure of the capacity to fantasize; affect word count, as a measure of the capacity for emotional expressiveness; and affect variability, as a measure of the range of affective vocabulary. Only the correlation between total word count and the BIQ reached significance.

Partial support for the validity of the BIQ was provided also by a study examining its factor structure (Gardos *et al.*, 1984). However, the study failed to report inter-rater reliability among the three clinicians who had scored the BIQ. Furthermore, the inclusion of items associated with, but not conceptually a part of, the alexithymia construct made the results of the factor analysis difficult to interpret.

In a recent review, Linden, Wen and Paulhaus (1994) reported that six of the eight studies examining the inter-rater reliability of the BIQ produced acceptable levels of reliability. In five of these six studies, however, reliabilities were obtained from independently rated audio- or videotapes of a single interview (Federman & Mohns, 1984; Kleiger & Jones, 1980; Kleiger & Kinsman, 1980; Paulson, 1985; Postone, 1986). This procedure fails to take into account the contribution of examiner–examinee variance that can be attributed to the specific interactional nature of the interview, an important variable in the affective expression of most patients (Lolas, von Rad & Scheibler, 1981; Schneider, 1977; Wolff, 1977). In contrast, Lolas *et al.* (1980) and Taylor, Doody and Newman (1981) reported unacceptably low inter-rater reliability when using separate interviews to rate the same patients. Only Sriram, Pratap and Shanmugham (1988) have reported adequate inter-rater reliability of the BIQ using live interviews; these researchers probably enhanced the reliability by attempting to standardize the administration and scoring of the eight 'key' items. The test–retest reliability of the BIQ is also uncertain; while Sriram *et al.* (1988) obtained a high and significant correlation coefficient in a normal sample after a three-month interval, Keltikangas-Järvinen (1987) reported rather low correlation coefficients in a study that retested several different groups of somatically ill patients after intervals of 18 to 24 months.

Although the above studies provide only minimal support for the validity of the alexithymia construct, and for the reliability of the BIQ, the results of recent studies examining the concurrent validity of the BIQ and the self-report Toronto Alexithymia Scale (TAS) are more encouraging. The BIQ has shown moderate to strong correlations not only with the English version of the TAS (Jimerson *et al.*, 1994), but also with Indian dialect (Sriram *et al.*, 1987*a*), Finnish (Kauhanen, Julkanen, & Salonen, 1992a), and Japanese (Fukunishi, Saito & Ozaki, 1992) translations of the TAS. As will be outlined later in this chapter, the psychometric properties of the TAS provide considerable empirical support for the validity of the alexithymia construct.

Following the suggestions of Sriram *et al.* (1988) for enhancing the psychometric properties of the BIQ, we recently developed a modified version by adding four new items for rating alexithymia and eliminating nine of the original 17 items that are less relevant to the construct (Bagby, Taylor & Parker, 1994*b*). We also changed the rating scale from a dichotomous format to a 7-point Likert type format. The resulting 12-item questionnaire (see Appendix) comprises six items pertaining to the ability to identify and verbally communicate feelings (i.e., affect awareness), and six items pertaining to imaginal activity and externally oriented thinking (i.e. operatory thinking, or *pensée opératoire*).

Preliminary testing of the 12-item modified BIQ has yielded results that encourage its further use in assessing the alexithymia construct. With a sample of patients attending a behavioural medicine outpatient clinic, the interrater agreement among three clinicians for the 12-item BIQ was satisfactory (Bagby *et al.*, 1994*b*). The mean score of the three clinicians for the modified BIQ correlated significantly with patients' scores on the revised Twenty-Item Toronto Alexithymia Scale (TAS-20) (which is described later) and was stronger than the correlation of TAS-20 scores with the mean score of the three clinicians for the eight 'key' items of the original BIQ.

### The Alexithymia Provoked Response Questionnaire

Recognizing the need for a standardized interview to minimize interviewer bias, Krystal, Giller and Cicchetti (1986) developed the Alexithymia Provoked Response Questionnaire (APRQ). The 17 questions on the APRQ are derived directly from a self-rated version of the BIQ that was used in a single study by Sifneos, Apfel-Savitz and Frankel (1977). Rather than rating the patient on information obtained from a clinical interview, the clinician administering the APRQ elicits responses to questions that are specifically designed to assess the subject's capacity for using affective language while imagining himself in a variety of potentially stressful situations. To date, only two studies have been published on the validity and reliability of the APRQ. Using a mixed sample of psychiatric and medical patients suffering from either posttraumatic stress disorder, major depressive disorder, or a somatic disease, Krystal *et al.* (1986) reported high levels of interrater agreement both for the presence of alexithymia and for the absence of alexithymia. Pierce *et al.* (1989) also reported a high level of interrater agreement when the APRQ was administered to a group of patients suffering from chronic pain. Although the APRQ has been found to correlate highly with the BIQ (concurrent validity), it showed a low magnitude correlation with the TAS and no relationship with other self-report measures of alexithymia other than with an analogue version of the Schalling–Sifneos Personality Scale (Krystal *et al.*, 1986; Pierce *et al.*, 1989).

Although the APRQ requires subjects to imagine themselves in a variety of situations, the responses are scored for affective content only, and not for the ability to fantasize, which is an important component of the alexithymia construct. Given the absence of studies evaluating the relationships between the APRQ and measures of imaginal activity and other personality constructs, the APRQ provides minimal empirical support for the validity of the alexithymia construct and cannot yet be recommended for clinical or research purposes.

### Self-report measures

#### The MMPI Alexithymia Scale
One of the most widely used self-report measures in early alexithymia research was the MMPI Alexithymia scale (MMPI-A). This 22-item scale was developed by Kleiger and Kinsman (1980) using an empirical criterion method of scale construction (Meehl, 1945). The entire 566-item Minnesota Multiphasic Personality Inventory (MMPI) was administered to 100 patients suffering from chronic respiratory diseases who were also interviewed and rated on the BIQ. Items on the MMPI were retained for the MMPI-A if they differentiated between alexithymic and non-alexithymic patients as classified by BIQ scores.

The empirical criterion method of scale construction has several liabilities. For example, using a significance level of 0.05, one can expect 28 of the 566 MMPI items to be selected by chance. Although Kleiger and Kinsman (1980) controlled for chance effects by splitting their sample in half and selecting only those items that produced significant differences in both sample halves, they never cross-validated their results in another separate, independent sample. In five subsequent studies that examined the relationship between the BIQ and MMPI-A across a diverse set of samples, including chronic pain patients (Demers-Desrosiers *et al.*, 1983; Postone, 1986), migraine headache patients (Federman & Mohns, 1984), Vietnam veterans (Krystal *et al.*, 1986), and hypertension patients (Paulson, 1985), only the study conducted by Postone reported a significant correlation. The lack of concurrent validity of the MMPI-A has been demonstrated also by non-significant correlations with the APRQ (Krystal *et al.*, 1986), and with other self-report measures of alexithymia (Bagby, Taylor & Atkinson, 1988*a*; Krystal *et al.*, 1986; Norton, 1989; Paulson, 1985).

Several different studies have demonstrated consistently low estimates of internal reliability for the MMPI-A across a variety of samples (Bagby *et al.*, 1988*a*; Bagby, Parker & Taylor, 1991*a*, 1991*b*; Kinder & Curtiss, 1990). In addition, several attempts to uncover the inherent underlying dimensionality of the MMPI-A through factor analysis have failed to extract thematically meaningful factors related to the alexithymia construct (Bagby *et al.*, 1991*a*, 1991*b*; Norton, 1989). This is not surprising given the atheoretical method of item selection used by Kleiger and Kinsman (1980) in developing the scale.

Given its poor psychometric properties, the MMPI-A provides no support for the validity of the alexithymia construct and cannot be recommended for clinical or research purposes.

**The Schalling–Sifneos Personality Scale**

The Schalling–Sifneos Personality Scale (SSPS) is a 20-item self-report measure, which also was used extensively in early empirical research on alexithymia (Apfel & Sifneos, 1979). Each item is rated on a four-point Likert scale, and the content of many of the items corresponds closely to the content of 'key' items on the BIQ. However, though the items were written to reflect the substantive domain of the alexithymia construct, the SSPS was not subjected to item analyses or assessed for internal consistency prior to its use in clinical research.

Subsequent investigations demonstrated that the SSPS has minimal response set bias and good test–retest reliability over a two-week interval (Bagby *et al.*, 1988*a*; Shipko & Noviello, 1984). In addition, the scale is not unduly influenced by age, education, and socioeconomic status. However, other studies revealed poor item-total correlations, poor internal consistency, and an unstable factor structure (Bagby *et al.*, 1988*a*; Bagby, Taylor & Ryan, 1986*a*; Faryna, Rodenhauser & Torem, 1986; Norton, 1989). While several factor-analytic studies yielded three- or four-factor solutions congruent with the theoretical construct of alexithymia, very few of the SSPS items loaded significantly on any one factor, and different factor structures emerged in different studies using separate samples (Bagby *et al.*,

1986*a*; Bagby *et al.*, 1988*a*; Blanchard, Arena & Pallmeyer, 1981; Martin, Pihl & Dobkin,᾿ 1984; Norton, 1989; Shipko & Noviello, 1984). It is notable, however, that all of the factor analytic studies extracted a 'difficulty in describing feelings' factor, which is a central component of the alexithymia construct.

The SSPS has failed also to demonstrate adequate concurrent validity. In our own research, we found a significant correlation between the SSPS and the TAS (Bagby *et al.*, 1988*a*), but the correlation was of low magnitude; several other researchers have reported nonsignificant correlations with the BIQ (Kleiger & Jones, 1980; Krystal *et al.*, 1986; Paulson, 1985). In testing the convergent validity of the SSPS, however, Norton (1989) obtained a weak but significant negative correlation with the Absorption Scale (Tellegen & Atkinson, 1974), a finding that is consistent with the decreased fantasy involvement component of the alexithymia construct.

Sifneos (1986) later made several changes to the SSPS and introduced a revised version – the SSPS-R; seven of the original items were rewritten slightly, nine items were replaced by new items, and four items were left unchanged. In addition, the four-point Likert rating scale was replaced by a dichotomous scoring system.

In the only study examining the psychometric properties of the SSPS-R, we found no substantial improvement over the original SSPS (Parker *et al.*, 1991*b*). The factor structure of the SSPS-R was found to be reasonably congruent with the theoretical domains of the alexithymia construct; however, the scale lacked homogeneity and internal reliability. None the less, Jimerson *et al.* (1994) later reported a significant moderate correlation between the SSPS-R and the TAS and, consistent with predictions, women with bulimia nervosa scored significantly higher than healthy female control subjects on both of these self-report scales and on the BIQ.

Attempts by other researchers to improve the SSPS by changing the number of items (Martin *et al.*, 1984; McDonald & Prkachin, 1987), or by changing the Likert rating scales to an analogue scoring system (Faryna *et al.*, 1986), have also failed to enhance the psychometric properties of the scale. Thus, while the SSPS provides partial support for the validity of the alexithymia construct, the scale in both its original and modified versions lacks sufficient validity and internal reliability to be recommended for clinical or research purposes.

## Projective techniques

The use of projective techniques to evaluate alexithymic characteristics began with Ruesch (1948, 1957) who discovered that patients with 'infantile personalities' (see Chapter 2) produced only 'primitive, unimaginative and stereotyped' fantasies in response to the Rorschach and TAT. While these findings supported Ruesch's clinical impression of reduced symbolic self-expression in such patients, the kinds of responses that subjects give to projective techniques may be unduly influenced by the examiner and the examiner–examinee interaction, and the scoring and interpretation of responses are highly subjective.

In an attempt to increase the reliability of projective techniques in assessing alexithymic characteristics, several contemporary investigators have used quantitative scoring systems. For example, researchers in Canada, Germany, India, and the United States have calculated indices from responses to selected TAT cards (Abramson et al., 1991; Sriram et al., 1987b; Taylor & Doody, 1985; Taylor et al., 1981; von Rad et al., 1977). As noted in our discussion of the BIQ, the length of stories (total word count) is used as an index of the capacity for fantasy, the affect word count as an index of emotional expressiveness, and the affect vocabulary score as an index of the potential for expression of different affects. However, the relationship between these indices and other measures of alexithymia appear to be inconsistent. Whereas Sriram et al. (1987a) found the total word count in response to four TAT cards to correlate significantly with both the BIQ and the TAS, the correlations with the affect word count and affect vocabulary score failed to reach significance. In a study using responses to five TAT cards, Taylor and Doody (1985) and Taylor et al. (1981) found no relationships between the BIQ and all three indices; however, the affect vocabulary score correlated significantly with the TAT total word count and with the number of human movement responses on the Rorschach (another index of fantasizing ability), thus providing some support for the validity of the alexithymia construct.

### The Rorschach Alexithymia Indices

Drawing upon the unique capacity of the Rorschach to measure cognitive–perceptual style and capacities for fantasy, affective responsiveness, and adaptively integrating affect, Acklin and Bernat (1987) proposed a set of Rorschach alexithymia indices that were derived from the Comprehensive System developed by Exner (1986). Acklin and Bernat (1987) hypothesized the following profile for alexithymic individuals: Low response productivity (R) and low human movement percepts (M) as indices of an impoverished capacity for fantasy;

Restricted affective response (Sum C) and Poorly adapted use of colour (Low FC) as indices of reduced affective responsiveness and adaptively integrated affect; Concrete cognition (Low Blends) and Stereotypy (High Lambda) as indices of a constricted and concrete cognitive style; and Deficient ideational and affective assets (Low EA) as an index of limited adaptive resources.

Acklin and Alexander (1988) and Acklin and Bernat (1987) found that this set of indices could discriminate somatically ill patients from depressed patients and non-clinical subjects. Similarly, Clerici *et al.* (1992) found that a group of massively obese patients scored significantly lower than a non-patient reference group on all of the Rorschach alexithymia indices except for Stereotypy (Lambda) on which they scored significantly higher, as would be expected with an alexithymic profile. Despite these findings, however, there have been no published studies examining the validity and reliability of the specific Rorschach indices as a measure of alexithymia. In a recent unpublished study of a small sample of female incest victims, Hofmann-Patsalides (1994) found no relationship between the Rorschach alexithymia indices and the TAS-20. Further studies are needed to determine whether these two measures assess similar or different facets of the alexithymia construct.

**The Objectively Scored Archetypal Test**
Another projective technique that has been used to assess a central feature of the alexithymia construct is the Scored Archetypal Test with nine elements (SAT$_9$). Adapted from Durand's theory of the structure of the imagination by Demers-Desrosiers (1982) and her colleagues (Cohen *et al.*, 1985), the SAT$_9$ is a projective drawing technique which assesses an individual's symbolic function and capacity for creating fantasy. The individual is presented with a list of nine mythical items or symbols (a fall, a sword, a refuge, a devouring monster, something cyclical that turns or progresses, a character, water, an animal, and fire) and asked to make a drawing that will link together these nine symbols, and then to write a short story explaining the drawing. When the symbolic function is impaired, the individual is unable to create a myth; he or she is unable to defend against the anxiety evoked by certain symbols and unable to integrate the meaning (story) and image (drawing) of the symbols. In content and form, the drawings are said to lose their subtlety, originality, and cohesion as the degree of alexithymia increases. One would expect creative drawings and poetic stories to be found exclusively in non-alexithymic individuals.

The psychometric properties of the SAT$_9$ have been evaluated in a small number of studies. Though sample sizes were small, one study demonstrated good internal reliability (Cohen *et al.*, 1985), four studies reported good interrater reliability (Bourke, Taylor & Crisp, 1985; Cohen *et al.*, 1985; Cohen, Demers-Desrosiers & Catchlove, 1983; Demers-Desrosiers, 1985), and one study reported low inter-rater reliability (Norton, 1989); however, not all studies used the same method of scoring the test. The SAT$_9$ has demonstrated concurrent validity with the BIQ, but shows no relationship with any of the self-report measures of alexithymia including the TAS and TAS-20 (Catchlove *et al.*, 1985; Cohen, Auld & Brooker, 1994; Norton, 1989; Parker, unpublished data).

While the finding of no association between the SAT$_9$ and the well-validated TAS-20 (which is described later) might raise questions about the relation of reduced imaginal activity with other facets of the alexithymia construct, a study with a non-clinical sample found no relationship between the SAT$_9$ and the Absorption Scale (Norton, 1989), which is another index of fantasy. This is surprising given that the Absorption Scale is significantly and substantially related to the Openness to Experience score on the NEO Personality Inventory (McCrae & Costa, 1997), which, as will be discussed later in this chapter and in more depth in the next chapter, correlates negatively with the TAS-20.

Thus, while the SAT$_9$ demonstrates reliability as a projective technique, and appears to measure some aspect of the capacity for symbolization and creativity, there is presently an absence of empirical support for recommending its use even as a measure of one facet of the alexithymia construct. Further validational studies of the SAT$_9$ are needed including assessments of its relationship with TAT indices and the set of Rorschach alexithymia indices.

## Development of the Toronto Alexithymia Scale

Recognizing the limitations of the available measures of alexithymia, and the paucity of empirical support for the validity of the alexithymia construct, our research team embarked on a program of research aimed at assessing the validity of the construct through the development of a self-report alexithymia scale. As outlined in earlier contributions (Taylor, 1994; Taylor *et al.*, 1990*a*; Taylor, Ryan & Bagby, 1985), we employed a combined rational and empirical approach to scale construction (Nunnally, 1978).

After reviewing the literature on alexithymia, we defined five content areas thought to reflect the substantive domain of the construct

(Taylor *et al.*, 1985). These were (i) difficulty in describing feelings, (ii) difficulty in distinguishing between feelings and the bodily sensations that accompany states of emotional arousal, (iii) lack of introspection, (iv) social conformity, and (v) impoverished fantasy life and poor dream recall. Based on these content areas, we developed an initial pool of 41 items; 8 items were taken from the SSPS, 4 from the Interoceptive Awareness subscale of the Eating Disorder Inventory (Garner, Olmsted & Polivy, 1983*b*), and 4 from the Need For Cognition Scale (Cacioppo & Petty, 1982). Most of these items were rewritten so that there was uniformity of style for all of the items and to fit the requirements of a 5-point Likert scale ranging from 'strongly disagree' to 'strongly agree'; half of the items were negatively keyed and half positively keyed to control for acquiescent responding. The 41-item pilot scale was administered to a sample of 542 undergraduate university students.

Following a series of factor and item analyses, 26 items were retained that met pre-established criteria and clustered into four factors: (F1) difficulty identifying and distinguishing between feelings and bodily sensations; (F2) difficulty describing feelings; (F3) reduced daydreaming; and (F4) externally oriented thinking. These four factors were theoretically congruent with the alexithymia construct; the first two factors corresponded to the affective disturbance described by Nemiah and Sifneos (1970); the third and fourth factors corresponded to the *pensée opératoire* initially described by Marty and de M'Uzan (1963). Social conformity (one of the five theoretical domains which informed the basis of the initial item pool) did not emerge as a separate factor. Items inquiring about dream recall and the tendency to use action rather than reflection were eliminated on the basis of low item-total scale correlations and/or item-factor scale correlations. The 26-item scale was named the Toronto Alexithymia Scale (TAS), and its four-factor structure was subsequently cross-validated in clinical as well as non-clinical populations (Bagby *et al.*, 1990).

The internal reliability of the TAS was demonstrated also with clinical as well as non-clinical populations, and the scale showed good test–retest reliability over 1-week and 5-week intervals (Bagby *et al.*, 1990; Taylor *et al.*, 1985). Some scale developers may question the finding of adequate estimates of internal consistency in a multifactor scale. When evaluating the TAS, however, one must consider the theoretical conceptualization of alexithymia as a multifaceted construct composed of several logically related subordinate concepts. In measuring such a broad and multifaceted construct, 'a scale can reach generally acceptable levels of internal consistency and homogeneity and still yield multiple factors' (Briggs & Cheek, 1986, p. 110).

Subsequent studies have provided considerable support for the convergent and discriminant validity of the TAS, and thereby also for the validity of the alexithymia construct. For example, consistent with the descriptive features of the alexithymia construct, the TAS correlated negatively with the Psychological Mindedness (PY) Scale of the California Psychological Inventory (CPI) (Gough, 1969), negatively with the Anger-Expression Scale (Spielberger et al., 1985), and positively with the Poor Attentional Control Subscale of the Short Imaginal Processes Inventory (Huba et al., 1982) (Bagby et al., 1988b; Bagby, Taylor & Ryan, 1986b). The TAS also correlated negatively with the short form of the Need for Cognition Scale (NCS) (Cacioppo, Petty & Kao, 1984), which assesses an individual's tendency to engage in and enjoy effortful and analytical cognitive endeavors (Cacioppo & Petty, 1982). (The short form of the NCS contains only one of the four items that were taken from the longer version of the NCS in the development of the TAS; this particular item was deleted for the analysis.) Discriminant validity of the TAS was demonstrated by nonsignificant correlations with several subscales of the Basic Personality Inventory (BPI; Jackson, 1974), which assess constructs that are theoretically unrelated to the alexithymia construct, viz., denial (equivalent to social desirability on the BPI), interpersonal problems, alienation, and deviation (Bagby et al., 1986b).

Although alexithymia is generally regarded as a dimensional construct, preliminary cutoff scores were established for the TAS to facilitate comparative studies among diverse populations. Individuals scoring ≥74 are considered alexithymic; those scoring ≤62 are considered non-alexithymic (Taylor et al., 1988).

Evidence that alexithymia is not a culture-bound construct merely reflecting the emphasis of Western psychotherapy on psychological mindedness, as some critics have suggested (Kirmayer, 1987; Prince, 1987), was provided by investigators in several other countries who developed and evaluated translated versions of the TAS. For example, the four-factor structure of the TAS was replicated with Finnish (Kauhanen, Julkunen & Salonen, 1992a), German (Bach et al., 1996), Italian (Pasini et al., 1992), Indian dialect (Kannada) (Sriram et al., 1987b), and Spanish (Rodrigo & Lusiardo, 1992; Rodrigo, Lusiardo & Normey, 1989) translations of the scale. These versions of the TAS also showed adequate internal consistency. Support for the view that alexithymia is a stable trait was provided by the findings of a high 3-month test–retest reliability for the Kannada translation and a high 8-month test–retest reliability for the Finnish translation. Studies with Czech (Kondas & Kordacova, 1990), French (Loas et al., 1993), and Japanese (Miyaoka, 1992) translations of the TAS have also yielded empirical support for the view that alexithymia is not merely a reflection of culture-related differences in emotional expressiveness.

## Scale revision and construct refinement

Though the TAS demonstrated psychometric properties superior to those of other measures of the construct, construct validation is generally considered an ongoing process that may lead to revisions to a measure as well as to further understanding and refinement of the construct (Comrey, 1988; Golden, Sawicki & Franzen, 1984; Hogan & Nicholson, 1988).

Indeed, as Nunnally (1978) has indicated, the complete process of construct explication requires that results from correlational and experimental studies be used to re-evaluate the logical foundation initially used to define and operationalize the construct. This, in turn, should lead to revisions to the measurement instruments and to further validational studies. As Hogan and Nicholson (1988) point out, researchers 'must continually work back and forth between the indicators and the construct without being swallowed up by either' (p. 625).

As described earlier, the development of the TAS led to some refinement and clearer definition of the alexithymia construct as the characteristics of social conformity, low dream recall, and tendency to action rather than reflection did not emerge as essential facets of the construct. Similarly, in the course of evaluating the TAS, several observations prompted us to further examine its compositional structure as it related to some of the domain specifications of the construct. While the four-factor structure of the TAS was found to be replicable across samples, the first two factors were highly correlated and had several items that loaded significantly on both factors, thus questioning the independence of these two factors. In addition, on theoretical grounds, we expected that all of the TAS items and factors would be moderately and positively correlated; however, the items comprising the daydreaming factor had low magnitude corrected item-total correlations with the full TAS; this factor correlated *negatively* with the first factor (Taylor *et al.*, 1985). Further, using causal modelling procedures, Haviland *et al.* (1991) found negative correlations between the daydreaming factor and the factors assessing affect awareness and externally orientated thinking, suggesting that the items assessing daydreaming have little theoretical coherency with the other facets of the alexithymia construct. Given that an externally orientated cognitive style reflects, at least in part, an impoverished inner fantasy life

(Horney, 1952; Kelman, 1952), and that these facets were linked by Marty and de M'Uzan (1963) in the concept of *pensée opératoire*, we expected a higher correlation between the daydreaming factor (F3) and the externally-oriented thinking factor (F4).

The daydreaming items were included in the TAS in an attempt to assess the domain of the alexithymia construct pertaining to constricted imaginal processes. In our attempts to explain the apparent lack of theoretical relevancy, we speculated that: (a) the self-reporting of daydreaming activity might be confounded by a social desirability response bias, *viz.*, that daydreaming might be regarded as an undesirable behaviour reflecting a lack of initiative and/or drive; and (b) the assessment of daydreaming alone may not capture adequately the capacity for imaginal activities.

Finally, there was evidence that the four factors of the TAS display different patterns of correlation with measures of other constructs, in particular with anxiety, depression, somatization, and introspectiveness (Haviland *et al.*, 1991; Hendryx, Haviland & Shaw, 1991; Kirmayer & Robbins, 1993). These findings had led some researchers to question the interrelatedness of the various components of the construct, as measured by the TAS, and to suggest that it might be more appropriate to use separate factor scores rather than full-scale scores (Hendryx *et al.*, 1991; Kirmayer & Robbins, 1993).

With these observations in mind, we decided to re-examine the domain specifications of the alexithymia construct. We wrote an additional set of items and attempted to create a revised and improved version of the TAS taking into account the theoretical and statistical limitations of the original scale. As outlined in earlier contributions (Bagby *et al.*, 1994a; Taylor *et al.*, 1992a), a total of 17 additional items were written and added to the original 26 items to create a revised item pool of 43 items. Seven of these new items were written to reflect the imaginal processing component of the construct; five new items had content relevant to externally oriented thinking; and five new items had content related to communicating feelings to others.

The initial effort in scale reconstruction using the revised item pool led to the development of a 23-item scale (the TAS-R), which eliminated all items assessing imaginal activity (Taylor *et al.*, 1992a). Exploratory factor analysis of these 23 items yielded a two-factor solution: the first factor comprised items assessing both the ability to distinguish between feelings and bodily sensations associated with emotional arousal and the ability to describe feelings to others; the second factor comprised items assessing externally-oriented thinking. Subsequent testing of the factor structure using confirmatory factor analysis, however, indicated that the two-factor structure was not a good representation of the data, and that a three-factor solution was a much better match to the data. Given this finding, we attempted a second revision of the scale using the same 43-item pool.

### The Twenty-Item Toronto Alexithymia Scale

This later research resulted in the development of a 20-item version of the scale, which has been named the Twenty-Item Toronto Alexithymia Scale (TAS-20) (Bagby et al., 1994a,b). As occurred during item selection for the TAS-R, all items directly assessing daydreaming and other imaginal activity were eliminated because of low corrected item-total correlations and/or high correlations with a measure of social desirability. The TAS-20 demonstrated good internal consistency (Cronbach's alpha = 0.81) and test–retest reliability over a three-week interval ($r$ = 0.77), and a three-factor structure theoretically congruent with the alexithymia construct – (F1) difficulty identifying feelings; (F2) difficulty describing feelings to others; and (F3) externally oriented thinking. The stability and replicability of this three-factor structure were demonstrated with both clinical and non-clinical populations by the use of confirmatory factor analysis (Bagby et al., 1994a; Parker et al., 1993a). Although the first two factors of the TAS-20 still correlated highly, a three-factor model provided a better fit to the data obtained from several different samples than either a two-factor model or a unidimensional model. In fact the parameter estimates for the relationships among the three TAS-20 factors provided further evidence that the revised scale surmounts the limitations of the original TAS and that the three factors reflect separate, yet empirically related, facets of the alexithymia construct.

The convergent validity of the TAS-20 was assessed by examining the relationships of the scale with both the NCS (short form) and the Psychological Mindedness Scale (PMS) in a sample of undergraduate university students (Bagby et al., 1994b). Whereas the NCS was used in our studies evaluating the TAS, the PMS is a new measure developed by Conte et al. (1990, 1995) to assess four salient facets of psychological mindedness that were described in Chapter 2 and are considered relevant to evaluating suitability for analytically-oriented psychotherapy. As shown in Table 3.1, the TAS-20 and its three factors all correlated strongly and negatively with both the NCS and the PMS.

Additional data supporting the convergent validity of the TAS-20 was provided by Yelsma (1992, 1996), who examined the relationship between the TAS-20 and the self-report Affective Orientation Scale

(AOS; Booth-Butterfield & Booth-Butterfield, 1990) in a mixed sample of normal adults and victims and perpetrators of verbal and/or physical abuse. The AOS is a measure of the affective orientation construct which, as outlined in Chapter 2, is related to the emotional intelligence construct and refers to the extent to which individuals are aware of their affects and use this information to guide communication behaviour. According to Booth-Butterfield and Booth-Butterfield (1990), people who score low on the AOS seem to weigh logic and facts more heavily than affects in guiding their behaviour. Consistent with the alexithymia construct, the TAS-20 and its three factors all correlated significantly and negatively with the AOS (see Table 3.1). The findings that all three factors of the TAS-20 correlate significantly and negatively with the NCS, PMS, and AOS support the theoretical view that the alexithymia construct is composed of at least three lower-order concepts; as the factor structure of the TAS-20 shows, these subordinate concepts are part of a broader and more important superordinate construct.

Costa and McCrae (1987a) have argued that the evaluation of any new hypothetical personality construct should include an examination of the relationship of purported measures of the construct with a standard taxonomy of personality traits. With this in mind, we examined the relationships between the TAS-20 and the five basic dimensions of personality assessed by the NEO Personality Inventory (Costa & McCrae, 1985). The study was conducted with a sample of undergraduate university students (Bagby et al., 1994b). As the complete results of the study are discussed in Chapter 4, we will note here only that all correlations were as predicted; in particular, the TAS-20 correlated negatively and most strongly with the Openness to Experience dimension, which is consistent with the conceptual overlap between these two constructs. The finding of negative correlations between the TAS-20 and the subscales assessing openness to feelings

**Table 3.1** Correlations of the TAS-20 and factor scales with measures of psychological mindedness, need-for-cognition, and affective orientation

|  | N | TAS-20 | F1 | F2 | F3 |
|---|---|---|---|---|---|
| Psychological mindedness | 85 | −0.68 | −0.44 | −0.51 | −0.54 |
| Need-for-cognition | 85 | −0.55 | −0.40 | −0.36 | −0.44 |
| Affective orientation | 210 | −0.37 | −0.24 | −0.36 | −0.28 |

All correlations are significant; p <0.01.
Note: Factor 1 = difficulty identifying feelings; Factor 2 = difficulty describing feelings; Factor 3 = externally orientated thinking.

and openness to fantasy indicate that the scale is assessing deficiencies in emotional awareness and imaginal activity – salient features of the alexithymia construct. Indeed, the results provide evidence that the TAS-20 taps the reduced imaginal processing facet of the construct, despite the absence of items on the revised scale that directly inquire about daydreaming and other imaginal activity. Discriminant validity of the TAS-20 was supported by the findings of non-significant correlations with the personality dimensions of Agreeableness and Conscientiousness.

Given that significant correlations between the TAS-20 and self-report measures of related constructs could be partly accounted for by method variance (Wiggins, 1973), we conducted an additional investigation with a sample of 39 behavioural medicine outpatients in which we examined the level of agreement between TAS-20 self-report scores and alexithymia ratings by external observers (Bagby et al., 1994b). The patients were interviewed by one clinician, who was selected randomly from among three clinicians, all of whom rated the patient on the modified version of the BIQ that was described earlier in this chapter. Table 3.2 shows the correlations between the patients' TAS-20 total scores and factor scale scores and the mean scores of the three clinicians for the modified BIQ and its two subscales. The finding of strong positive correlations between the TAS-20 and the total BIQ and its two subscales provides compelling evidence for the concurrent validity of the TAS-20. Not surprisingly, Factor 1 (difficulty identifying feelings) correlated significantly with the BIQ subscale assessing affect awareness, and Factor 3 (externally oriented thinking) correlated significantly with the subscale assessing operatory thinking. Factor 2, which reflects difficulty in communicating feelings to others, showed strong correlations with both subscales of the BIQ. The high level of agreement between a self-report measure of alexithymia and an observer-rated measure provides considerable support for the consensual validity (McCrae, 1982) of the alexithymia construct.

As was done with the TAS, data from this last study were used to establish preliminary cutoff scores for the TAS-20. Individuals scoring ⩾61 are considered alexithymic; those scoring ⩽51 are considered non-alexithymic.

**Translations of the TAS-20**

Since its development, the TAS-20 has been translated into many languages including Cantonese, Dutch, Finnish, French, German, Greek, Hebrew, Hindi, Italian, Japanese, Korean, Lithuanian, Polish, Portuguese, Spanish, and Swedish. For each of the translated versions, back-translation methodologies were employed. To test the replicability of the three-factor structure of the TAS-20 in the translated versions, correlation matrices for diverse samples from different countries are factor analyzed and compared to the three-factor model using confirmatory factor analysis.

To date, the three-factor model of the TAS-20 has been cross-validated in samples from Brazil (Sandra Fortes, personal communication, April 4, 1995), Germany (Parker *et al.*, 1993*a*), Greece (Tanya Anagnostopoulou, personal communication, April 6, 1995); Finland (Juhani Julkunen, personal communication, May 5, 1995); Italy (Bressi *et al.*, 1996), India (Pandey *et al.*, 1996), Israel (David Rabinowitz, personal communication, February 26, 1993), Korea (Lee *et al.*, 1996), Lithuania (Beresnevaite *et al.*, 1998), Poland (personal communication, Marcin Ziółkowski, March 20, 1996) and Sweden (Sven Carlsson, personal communication, October 20, 1994). In these samples, the translated versions of the TAS-20 have also yielded Cronbach alpha coefficients of internal reliability comparable to those obtained with the English version of the scale. Consistent with the trait view of alexithymia, studies have shown a high 3-month test–retest reliability ($r = 0.83$) for the Hindi translation of the TAS-20, and a high 6-month test–retest reliability ($r = 0.95$) for the Italian translation.

## Conclusions and implications

The results from our own program of research, as well as findings provided by many other investigators, indicate that the shortcomings of the TAS have been largely overcome through the development of the revised TAS-20. The internal reliability of the TAS-20 is slightly better, the factor structure is more stable, and the three factors correlate in predictable ways with measures of other constructs. None the less, the development and validation of *both* scales has yielded considerable support for the validity of the alexithymia construct, and enabled

**Table 3.2** Correlations of the TAS-20 and factor scales with interviewer ratings on the modified Beth Israel Hospital Psychosomatic Questionnaire (N = 39)

| BIQ | TAS-20 | FI | F2 | F3 |
|---|---|---|---|---|
| Total score | 0.53** | 0.36* | 0.57** | 0.30* |
| Affect awareness | 0.53** | 0.43** | 0.52** | 0.26 |
| Operatory thinking | 0.48** | 0.26 | 0.58** | 0.30* |

\* $p < 0.05$. \*\* $p < 0.01$.

researchers to conduct a large number of empirical studies with reliable and valid self-report measures of the construct. These studies will be reviewed in later chapters.

Although the TAS-20 is the measure we currently recommend for both clinical and research purposes, it is essential to remember, as McCrae (1991) has pointed out, 'that all assessment devices are merely tools that must be thoughtfully used by the clinician' (p. 411). In our view, clinicians should use the TAS-20 as a screening device for alexithymia and evaluate the significance of an individual patient's score in the context of information from other sources including clinical observations, reports from close friends or relatives of the patient, and results from other personality tests. In our own clinical work, we often administer the Revised NEO Personality Inventory (Costa & McCrae, 1992) along with the TAS-20, as scores on the openness to feelings and openness to fantasy subscales of the Openness to Experience domain may be used to confirm or correct the information obtained with the TAS-20; examples of this are given in Chapter 4.

Empirical research is always enhanced by the use of a multi-method approach to measuring a construct. This is especially applicable to alexithymia research as a self-report measure alone may not adequately assess affective and cognitive capacities that alexithymic individuals may not know they lack. In addition to the TAS-20, investigators might wish to use interviews scored with the modified BIQ (preferably with two or more raters and assessments of inter-rater reliability). Projective techniques may also provide useful information in empirical studies. For example, our research has yielded preliminary evidence that individuals who score in the non-alexithymic range on the TAS-20 show a significantly greater range of affect words in response to TAT cards than individuals who score in the alexithymic range of the TAS-20. However, the Scale for Failures in Self-Regulation, which also uses TAT responses, may provide more useful information regarding preverbal as well as verbal components of failures in the self-regulation of affects and impulses (Wilson et al., 1989; Wilson, Passik & Faude, 1990). An additional benefit of including the Rorschach and the TAT is their ability to assess self- and object representations and patterns of attachment (Blatt & Lerner, 1983; Graves & Thomas, 1981; Thompson, 1986), which are expected to be impaired in alexithymic individuals.

## Experimental approaches to construct validation

While most of the support for the validity of the alexithymia construct is based on the results of correlational and factor analytic studies and the demonstration of consensual validity, there have been some attempts to explore the validity of the construct using experimental approaches. Indeed, some psychologists regard validation of the descriptive features of a personality construct as a relatively weak type of validity, and consider it essential also to produce experimental evidence that supports predictions as to ways in which people who score high on the construct should differ from those who score low (Eysenck & Eysenck, 1985).

In applying this approach to the alexithymia construct, we initially made the prediction that individuals who score high on the TAS should have more difficulty in distinguishing between different affective states than individuals who score low on the TAS. This prediction was tested using data collected by Marvin Acklin, who had administered the Profile of Mood States (POMS; McNair, Lorr & Droppleman, 1971/81), along with the TAS and several other measures of psychopathology, to a sample of 131 patients referred to the psychiatric outpatient department of a large metropolitan general hospital in Honolulu, Hawaii. The POMS is a 65-item, 5-point adjective rating scale designed to measure six factor analytically derived mood or affective states: tension–anxiety, depression–dejection, anger–hostility, vigor–activity, fatigue–inertia, and confusion–bewilderment. Only the five negative emotion scales were used in the analysis. Consistent with our prediction, patients scoring in the alexithymic range on the TAS ($\geqslant 74$; N = 54) showed no significant variation in the emotional states across the POMS scales, while patients scoring in the non-alexithymic range ($\leqslant 62$; N = 37) showed significant differences across the self-reported emotional states (Bagby et al., 1993). The alexithymic and non-alexithymic patient groups did not differ in age or in their overall level of symptoms and functioning, as measured by the DSM-III-R (Axis V) Global Assessment of Functioning Scale.

In another study, we tested the prediction that alexithymic individuals should differ from non-alexithymic individuals in the way they respond to emotion-activating stimuli. Specifically, because of their reduced ability cognitively to process emotions, we predicted that alexithymic individuals should be more distracted than non-alexithymic individuals by stimuli that are likely to evoke states of emotional arousal, and therefore be less able to attend to tasks at hand. To test this prediction we used a modification of the Stroop colour-naming task (Stroop, 1935). The sample comprised 16 undergraduate university students identified as alexithymic by TAS-20 scores ≥61 and 54 undergraduate students identified as non-alexithymic by TAS-20 scores ≤51. Consistent with our prediction, the alexithymic students took significantly longer than the non-alexithymic students to colour-name arousal words, but the groups did not differ in their ability to colour-name neutral words and baseline stimuli (Parker, Taylor & Bagby, 1993*b*).

While the results of the above studies support the view that alexithymia reflects a deficit in the cognitive–experiential domain of emotion response systems, experiments have been conducted to explore whether alexithymic individuals also show deficits in the motor-expressive domain. In a preliminary study using the SSPS, McDonald and Prkachin (1990) explored the relationship between alexithymia and the expression and perception of facial emotions in a small sample of male undergraduate students. Although alexithymic students were found comparable to non–alexithymic students in their ability to recognize posed human facial expressions of emotions, they showed deficits in spontaneous displays of negative emotion and in their ability to pose the emotions of happiness and anger. In a later study that used the TAS to categorize undergraduate students into high, moderate, and low alexithymia groups, we found that students in the low alexithymia group were able to more accurately identify posed facial expressions of emotion than students in the high alexithymia group (Parker *et al.*, 1993*c*).

Another experimental approach to evaluating the validity of the alexithymia construct has been to test the prediction that alexithymic individuals should show a decoupling of the physiological component of emotional arousal from the subjective feeling state in response to stress. Although two experimental studies have yielded results that support this prediction, the findings must be considered preliminary as subjects were categorized into high and low alexithymia groups on the basis of scores on the SSPS (Martin & Pihl, 1986; Papciak, Feuerstein & Spiegel, 1985). Attempts should be made to replicate these studies using more reliable and valid measures to assess alexithymia. Such studies may not only provide support for the validity of the alexithymia construct, but also help explain the association between alexithymia and certain medical and psychiatric disorders.

# 4] Relations between alexithymia, personality, and affects

While the results of measurement-based research and experimental studies have yielded considerable empirical support for the validity of the alexithymia construct, the evaluation of any new hypothetical construct should include an examination of the relationships of the construct with higher-order traits or basic dimensions of personality (Costa & McCrae, 1987a). This may be accomplished by examining the relation of reliable and valid measures of the construct with measures of standard taxonomies of personality dimensions. Such taxonomies also provide frameworks for examining the relation between personality and subjective affective experience (Watson & Clark, 1992).

In this chapter, we first describe some currently employed theoretical models of personality, and then review empirical research that has investigated the relations between the alexithymia construct, dimensions of personality, and affects. Because psychological defense mechanisms are aspects of personality that play an important role in the regulation of affects, we also review theoretical conceptions and some recent empirical research on alexithymia and defense style. As with most personality traits, alexithymia is conceptualized as a dimensional construct throughout the chapter.

## Personality structure

A central problem in the field of personality psychology has been determining the basic structure of personality. Allport and Odbert (1936) observed long ago that the English language alone has close to 18 000 potential trait terms for possible use in personality research. Important choices obviously have to be made about what constitute the essential or core traits of personality. In recent years, as Watson, Clark and Harkness (1994) have noted, there have been three basic approaches to the problem of organizing and understanding personality structure: a *multidimensional* approach, the use of a *three-factor model*, and the use of a *five-factor model*. Most of the empirical research examining the relationship between alexithymia and personality structure has used constructs that belong to one of these three personality trait models.

Advocates of the multidimensional approach to personality structure acknowledge that there are a great variety of potential trait concepts that can be studied, although usually they focus attention on a more restricted number of constructs. A variety of omnibus personality inventories have been developed to assess different sets of important trait dimensions. The California Psychological Inventory (Gough, 1987), for example, was developed to assess 20 different traits; the Sixteen Personality Factor Questionnaire (Cattell, Eber & Tatsuoka, 1980) was constructed to assess 16 basic personality traits; and the Basic Personality Inventory (Jackson, 1974) was developed to assess 12 'sources of maladjustment and personal strengths'.

The second influential trait model in the personality area focuses on three dimensions of personality: Neuroticism, Extraversion, and Psychoticism (Eysenck, 1991a). The Neuroticism dimension (N) is viewed to be 'indicative of emotional lability and overreactivity. High-scoring individuals tend to be emotionally overresponsive and to have difficulties in returning to a normal state after emotional experiences' (Eysenck & Eysenck, 1968, p. 6). Individuals high on the Extraversion dimension (E) are described as 'outgoing, impulsive and uninhibited, having many social contacts and frequently taking part in group activities' (Eysenck & Eysenck, 1968, p. 6). Individuals scoring high on the Psychoticism dimension (P) are described as 'egocentric, aggressive, impersonal, cold, lacking in empathy, impulsive, lacking in concern for others, and generally unconcerned about the rights and welfare of other people' (Eysenck, 1982, p. 11). Given the traits that define P, some theorists have suggested the term *psychopathy* as a more appropriate label than psychoticism (Zuckerman, Kuhlman & Camac, 1988).

Consistent with the view that biological factors underly the basic dimensions of personality, Eysenck (1990) has presented some evidence that N, E, and P are determined by genetic factors. There is evidence also that high and low levels of N and E may be associated with individual differences in brainstem arousal and autonomic nervous system reactivity to sensory stimulation. These associations have implications for understanding aspects of affect regulation; for example, the lability of the autonomic nervous system in neurotic individuals may prolong states of affective dysregulation evoked by stress; and extraverts may seek out certain types of stimulation that introverts tend to avoid.

Although the three-factor personality model is best identified with the work of Hans Eysenck (1982; Eysenck & Eysenck, 1975; Eysenck & Eysenck, 1985), similar models have been proposed by Tellegen (1985) and by Watson and Clark (1993). These other personality psychologists emphasize emotional experience and the temperamental underpinnings of higher-order personality traits, and they prefer to interpret N and E as Negative Affectivity and Positive Affectivity, respectively (Watson & Tellegen, 1985). Later in this chapter, we will refer to some empirical research that has shown a clear convergent/ discriminant pattern of correlations between measures of positive and negative affects and measures of N and E.

The third influential trait model, the five-factor personality model, identifies five basic personality dimensions (Digman, 1990; Goldberg, 1993; McCrae & Costa, 1987). Although researchers have given different names to the five basic dimensions, there appears to be a growing consensus about the structure of the five-factor model (Digman, 1990; Goldberg, 1993). Along with the dimensions of N and E, the five-factor model includes the dimensions of Conscientiousness (C), Agreeableness (A), and Openness to Experience (O) (sometimes labeled Culture or Intellect). Individuals high on A are described as honest, sincere, and willing to help others; individuals high on C are described as being well organized, reliable, and determined; individuals high on O are described as being curious about both inner and outer worlds, and open to new ideas and experiences (McCrae & Costa, 1987; McCrae & John, 1992). It is important to recognize that O is not equivalent to intelligence, and that 'many people score high in O without having a corresponding high IQ' (McCrae & John, 1992, p. 198). Some researchers are of the opinion that the five- and three-factor models are not incompatible, but merely different levels in a hierarchical model (Zuckerman et al., 1988); for example, low A combined with low C seems to correspond to P in Eysenck's three-factor model (McCrae & John, 1992).

Although the five-factor model is not a complete theory of personality and has certain recognized limitations (McAdams, 1992), it has become an important and useful model for evaluating new constructs and for exploring the relationships among affects, personality, and physical and mental health (Costa & McCrae, 1987a; Marshall et al., 1994; Smith & Williams, 1992; Watson & Clark, 1992). Some personality psychologists, who view affects as central organizing elements in the structure of personality, even contend that 'the five dimensions of personality rendered by factor-analytic studies are more legitimately seen as being related to emotion traits' (Magai & McFadden, 1995, p. 228). Of course the interaction between personality traits and situational variables must also be considered in research exploring the effects of personality and emotions on health or related outcomes (Smith & Williams, 1992).

### Alexithymia and personality structure

### The multidimensional approach

Given the plethora of measures that have been developed by researchers employing the multidimensional approach to personality, it is not surprising that a broad range of constructs have been used to study the relationship between alexithymia and personality structure. In some of the early research, alexithymia was found to be unrelated to several personality traits including neuroticism, trait anxiety, repression-sensitization, and the Type A behaviour pattern (Fava, Baldaro & Osti, 1980; Martin & Pihl, 1986; Mendelson, 1982; Schiraldi & Beck, 1988). It is likely that these findings reflect measurement error rather than the true relationship between alexithymia and these diverse personality traits, as alexithymia was measured with self-report scales that have been shown subsequently to lack reliability and validity, *viz.*, the SSPS, the Revised SSPS, and the MMPI-A (see Chapter 3).

Using the more reliable and valid BIQ to measure alexithymia, Keltikangas-Järvinen (1990) investigated a group of 164 surgical patients in Finland and found no association between alexithymia and the Type A behaviour pattern. In the same study, however, a pattern of relationships was found between the BIQ and the Lazare–Klerman–Armor Trait Scales (LKATS; Lazare, Klerman & Armor, 1970) that was consistent with some aspects of the alexithymia construct. The BIQ showed significant positive correlations with the LKATS compulsive personality traits of perseverance, rigidity, and orderliness, and a significant negative correlation with the emotionality scale, indicating emotional constriction. Bach *et al.* (1994*a*) also found a moderate association between alexithymia (assessed with the TAS) and the trait of obsessive–compulsiveness, which was assessed with a subscale of the Revised Version of the Hopkins Symptom Checklist 90 (SCL-90R; Derogatis, 1977), in a group of 45 Austrian psychiatric inpatients with functional somatic symptoms. Bach and his colleagues (1994*a*) accounted for this finding by noting the 'similarities in the restricted affective structure and the rigid, externally oriented cognitive structure between alexithymic and obsessive subjects' (p. 535). It is important to note, however, that the correlations reported in the Finnish and Austrian studies were with obsessive–compulsive traits and not with obsessive–compulsive disorder with which alexithymia appears to have a low association (Zeitlin & McNally, 1993) (see Chapter 7).

In a study aimed at evaluating the convergent and discriminant validity of the TAS (which was mentioned in Chapter 3), Bagby *et al.* (1986*b*) obtained data pertaining to the relationships between alexithymia and a broad range of personality traits and psychopathology measured by the Basic Personality Inventory (BPI; Jackson, 1974). In a sample of undergraduate university students, alexithymia was unrelated to denial (which in the BPI is equivalent to social desirability), interpersonal problems, alienation, and deviation, but related weakly to anxiety, persecutory ideation, thinking disorder, impulse expression, social introversion, and self-depreciation. Stronger relationships were found with hypochondriasis and depression.

Several subsequent studies have also found weak to moderate correlations between the TAS or TAS-20 and measures of anxiety and depression. While in some instances it has not been clear whether a state condition is influencing the response to a trait measure, one would expect alexithymic individuals to manifest a tendency to experience emotional distress (such as anxiety and depression) if, as has been theorized, alexithymia reflects a deficit in the cognitive processing and regulation of emotions (Lane & Schwartz, 1987). Conversely, one would expect an inverse relationship between alexithymia and dysphoria if alexithymia was functioning as a defense, as several investigators have suggested (Haviland, MacMurray & Cummings, 1988*a*; Haviland *et al.*, 1988*c*). Though alexithymic individuals are able to report emotional distress when responding to very specific, highly structured self-report measures (such as the Beck Depression Inventory), as was noted in Chapter 2, intensive questioning in clinical interviews reveals that they know very little about their own feelings and, in most instances, are unable to link them with memories, fantasies, or specific situations. The difficulty that alexithymic individuals experience in distinguishing between different affective states was demonstrated in a study that was described in Chapter 3 (see p. 65). The consistently found relationship between alexithymia and measures of depression or other types of emotional distress has led a number of researchers to suggest that measures of alexithymia, such as the TAS, may assess aspects of neuroticism or depression rather than a unique personality construct. Mayer, DiPaolo and Salovey (1990), for example, suggest that 'it is probably best to group the TAS and Neuroticism scales together as measures of distress' (p. 779). In more recent work, however, as was noted in Chapter 2, Salovey *et al.* (1993) conceptualized alexithymia as an extreme pole of the emotional intelligence construct, which they propose as a framework for understanding affect regulation. Another group of investigators (Rubino *et al.*, 1991) concluded that alexithymia should be considered part of the neurotic personality dimension on the basis of a study in which the mean TAS score in a group of psychiatric (psychoneurotic and delusional) patients was significantly higher than the mean TAS scores in a normal control group and a group of somatically ill patients. However, as we outlined in an earlier contribution (Taylor *et al.*, 1993), Rubino and his associates confused neuroticism (a personality dimension) with psychoneurotic disorder (a psychiatric diagnosis), and ignored findings from several other studies that suggest an independence of alexithymia from psychoneurotic pathology. And, despite several reports of moderate correlations between the TAS and the Beck Depression Inventory (BDI) (Haviland *et al.*, 1988c; Hendryx, Haviland & Shaw, 1991), a factor analysis of the combined items from these two measures has provided evidence that alexithymia is a construct that is separate and distinct from the construct of depression (Parker *et al.*, 1991a).

*Alexithymia as a personality trait*
The relationship between alexithymia and depression or other psychological distress has been explored also in several prospective studies that have yielded strong support for alexithymia being a stable personality trait in many individuals. For example, Salminen *et al.* (1994) administered the Brief Symptom Inventory and the TAS to a group of 54 patients at the time of admission to a general psychiatric outpatient clinic and again one year later. The majority of patients received diagnoses of anxiety or depressive disorders and 65% of them received some kind of active psychiatric treatment. For all patients there was a significant decrease in psychological distress over the one year period but there was no significant change in the mean alexithymia score.

Similar results were obtained by Porcelli *et al.* (1996) who conducted a longitudinal study with a group of 104 medical outpatients suffering from inflammatory bowel diseases. These patients were clinically assessed for level of disease activity and administered the TAS-20 and the Hospital Anxiety and Depression Scale prior to the initiation of treatment (Time 1) and after six months of treatment (Time 2). Based on a comparison of levels of disease activity between Time 1 and Time 2, patients were categorized into unchanged, improved, or worsened groups at Time 2. The test–retest reliability of the alexithymia scale for the total group of patients regardless of outcome status was 0.95, which strongly suggests that alexithymia is a stable personality trait in these patients. For the improved group of patients, there were significant reductions in anxiety and depression scores between Time 1 and Time 2, but there was no corresponding reduction in mean alexithymia scores.

In another longitudinal study, Della Chiaie (personal communication, April, 1994) administered the TAS, Spielberger's state and trait anxiety scales, and the BDI to a group of 63 inpatients with major depressive disorders. The patients were treated with either tricyclic antidepressant medication or electroshock therapy and completed the scales at the beginning of hospitalization and again two days prior to discharge. A comparison of test scores before and after treatment showed statistically significant reductions in trait and state anxiety scores and depression scores, but there was no significant change in the mean alexithymia score.

Several other prospective studies have been conducted with groups of patients with substance use disorders and have demonstrated a similar stability of alexithymia scores over time despite significant reductions in depression. These studies will be reviewed in Chapter 8. While there is some shared variance between measures of depression, anxiety and alexithymia, the data from the prospective studies with various medical and psychiatric patient populations indicate that alexithymia is not simply a secondary response to anxious or depressed states.

**The three-factor model**

In some of our earlier work with the TAS, we examined the relationship of alexithymia with Eysenck's three-factor model of personality, which was assessed with the Eysenck Personality Questionnaire (EPQ; Eysenck & Eysenck, 1975; Parker et al., 1989a). In a sample of 190 undergraduate university students, the TAS had a low to moderate correlation with N ($r = 0.29$, $p < 0.01$), a moderate negative correlation with E ($r = -0.37$, $p < 0.01$), and a low correlation with P ($r = 0.17$, $p < 0.05$). Similar results were reported by Mayer et al. (1990), who administered the TAS and a brief form of the Eysenck Personality Inventory to a sample of 139 college students; the correlation between the TAS and N was 0.34, the correlation between the TAS and E was −0.24.

The finding of a positive association between alexithymia and N is consistent with clinical and empirical evidence that both neurotic individuals and alexithymic individuals are prone to somatization and generalized dysphoria (Eysenck & Eysenck, 1975; Lesser, 1985; Taylor et al., 1992b). The finding of a negative association between alexithymia and E is also not unexpected as both alexithymic individuals and introverted individuals have difficulty communicating feelings to other people, and are frequently regarded by others as emotionally distant. It is important, however, to recognize differences between the alexithymia construct and the constructs of N and E. Neurotic individuals are quickly aroused physiologically by all types of stimuli and readily express their emotions verbally (Eysenck & Eysenck, 1975). In contrast, while alexithymic individuals also may easily be aroused physiologically by a variety of stimuli, they are less able to identify the subjective 'feeling' component of emotional arousal and therefore have difficulty expressing their emotional states verbally. Similarly, introverts are typically thoughtful and introspective about their emotions, whereas alexithymic individuals tend to be preoccupied with external events and rarely reflect on their inner subjective lives. Thus, while alexithymia shows some relation to N and E, these broader personality dimensions do not capture some of the more specific and crucial aspects of the alexithymia construct.

To further explore the relationship between alexithymia and the three-factor model of personality, we reanalysed the data from our earlier study with university students (Parker et al., 1989a), this time using confirmatory factor analysis. As the students in that study had completed a pilot scale containing items for both the TAS and TAS-20, we were able to conduct the analysis using TAS-20 scores as well as EPQ scores. Because we consider alexithymia to be distinct from the three personality dimensions measured by the EPQ, we constructed a hypothetical four-factor model with the four factors corresponding to N, E, P, and alexithymia. To reduce error variance and the possibility of spurious associations due to the modest sample size, we collapsed the number of indicators for the alexithymia and personality dimensions from 87 items (the TAS-20 has 20 items and the EPQ has 67 items) to 12 parcels by using a variation of Cattell and Burdsal's (1975) parcelling technique. By reducing the number of indicators, parcelling improves the ratio between sample size and number of indicators (in this study from 190/87 to 190/12). For each of the three EPQ scales, items were randomly divided into three parcels; for the TAS-20, items were divided into the three factor scales. Thus, the four-factor model we tested had a total of 12 indicators (3 alexithymia, 3 neuroticism, 3 psychoticism, and 3 extraversion).

Using the goodness-of-fit indicators recommended by Cole (1987) and described in our initial report on the development of the TAS-20 (Bagby et al., 1994a), confirmatory factor analysis indicated that the hypothesized four factor model was a good fit to the data. The parameter estimates for the relationships among the four factors are presented in Fig. 4.1. Alexithymia is related moderately to N, moderately and inversely to E, and only weakly to P. The good fit of the model provides additional support for the view that the alexithymia construct is relatively distinct from N, E, and P.

## The five-factor model

The relationship between alexithymia and the five-factor model of personality was explored first by a group of investigators in the United States. In an initial study, Wise, Mann and Shay (1992) administered the TAS and the NEO Five Factor Inventory (NEO-FFI; Costa & McCrae, 1985) to a diagnostically heterogeneous group of 114 psychiatric outpatients (57 men and 57 women) and to 71 adult hospital volunteers screened for psychiatric distress. Designed to be a brief self-report instrument for assessing the five basic dimensions of the five-factor personality model, the 60-item NEO-FFI is a short form of the NEO Personality Inventory which will be described later. Wise *et al.* (1992) ran a series of stepwise multiple regression analyses, separately

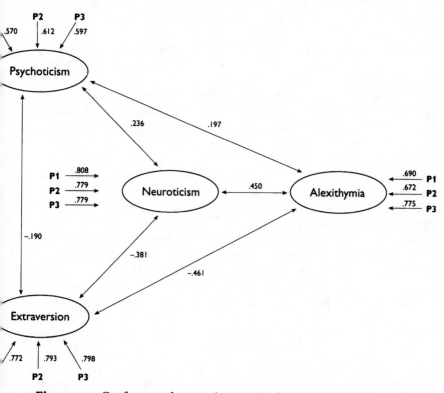

**Figure 4.1** *Confirmatory factor analytic model of alexithymia and basic dimensions of personality* (**P** = parcel).

for clinical and non-clinical groups, to predict TAS scores from the five NEO-FFI scales. For the normal adult sample, 38.1% of the variance in predicting TAS scores was explained by E (26.4%), O (8.3%), and N (3.6%). For the outpatient sample, 57.1% of the variance in predicting TAS scores was explained by N (35.1%), O (16.3%), and E (5.7%).

In a later study, Wise and Mann (1994) administered the TAS and NEO-FFI (along with several other measures) to a group of 101 psychiatric outpatients (53 men and 48 women) most of whom had a depressed or anxious mood. Partial correlation coefficients controlling for depression revealed the TAS to correlate positively with N ($r = 0.38$), and negatively with E ($r = -0.40$), O ($r = -0.40$), and C ($r = -0.32$); the TAS did not significantly correlate with A.

The results of these studies are consistent with the research using the three-factor model that found a low to moderate positive association between alexithymia and N, and a low to moderate negative association between alexithymia and E. However, the results also indicate an association between alexithymia and O, and possibly also with C. The finding of an association between alexithymia and O is not surprising; as Costa and McCrae (1987a) have pointed out, there is considerable conceptual overlap between the alexithymia construct and the openness to experience dimension (which should not be confused with self-disclosure). The elements of O include 'active imagination, aesthetic sensitivity, attentiveness to inner feelings, preference for variety, intellectual curiosity, and independence of judgement' (Costa & McCrae, 1992; McCrae & Costa, 1985, 1997). Furthermore, O encompasses the construct of psychological mindedness, as was noted in Chapter 2, and has been shown to be associated positively with divergent thinking, creativity, and absorption (the ability to become immersed in fantasy, memories, and other imaginative activity) (McCrae, 1987; Mutén, 1991), characteristics that are lacking in alexithymic individuals.

To investigate these relationships further, we examined correlations between the TAS-20 and the self-report version of the NEO Personality Inventory (NEO PI; Costa & McCrae, 1985) using data collected from a group of 83 college students (22 men and 61 women) (Bagby et al., 1994b). The NEO PI is a 181-item measure that provides a comprehensive assessment of the five basic dimensions of personality including six specific facets in the domains of N, E, and O. Pearson product–moment correlations between the TAS-20 and the NEO PI scales are presented in Table 4.1.

As expected, a moderate positive association was found between alexithymia and N and the subscales reflecting the tendency to experience the negative affects of Anxiety, Depression, and

**Table 4.1.** *Correlations between the TAS-20 and the NEO Personality Inventory in an undergraduate university student sample*

| NEO PI | TAS-20 |
|---|---|
| *Neuroticism* | .27* |
| Anxiety | .25* |
| Hostility | −.05 |
| Depression | .36** |
| Self-consciousness | .30** |
| Impulsiveness | −.10 |
| Vulnerability | .35** |
| *Extraversion* | −.21 |
| Warmth | −.08 |
| Gregariousness | −.08 |
| Assertiveness | −.22* |
| Activity | −.19 |
| Excitement seeking | .07 |
| Positive emotions | −.36** |
| *Openness to Experience* | −.49** |
| Fantasy | −.30** |
| Aesthetics | −.29** |
| Feelings | −.55** |
| Actions | −.24* |
| Ideas | −.33** |
| Values | −.17 |
| *Agreeableness* | −.09 |
| *Conscientiousness* | −.21 |

\* $p < 0.05$. \*\* $p < 0.01$.

Self-consciousness (i.e. shame and embarrassment). Alexithymia was associated positively also with Vulnerability to stress, suggesting that alexithymic individuals tend to become dependent, hopeless, or panicky when facing emergency situations.

Although the correlation between the TAS-20 and E did not quite reach a level of significance, within the domain of E alexithymia was associated significantly and negatively with the tendency to experience Positive Emotions. Such a finding is consistent with the clinical reports discussed in Chapter 2 that alexithymic individuals show a limited ability to experience positive affects such as joy, happiness, and love (Krystal, 1988; Sifneos, 1987). Although one would predict that alexithymic individuals would also score low on the Warmth and

Gregariousness facets of E, the TAS-20 did not correlate with these subscales in our college student sample. As will be shown later in some clinical vignettes, however, NEO PI results from alexithymic patients with psychiatric disorders usually reveal low scores on the Warmth and Gregarious subscales of E as well as low scores on the Positive Emotions subscale.

Alexithymia was again found to be negatively related to O, as Costa and McCrae (1987a) had predicted, and to all of its facet scales except Openness to Values. There was no relationship with A and C.

Overall, the results of the empirical research employing the five-factor model of personality extend the findings obtained with the three-factor model and suggest that the alexithymia construct combines elements of N, E, and O, in particular a tendency to experience emotional distress, a low proneness to experience positive emotions, and a limited imagination and failure to give importance to subjective feelings. Given these findings, one may ask whether alexithymia should be conceptualized as a unique construct with explanatory power, or whether it is adequately represented by, and therefore redundant with, existing dimensions of personality. This question relates to a larger controversy in personality psychology as to whether researchers should focus primarily on the broad dimensions of personality, or sharpen their focus on the elements that comprise these dimensions (Briggs, 1989; Costa & McCrae, 1987a; Eysenck, 1991a; Marshall et al., 1994; McAdams, 1992; Smith & Williams, 1992). Briggs (1989) considers the two approaches 'complementary, but quite distinct' and argues that the study of personality should focus on both broad dimensions and personal tendencies. The former focus is basically descriptive in its emphasis on tendencies that define people generally; the latter focus identifies individual differences that are more specific and have greater utility for generating hypotheses and predicting criteria (Briggs, 1989; Smith & Williams, 1992). Moreover, it is now known that many traits that have been of central importance in personality and health research are blends of two or more of the five basic dimensions (Marshall et al., 1994; McCrae & John, 1992).

### Alexithymia, personality, and affects

The demonstration that the alexithymia construct converges with the first three dimensions of the five-factor model of personality is consistent with our view that alexithymia reflects a deficit in the ability cognitively to process and regulate emotions. Indeed, as noted earlier, some personality theorists conceptualize N and E as two dominant dimensions of emotional experience: Negative Affectivity and Positive Affectivity, respectively (Watson & Clark, 1984; Watson & Tellegen, 1985). This conceptualization is supported by evidence that measures of negative affects correlate strongly with N, and only weakly or modestly with E, whereas measures of positive affects correlate significantly with E, but only modestly with N (Costa & McCrae, 1980; Meyer & Shack, 1989; Watson & Clark, 1992). Furthermore, there is evidence from human infancy research, as well as from correlational and factor analytic studies, that negative emotions and positive emotions are largely independent of one another, rather than being opposite poles of a single dimension of personality (Emde, 1991; Watson & Clark, 1984, 1992).

Most studies examining the relations between affects and the five-factor model of personality report low positive correlations between O and measures of both positive and negative affects, suggesting that 'O does not have an affect-biasing influence as E and N do', and that open people experience affects more intensely (McCrae & Costa, 1991, p. 228). Some recent studies, however, have found negative affects to be related negatively to O (Watson & Clark, 1992). There is some evidence also that individuals who are high on A and C experience more positive affects and less negative affects (McCrae & Costa, 1991); but it may be a disposition to experience positive affects that promotes agreeable interpersonal behavior and achievement striving rather than the reverse (Watson & Clark, 1992).

Personality psychologists generally include *interest* among the positive affects (along with enthusiasm, joy, excitement, attentiveness, happiness, etc.) and therefore link it with the E dimension of personality (Watson & Clark, 1992; Watson, Clark & Tellegen, 1988). Within the broad dimension of O, however, several lower-order traits seem to refer to the affect of interest. Indeed, McCrae and Costa (1985) point out that individuals who score low on O 'are not so much resistant to new ideas and feelings as they are uninterested. *Dull*, rather than *dogmatic*, seems to capture the essence of closedness' (p. 161).

Although empirical studies are needed to clarify whether measures of the specific affect of interest correlate significantly with O, it is possible that the finding of an association between alexithymia and low O reflects a temperamental deficiency in the innate affect of interest as well as a limited ability to engage in imaginative and divergent thinking (McCrae, 1987). Reports that alexithymic patients receiving psychotherapy tend to evoke feelings of boredom and dullness in their therapists (Nemiah & Sifneos, 1970; Sifneos, 1974; Taylor, 1977, 1984*b*) also suggest a deficiency in the interest affect system of these patients, as low interest is contagious. High interest makes people both more interested and interesting to others, and generally triggers other positive emotions as well (Nathanson, 1992; Tomkins, 1962).

The relationships between alexithymia and negative and positive affects have been examined directly in several recent studies. In one of our own studies, we administered the Expanded Form of the Positive and Negative Affect Schedule (PANAS-X; Watson & Clark, 1991) to a group of 82 undergraduate university students, who were asked to respond on the basis of how they generally feel (i.e. the PANAS-X was used as a 'trait' measure). The students had been categorized previously into alexithymic and non-alexithymic groups on the basis of TAS-20 cutoff scores. The alexithymic group scored significantly higher on total negative affects (mean = 9.9, SD = 3.6) than the non-alexithymic group (mean = 6.3, SD = 2.3) ($t$ = 5.39, $df$ = 81, $p$ <0.01), and also significantly lower on total positive affects (mean = 8.1, SD = 1.9) than the non-alexithymic group (mean = 9.2, SD = 2.3) ($t$ = 2.44, $df$ = 81, $p$ <0.05).

Additional findings have been reported by Paul Yelsma (1996), who administered the TAS-20, the Positive Feelings Scale (PFS), and the Expression of Emotions Scale (EES; Balswick, 1988) to a mixed group of normal adults and victims and perpetrators of verbal and/or physical abuse (N = 206). The PFS, which is taken from the Communication Conflict Instrument developed by Brown, Yelsma and Keller (1980), assesses the extent to which individuals report having positive feelings about their lives. The EES assesses emotional expressiveness to one's spouse; subjects rate on a 4-point Likert scale the extent to which they express positive (love and happiness) and negative (sadness and anger) emotions.

The correlation between the TAS-20 and PFS was −0.46 ($p$ <0.01). The expression of positive emotion also correlated negatively and significantly with the TAS-20 ($r$ = −0.33, $p$ <0.01), as did the expression of negative emotion, although rather weakly ($r$ = −0.16, $p$ <0.05). This last finding, however, is consistent with earlier research with a group of college students in which the original TAS was found to negatively and significantly correlate with the Anger Expression Scale ($r$ = −0.35, $p$ <0.01) (Bagby, Taylor & Parker, 1988b), which assesses individual differences in anger expression as a personality trait (Spielberger et al., 1985). Thus, while alexithymic individuals show tendencies to experience negative affects and minimal positive affects, consistent with the theoretical construct, they tend not to communicate their feelings to other people. Consequently, as discussed in Chapter 2, they are deprived of the affect regulation that can be provided by important interpersonal relationships.

## Clinical illustrations

The following two clinical examples illustrate some associations between alexithymia, personality traits, and problems with the cognitive processing and regulation of affects.

### Case 1

Mr J, a 31-year-old store manager, sought psychiatric treatment because of a life-long tendency to experience high levels of emotional distress and an absence of pleasurable feelings. When questioned, Mr J indicated that his only pleasurable times were the occasions when he experienced a temporary absence of negative emotions. He suffered from frequent migraine headaches, had a past history of duodenal ulceration (one of the 'classical' psychosomatic diseases), and had been treated with a tricyclic antidepressant for an episode of major depression. The patient had been referred by a general psychiatrist to a senior psychoanalyst who recommended intensive psychoanalytic treatment. Mr J sought a second opinion because he was uncertain about taking the necessary time from his job.

In the initial consultation, the patient manifested extreme difficulty in identifying and describing specific feelings, including an inability to distinguish between anxiety, sadness, and depression. Mr J also reported an almost total absence of fantasies and that he had never recalled a dream in his entire life. Although he had decided recently to live with his girlfriend, upon whom he was very dependent, the patient was unable to feel emotionally intimate with her. He had few memories from his early childhood, but those he was able to recall suggested that relationships with parents had been emotionally impoverished.

Mr J obtained a score of 64 on the TAS-20, which is in the high range for alexithymia. As shown in Fig. 4.2, he also scored in the very high range on the N scale of the NEO PI (Costa & McCrae, 1985), particularly on the subscales of Anxiety, Depression, Self-Consciousness, and Vulnerability to Stress. Mr J also obtained a very low score on E, which was accounted for by scores in the very low range on the subscales of Positive Emotions, Gregariousness, and Warmth (capacity for intimacy). The patient also scored in the very low range on O, with very low scores on Feelings, Fantasy, and Actions, but with higher scores on the other Openness subscales. On the dimensions of A and C, Mr J scored in the average and high range, respectively. His score on the Beck Depression Inventory was 11, which is below the cut-off score for clinical depression.

These test results confirmed our clinical impression that the patient was alexithymic, and that his lack of psychological mindedness would render him a poor candidate for traditional psychoanalytic treatment. His high levels of neuroticism and anhedonia, however, coupled with low O, indicated a serious problem with affect regulation. This was evidenced also by his presenting symptoms, his tendency to somatize, and by a prior history of abusing alcohol and marijuana to regulate dysphoric states. Our recommendation was that Mr J was not a good candidate for psychoanalysis, and was more likely to benefit from a modified psychotherapeutic approach that sought to repair deficits in

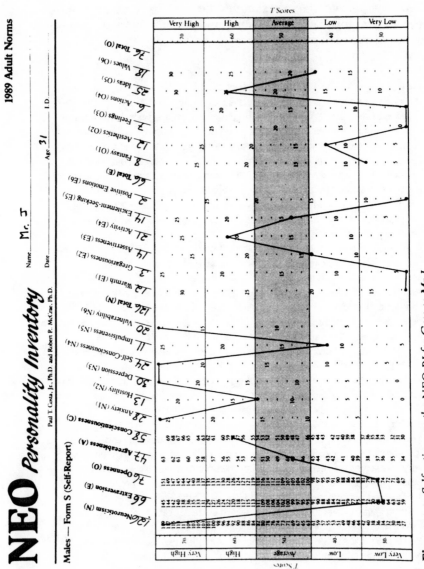

**Figure 4.2** *Self-ratings on the NEO PI for Case 1: Mr J.*

the cognitive–experiential and interpersonal domains of emotion regulation. This type of psychotherapy is described in Chapter 11.

### Case 2

Mr W, a 25-year-old university student, sought psychiatric treatment when he realized that his wife was likely to discover his compulsive habit of buying pornographic magazines and masturbating. Although he enjoyed a satisfying sexual relationship with his wife, Mr W indicated that for many years he had experienced the urge to masturbate whenever he was feeling lonely and emotionally tense. He thought that he probably had a tendency to 'bottle-up his emotions' and to not communicate his feelings adequately to his wife or other people. During the initial psychiatric consultation Mr W did not appear to be emotionally distressed. Indeed, he smiled often and, when questioned, acknowledged that this was a frequent behaviour in stressful interpersonal situations.

Mr W obtained a very high score of 76 on the TAS-20. As shown in Fig. 4.3, testing with the Revised NEO Personality Inventory (NEO PI-R; Costa & McCrae, 1992), which includes six subscales for all five dimensions of personality, yielded a personality profile consistent with some of the empirical research findings reported earlier. Mr W obtained very high scores on N and most of the subscales of N, and a very low score on the Positive Emotions subscale of E. He also obtained very low scores on the Warmth and Gregariousness subscales of E, which indicated a reduced ability to relate warmly and intimately in interpersonal relationships. He rated himself as somewhat open and generally agreeable, but as very low on C. Although he scored very low on the receptivity to Feelings subscale of O, the patient did score in the high range on the Fantasy subscale. It became evident later, in the course of psychotherapy with Mr W, that it was only through his use of pornographic material that he was able to demonstrate a capacity for crude fantasy elaborations of affect. In a style described by Spezzano (1993), the patient probably turned to such fantasy because of an inability to use relationships with other persons for the imaginative elaboration of his excitement and desire, or for regulation of his pain, loneliness, and anxiety.

It is important to recognize that individuals can show tendencies to experience negative affects (high N) and low levels of positive affects without being alexithymic. This is illustrated in two additional clinical vignettes, which further indicate that elements of the O dimension of the personality are an essential component of the alexithymia construct.

### Case 3

Mrs K, a 36-year-old married secretary, was referred for psychiatric consultation by her family physician because of frequent and prolonged episodes of feeling anxious and depressed. These episodes had occurred since her mid-adolescence and were associated with irritability, malaise, lack of motivation, and a high sensitivity to criticism. The patient gave no history of hypomanic episodes, and

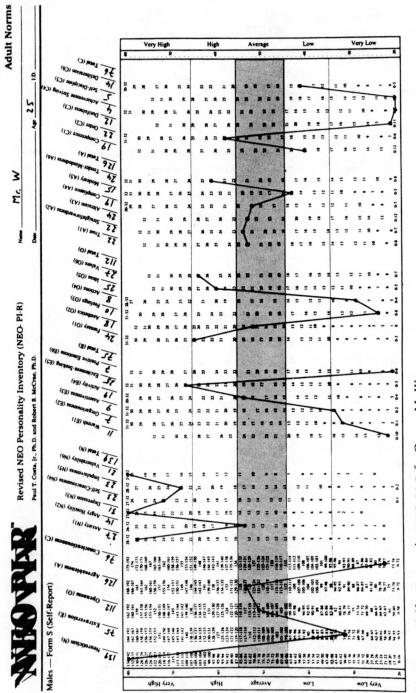

**Figure 4.3** *Self-ratings on the NEO PI-R for Case 2: Mr W.*

reported that her life was generally joyless. Although she had received psychotherapy from three different therapists for the greater part of the past 12 years, Mrs K had never been treated with psychotropic medication. In the consultation interview, she reported an active fantasy life and used a variety of different emotion words to convey the nature of her affective experience.

On psychological testing, Mrs K obtained a score of 24 on the Beck Depression Inventory, indicating a mild to moderate level of clinical depression. On the TAS-20 she obtained a score of 57, which is below the cutoff score for alexithymia. Figure 4.4 shows the NEO PI-R profile results of Mrs K's self-reports. The results indicate a strong tendency to experience negative emotions (high N), and a very low disposition to experience positive emotions. In contrast to the typical alexithymic patient, however, Mrs K scored in the high range on O with very high scores on the sub-scales assessing fantasy and receptivity to her own feelings. She scored in the average range on A and in the very low range on C.

### Case 4

Mr M, a man of 41, sought psychotherapy because of chronic unhappiness and a generally negative outlook on life. He described himself as a cynical, bitter, and shy person, and indicated that he was prone to experiencing 'black moods' and to having frequent outbursts of anger. The patient indicated also that he rarely expressed affectionate feelings or other positive emotions, and he stated that his wife complained of his lack of cheerfulness and joy. Mr M was very interested in philosophy and metaphysics, however, and pursued several hobbies. A score of only 42 on the TAS-20 indicated that Mr M was not alexithymic. His profile results on the self-report NEO PI-R are shown in Fig. 4.5. He rated himself as very high on N (especially prone to anxiety and depression) and very low on E. His introversion included an absence of interpersonal warmth, a failure to enjoy groups of people, and the experiencing of very little joy and happiness. Consistent with his score on the non-alexithymic range of the TAS-20, however, Mr M rated himself as somewhat open with an average imagination and receptivity to his own inner feelings. He scored a little below average on both A and C.

### Affect regulation and defense style

A substantial body of theory and research on personality structure and affect regulation can be found in the literature on psychological (ego) defense mechanisms (see Vaillant, 1992, 1994). The concept of defense mechanisms was developed originally by Freud (1926), and refined later by his daughter Anna Freud (1936), both of whom recognized that psychological defenses are a major means of managing affects and instinctual drives. Subsequent psychoanalytic theorists have also emphasized the adaptive function of defenses (e.g. Hartmann, 1939), and

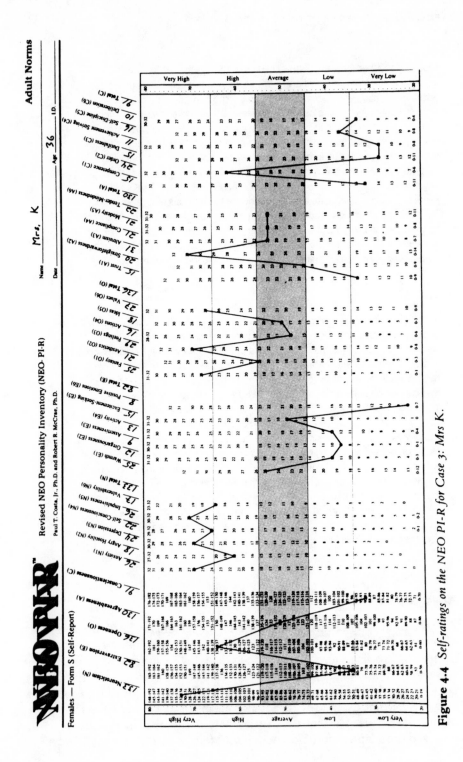

**Figure 4.4** *Self-ratings on the NEO PI-R for Case 3: Mrs K.*

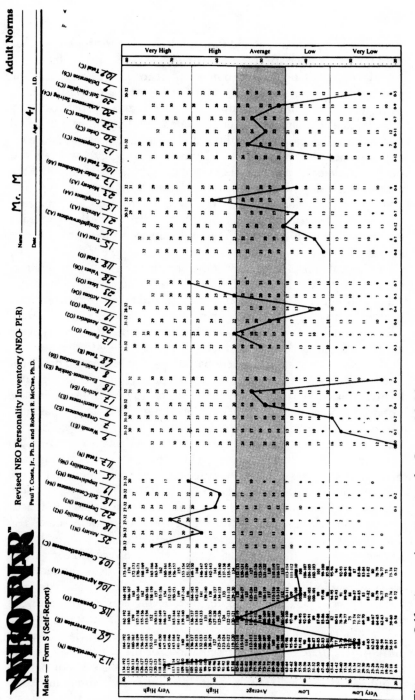

Figure 4.5 Self-ratings on the NEO PI-R for Case 4: Mr M.

nowadays recognize that an individual's defensive functioning is influenced not only by the affects associated with unconscious conflicts, but also by the status of one's ego and superego development and the psychic consequences of trauma and developmental defects (Dorpat, 1985). It is important to recognize, however, that while defenses may be mobilized to manage affects generated by conflicts, trauma, and developmental defects, affects themselves 'play a central role in organising and integrating cognition' (Ciompi, 1991, p. 97), and can also function as defenses against other more disturbing affects, as with the manic defense described by Klein (1935) and Winnicott (1935).

Much of the recent work in this area has focused on exploring individual differences in the defense mechanisms and other cognitive processes used by individuals faced with situations likely to generate unpleasant affects. According to recent theorists like Vaillant (1994), psychological defenses counteract the negative consequences of affective states by allowing the individual 'to reduce cognitive dissonance and to minimize sudden changes in internal and external environments by altering how these events are perceived' (p. 44).

During the past few decades a rather extensive literature has evolved on the classification of defense mechanisms according to the potential for affect dysregulation and psychopathology. Some theorists have proposed models that distinguish between 'adaptive' and 'non-adaptive' defenses (Haan, 1963; Kroeber, 1963; White, 1974), while others have proposed models that organize defenses along a hierarchy of potential psychopathology (Bond et al., 1983; Perry & Cooper, 1989; Vaillant, 1992). One of the more widely used models is Vaillant's (1971, 1992) hierarchical model, which is derived from psychodynamic theory and categorizes defenses along a 'mature/immature' continuum. Mature defenses are behaviours such as sublimation, humour, and suppression; immature defenses are behaviours such as projection, hypochondriasis, passive aggression, denial, dissociation, and acting out. Vaillant also identifies an intermediate category of 'neurotic' defenses including repression, intellectualization, displacement, and reaction formation.

Implicit in Vaillant's model, as with most other defense models, is the view that individuals with mature defense styles are likely to have better psychological health and more gratifying personal relationships than individuals with immature defense styles. As Aronoff, Stollak and Woike (1994) have noted, mature defenses are associated with 'a more differentiated set of representations of the self in the world in which the cognitive organization can form symbolic transformations of individual wishes, emotions, and thoughts and, simultaneously, maintain and manipulate similarly complex representations of the intentions of others' (p. 106).

Not surprisingly, given some of the defining characteristics of alexithymia, the relationship between this personality construct and immature (or 'primitive') defenses has long been the subject of speculation in the alexithymia literature. McDougall (1982a) and Taylor (1984b), for example, as was noted in Chapter 2, have suggested that alexithymic individuals may be prone to using the primitive defenses of splitting and projective identification that are associated with the paranoid–schizoid position of mental functioning described by Kleinian psychoanalysts. Knapp (1981, 1983) also recognized an association between alexithymia and immature defenses such as denial, avoidance, and externalization; as also noted in Chapter 2, however, he believed that alexithymia could be explained fully by ego defenses. More recently, Kuchenhoff (1993) has linked alexithymia with the defense of 'primitive denial', which is similar to Freud's (1918) concept of 'foreclosure' and is defined by Kuchenhoff as 'a radical exclusion of unbearable thoughts and affects from the intrapsychic experience' (p. 417). As Kuchenhoff (1993) explains, 'Such an exclusion of psychic representation brings about psychic stress that cannot be symbolized' (p. 418).

According to Dorpat (1985), primitive denial also corresponds to the defense of 'primal repression' which, as outlined in Chapter 2, was conceptualized initially by Freud (1915a) as a stage in the development of ordinary repression, or 'repression proper'. While primal repression may function together with repression proper, '[this] primitive defense prevents the formation of verbal representations of experiences' (Dorpat, 1985, p. 104), and may well account for the psychic structural defect and many of the clinical features associated with the alexithymia construct. These include the absence of normal affect and object representations, an absence of wish-fulfilling dreams, and a tendency to enact, rather than remember, early affective experiences, which are encoded as sensorimotor schemata and organized on a preconceptual level (Dorpat, 1985; Frosch, 1995; Kinston & Cohen, 1986).

### Alexithymia and defense style

Although several clinicians have written about the theoretical relationship between alexithymia and various defense mechanisms, there is a sparse empirical literature on this topic. One reason for this discrepancy may be the poor psychometric properties of many defense measures (Endler & Parker, 1995). In addition, there is little consensus in the literature about which defenses should be assessed and how these particular defenses might be defined.

In an attempt to overcome some of the psychometric weaknesses of earlier defense measures, Bond et al., (1983) developed a 67-item self-rated *Defense Style Questionnaire* (DSQ) to assess a cross-section of defenses. Bond (1986) subsequently introduced an 88-item revised version of the DSQ which, like the original version, yields four factors: maladaptive action patterns (withdrawal, regression, acting out, inhibition, passive aggression, and projection); image-distorting defenses (omnipotence, splitting, primitive idealization); self-sacrificing defenses (reaction formation, pseudoaltruism); and adaptive defenses (suppression, sublimation, humour). More recently, Andrews, Pollock, and Stewart (1989) used a group of clinicians to categorize the DSQ items into 20 defense scales that conformed to the glossary of defense mechanisms developed for the DSM-III-R (see Vaillant, 1986). A second order factor analysis with the 20 defense scales produced a three-factor model (mature defenses, neurotic defenses, and immature defenses) that proved to be more stable than the four-factor model developed by Bond et al. (1983).

Wise, Mann and Epstein (1991) used the 88-item revised version of the DSQ to examine the relationships between ego defense styles and alexithymia (assessed with the TAS) in a sample of 56 mildly depressed psychiatric outpatients. Consistent with some of the theoretical literature on alexithymia and defense (e.g. McDougall, 1982a,b; Warnes, 1985), Wise et al. (1991) found alexithymia to be positively associated with Bond et al.'s (1983) maladaptive or immature defense factor ($r = 0.42$, $p < 0.01$), and negatively associated with the adaptive or mature defense factor ($r = -0.40$, $p < 0.01$). The correlations between the TAS and the image-distorting and self-sacrificing defense factors were non-significant.

Similar findings were reported by Schaffer (1993), who administered the 88-item DSQ and the TAS to 176 adult outpatients (130 women, 46 men) receiving weekly individual psychotherapy. The TAS correlated positively with the maladaptive defense factor ($r = 0.46$, $p < 0.01$), and negatively with the adaptive defense factor ($r = -0.37$, $p < 0.01$). Although there was a non-significant correlation with the self-sacrificing defense factor, the TAS correlated weakly but significantly with the image-distorting defense factor ($r = 0.22$, $p < 0.01$). These results were reported as part of a larger study (which was discussed in Chapter 2), in which Schaffer (1993) examined the role of adult attachment in the experience and regulation of affect.

More recently, we examined the relationships between alexithymia and defense styles in a group of 287 normal adults. The mean age for men (N = 139) was 32.71 years (SD = 11.13); the mean age for women (N = 148) was 33.02 years (SD = 10.28). The subjects were non-student friends and parents of a group of undergraduate students enrolled in a psychology course at a large Canadian university. We used the TAS-20 to measure alexithymia and the three-factor model of defenses proposed by Andrews *et al.* (1989) for scoring the 88-item DSQ. The TAS-20 correlated most strongly with the immature defense factor ($r = 0.55$, $p < 0.01$), weakly with the neurotic defense factor ($r = 0.23$, $p < 0.01$), and negatively with the mature defense factor ($r = -0.25$, $p < 0.01$).

### Deficits and defenses

Although the results of the empirical studies indicate that alexithymia is associated most strongly with immature defenses, this does not mean that alexithymia itself should be conceptualized merely as a primitive defense, as some authors have mistakenly suggested (e.g. Haviland *et al.*, 1988*a*; Hogan, 1995; Knapp, 1981, 1983; McDougall, 1982*b*). Rather, one must view alexithymia as a more complex construct and ask what are the developmental and psychic structural elements that prevent an alexithymic individual from employing more neurotic or mature defenses to manage affects.

In this regard it is important to recall Dorpat's (1985) comment that 'An individual's defensive functioning is influenced by many causes, including the status of one's ego and superego development, unconscious conflicts, and the psychic consequences of trauma and developmental deficits' (p. 186). As we have shown in this chapter, the alexithymia construct demonstrates a particular pattern of relationships with other traits and basic dimensions of personality that suggests a fundamental disturbance in the area of affects. Furthermore, the reliance on immature defenses to regulate affects is consistent with the view outlined in Chapter 2 that alexithymia reflects a lower level of functioning in a hierarchical model of affect development and self-organization (Lane & Schwartz, 1987; Wilson *et al.*, 1990). This lower level of functioning involves deficits in ego development, including a failure to develop adequate higher-level defenses and other cognitive capacities to regulate affects. As Grotstein (1986) has elaborated, there are deficits not only in the capacity to regulate affects by way of mature ego defenses, but also in the capacity to mythicize primitive affects and drives into dreams or fantasies. Instead, immature defenses are employed in an attempt to organize the internal chaos that accompanies intense but poorly differentiated affective and drive arousal.

In Chapter 2, we outlined some of the ways whereby infantile trauma or deficiencies in early object relations might account for the deficits and primitive defenses associated with the alexithymic personality trait. As with other personality traits, however, one must also consider the biological processes underlying alexithymia, including possible hereditary factors and variations in the central nervous system that might dispose to the affective and cognitive behaviours that characterize the trait. These biological processes are considered in the next chapter.

# 5] The neurobiology of emotion, affect regulation, and alexithymia

In recent years, several personality theorists have emphasized the influence of genetic factors on adult personality traits and the need for linking personality constructs with neurobiological processes that might underlie individual differences in personality (Buss, 1990; Eysenck, 1991a; Gray, 1994; Cloninger, Svrakic & Przybeck, 1993; Zuckerman, 1992). Given the plethora of personality constructs that have appeared in the scientific literature, and the considerable overlap among various personality models, Eysenck (1991a) and Zuckerman (1992) have suggested that the most important and meaningful personality variables for future research will be those traits that show at least moderate heritability and that can be linked to underlying anatomical, physiological, or hormonal factors.

To date (and to the best of our knowledge), there has been only one attempt to investigate the heritability of alexithymia. This was a Norwegian study in which Heiberg and Heiberg (1977) measured alexithymia with the interviewer-rated BIQ and compared the similarity of identical (monozygotic) twins with that of fraternal (dizygotic) twins. The data yielded evidence for a strong genetic effect on the alexithymia trait. As Lesser (1981) has pointed out, however, only a small number of twins were studied (33 pairs), and since the twins were raised in their own families, they were exposed to similar environmental influences.

While much more genetic research is needed, using both twin design and adoption design methods, over the past two decades there has been a growing research interest in exploring the neurobiology of alexithymia. This research has drawn heavily on the work of several disciplines that have attempted to delineate the neural substrates of emotion and the brain mechanisms involved in affect regulation. As space permits discussion of only a small portion of this interdisciplinary work, we refer the interested reader to several excellent reviews (e.g. Borod, 1992; Davidson, 1993; Derryberry & Tucker, 1992; Ekman & Davidson, 1994; Schore, 1994; Schwartz, 1987).

In this chapter, we first present a brief overview of the neurobiology of emotion, with an emphasis on the roles of the two cerebral hemispheres in the experience, expression, and regulation of affects. We then review studies that have linked alexithymia either with a dysfunction in the right hemisphere, or with a deficiency in communication between the two cerebral hemispheres.

## The neurobiology of emotion

As mentioned in Chapter 1, Darwin (1872) addressed a number of important questions about the social and biological nature of emotion that have continued to interest researchers. Darwin noted, for example, that the face is the primary body part for the communication and expression of emotion in human and non-human primates and in other species. Not surprisingly, given the important role of facial expressions in human social interaction, the musculature of the face has been found to be more highly developed in humans than in any other species (Bradshaw, 1989). Darwin (1872) noted also that certain primary or basic emotions are expressed and understood across cultures, thus suggesting that primary emotions (including anger, fear, panic, sadness, surprise, interest, happiness, and disgust) are universal and have an innate neural basis. The idea that human behaviour is motivated largely by a set of primary innate emotions was elaborated subsequently by Tomkins (1962, 1963), who also regarded the face as the display board for the affect system. The search for emotion-specific physiology has occupied the attention of subsequent generations of emotion researchers (e.g. Davidson, 1994; Gray, 1994).

In the early decades of the present century, much of the research on the neurobiology of emotion focused on the brainstem and hypothalamus. These regions, which regulate basic vital functions (such as respiration, body temperature, sleep–waking rhythm, arousal, and orientation) and the autonomic and endocrine systems of the body, were thought also to be the central brain structures involved in the generation and regulation of emotions. This is evidenced, for example, in Cannon's (1929) work on the role of the hypothalamus in affective experience, and in Bard's (1934) discovery that slight provocations evoke violent 'sham rage' in dogs and cats, following removal of the cerebral cortex, which can be abolished by transection of the brainstem behind the hypothalamus. As research continued, however, the brainstem and hypothalamus were found to be associated only with the regulation of instinctive or basic emotion processes such as primitive rage and fight/flight behaviour. The study of emotion-specific physiology shifted to other parts of the brain, first to those structures comprising the limbic system, and later to the cerebral hemispheres.

**The triune brain**

The primate brain, as described by MacLean (1949, 1990, 1993), has evolved and expanded along a caudal–rostral axis to form a hierarchy of three brains in one (what he terms the 'triune' brain) comprising reptilian, paleomammalian, and neomammalian portions. As already noted, the brainstem, or reptilian brain structures, are involved in the regulation of autonomic, endocrine, and instinctive activities, all of which contribute to the experience of emotion. The intermediate and less primitive paleomammalian brain is the limbic system, which comprises the cingulate gyrus, the hippocampal formation, the fornix, the mammillary body, the septal region, the amygdala, and the dorsomedial nucleus. Extending an earlier proposal of Papez (1937) that these structures provide a mechanism for the elaboration and expression of the emotions, MacLean (1949) inferred that the limbic system functions as a crude analyzing mechanism that derives information and interprets experience in terms of emotional states instead of symbolic thought. MacLean (1949, 1993) sometimes refers to the limbic lobe as the 'visceral brain' not only because of its important connections to the hypothalamus and thereby with the entire endocrine and autonomic nervous system, but also to emphasize its association with strong inner emotional states and their associated visceral manifestations. In early mammals, such emotional states guide self-preservative and species-preservative behaviours.

The neomammalian brain, or neocortex, is responsible for cognitive functions including symbolization, and is referred to by MacLean (1949) as the 'word brain' (as was noted in Chapter 2). It is assumed to have evolved to provide higher level mental representations of the external and internal environments, as well as more finely tuned emotional responses and enhanced cognitive capacities related to anticipation and planning (Derryberry & Tucker, 1992). Although non-human primates may show a limited ability to conceptualize, it was the evolutionary development of a capacity to use symbols and language that separated humans from animals. Language, as Lynch (1993) has recently emphasized, 'gives men the unique potential to do what no animal can do . . . distinguish the difference between emotions and feelings' (p. 368). Numerous neural connections between the limbic system and the neocortex allow not only for emotions to evoke thoughts and a knowledge of what we feel, but also for cognitions to arouse emotions and to have modulating influences. The capacity for thought and reflection also allows humans to have some degree of voluntary control over their emotions (Ciompi, 1991).

### The amygdala and hippocampal system

In recent years, specific components of the limbic system have been the target of an increasing amount of attention in research on the neurobiology of emotion. LeDoux (1992, 1994), for example, has reviewed a large body of human and animal research that suggests that the amygdala plays a prominent role in endowing sensory input with affective and experiential tone. In addition, it is thought to integrate memory images of the external world with emotional experiences associated with those memories (Calvin, 1990). The amygdala also appears to play an important role in regulating some species-specific involuntary responses to emotional stimuli (e.g. fear responses), and in mediating between the cerebral cortex and the musculature of the face involved in facial expressions of emotion.

The hippocampal system has also received considerable attention in the emotion literature, particularly as it appears to be involved in both cognitive and emotional functions (Derryberry & Tucker, 1992). The hippocampus is involved in the important cognitive functions of spatial mapping and consolidating sensory information into memory, and contributes also to the interpretation of environmental cues likely to produce an emotional response. As summarized by Derryberry and Tucker (1992), '[the hippocampus] compares incoming information with generated predictions, and if a discrepancy is detected, it facilitates attention and inhibits ongoing motor behavior' (p. 332).

In contrast to the amygdala, which matures earlier and provides the affective quality to experience, the hippocampus is not fully myelinated until the third or fourth year of life, thus explaining infantile amnesia (van der Kolk, 1993, 1994). The maturation of the brain allows memory storage to shift 'from primarily sensorimotor (motoric action), to perceptual representations (iconic), to symbolic and linguistic modes of organization of mental experience ' (van der Kolk, 1993, p. 231), as conceptualized in Piaget's (1962) theory of cognitive development and in Lane & Schwartz's (1987) model of an epigenetic sequence of affect development.

The study of brain systems that appear to mediate both emotions and cognitions has led to the realization that the amygdala and hippocampus are part of a complex neural network in which these and other parts of the limbic system are responsible for generating emotional and other experiential states and for organizing related displays, while the neocortex is involved in the modulation and verbal communication of emotions. As elaborated by Ross, Homan and Buck (1994), extrapersonal sensory information is initially processed by the somesthetic, auditory, and visual areas of the cortex, which then relay the sensory-specific information to the medial temporal limbic system, where it is suffused with intrapersonal affective tone and subsequently consolidated into memory in the neocortex. That is, affects play a central role in the storage and categorization of sensory input into memory, and are involved also when memories of past events are retrieved.

As conceptualized by Ciompi (1991), the experience of particularly strong or repeated affects in similar circumstances leads to the development of stable cognitive–affective schemata or operational 'programmes' of feeling, thinking, and behaviour, which have corresponding networks of neuronal pathways that are established by repetitive actions according to the concept of neuroplasticity. Having past experience stored in their structure, such schemata and corresponding neuronal pathways are thought to represent probably the most important form of memory, and to function as internal systems of reference that influence the perception and cognitive processing of future experiences.

It has been shown that excessive stimulation of the amygdala, as might occur from increased secretion of neurohormones under conditions of severe stress and intense affective arousal, interferes with hippocampal functioning and thus with memory storage and categorization (van der Kolk, 1994). The cognitive evaluation and semantic representation of experience is inhibited; memories are then processed outside of the hippocampal system and organized on a preconceptual sensorimotor or iconic level as somatic sensations and visual images that can produce somatic symptoms, behavioural enactments, nightmares, and flashbacks (Frosch, 1995; van der Kolk, 1993, 1994). There may be lasting changes in neuronal excitability that render these emotional memories relatively indelible (Kolb, 1987; van der Kolk, 1994). These considerations have important implications for understanding the psychobiology of posttraumatic stress disorder and other disorders of affect regulation.

### Ascending and descending regulatory systems

Although the limbic system and other primitive parts of the brain continue to interest emotion researchers, over the past two decades, greater attention has been given to the role of the cerebral hemispheres in emotional processing. In contrast to the early neurobiological research, however, which focused almost exclusively on localizing particular emotion processes to specific parts of the brain, recent work on the neurobiology of emotion has stressed the importance of studying the interrelations of the different brain systems. Not only do the brainstem, limbic system, and neocortex play unique roles in various emotion processes, but ascending and descending connections among these structures allow them to play a collective role in the processing and regulation of emotion. Descending connections, as Derryberry and Tucker (1992) have outlined, 'allow the cognitive processes of the cortex to regulate the emotional functions of the limbic system and brainstem . . . [and also] allow for finely tuned peripheral responses' (p. 329).

This 'top-down' hierarchical organization is consistent with the view that cognitive attributions and appraisals can influence human emotion, and that states of emotional arousal 'take the form of patterns orchestrated within and across the autonomic, endocrine, and motor systems' (Derryberry & Tucker, 1992, p. 329). Each emotion tends to trigger its own complex pattern of motor and hypothalamic-autonomic responses, which appear to be preprogrammed and relatively 'hard-wired', and which, through facial expression, posture, gestures, and tone of voice, transmit the physical data that underlie empathy and emotional communication (Schwartz, 1987, 1992). That is, emotions involve the whole body and can be perceived directly by others without the aid of verbal communication and even before an individual is aware of his or her own subjective feeling state (Buck, 1994; Schwartz, 1987). While others are generally able to 'decode' and know the meaning of an individual's spontaneous, non-verbal expressions of emotion, there are times when one might unwittingly become a 'container' for, and react to, the individual's unacknowledged emotion, a phenomenon encompassed by the psychoanalytic concept of projective identification (Buck, 1994; Schwartz, 1987). During early development, however, as was outlined in Chapter 1, the parents' attunement to their young child's emotional signals, and their ability to contain and transform primitive emotions, facilitates the establishment of an interpersonal affect regulating system that evolves gradually into a capacity to self-regulate affects as the child learns to identify, distinguish, and label his or her own emotions and to be the bearer and container of his or her own feelings.

Ascending connections within the brain permit a 'bottom-up' modulation whereby different emotional states 'might influence learning and cognition' and thereby have 'important effects on attention and memory' (Derryberry & Tucker, 1992, p. 329). Interoceptive information from the musculature and viscera is also conveyed to higher levels via ascending pathways, thereby enabling peripheral physiological activity to contribute to our mental picture of affective states, though it is not essential for, or the primary cause of, emotional experiences as proposed in the James–Lange theory. Indeed, the physiological sensations that accompany emotional states promote our learning to identify, distinguish, and label our own feelings. For instance, as Schwartz (1987) points out, 'we learn with time . . . that when our heart pounds, we are likely to be feeling excited or afraid' (p. 474). This conception of feedback mechanisms in the regulation of emotion is consistent with a contemporary view of the brain as a homeostatic, self-organizing system in which the activity of neuromodulator systems regulates the flow of information through neural subsystems and thereby helps maintain stability of the behavioural output (Cicchetti & Tucker, 1994; Schwartz, 1979; Spoont, 1992).

Some of the major brainstem neuromodulator projection systems use norepinephrine, dopamine, or serotonin as neurotransmitters, and others use glutamate, gamma-aminobutyric acid, or acetylcholine. These neurotransmitters play an important role in mediating the regulation of emotional states, and have been implicated in the pathogenesis of a growing number of psychiatric and medical disorders including those we conceptualize as disorders of affect regulation (Akiskal, 1992; Dubovsky & Thomas, 1995a; Siever & Davis, 1985; Soloff, 1994; van der Kolk, 1994). Whereas much research has attempted to link certain disorders or temperaments with levels of activity of specific neurotransmitter systems that are either too high or too low, there is increasing evidence that the activities of the various neurotransmitters overlap and that 'most cerebral functions are the result of converging actions of many different neurotransmitters' (Dubovsky & Thomas, 1995a, p. 38). In addition, some researchers postulate that alterations in neurotransmitter functioning may not directly elicit specific abnormal emotional states, but instead dysregulate neurobiological subsystems, resulting in altered neural information processing and a decoupling of affect, cognition, and behaviour (Cicchetti & Tucker, 1994; Spoont, 1992).

Given the breadth and complexity of the field of neurochemical research, a detailed review of neurotransmitter mechanisms is beyond the scope of this book. However, we consider medications that influence neurotransmitter functions an important aspect of treatment for many patients with disorders of affect regulation and will discuss this approach in Chapter 11.

**Cerebral laterality and emotion**

Current thinking about the role of the cerebral hemispheres in emotional processing is based on findings from four main sources: (i) studies examining the consequences of damage or lesions in one or other of the cerebral hemispheres; (ii) observations of individuals with damage to the corpus callosum (the large central fibre tract connecting the two cerebral hemispheres and providing the major pathway for interhemispheric communication); (iii) observations of epileptic patients who have undergone cerebral commissurotomies (so-called 'split-brain' patients whose corpus callosum has been divided surgically); and (iv) studies of perceptual laterality in neurologically intact individuals.

The reader will recall that sensory pathways are relayed from one side of the body to the contralateral (opposite) cortex. In the human visual system, for example, information coming from one side of the visual field is sent to the contralateral cerebral hemisphere. Similarly, tactile information from the fingers of the left hand are projected to the right cerebral hemisphere; the opposite pattern is found for the fingers of the right hand. If different auditory stimuli are presented simultaneously to the left and right ears, information from each ear goes to the contralateral cerebral hemisphere (Bradshaw, 1989). Researchers have taken advantage of both perceptual laterality and interhemispheric transfer to study the unique functions of the two cerebral hemispheres.

The findings from numerous studies over many years have established that the right and left hemispheres have different roles in mediating a wide variety of behaviours and higher mental processes. Our emphasis, however, will be on hemispheric specialization and integration in the processing of emotions.

An association between linguistic abilities and the left cerebral hemisphere has been one of the most consistent findings from research that has used either brain-damaged or neurologically intact individuals (Bradshaw, 1989). Severe disturbances in the semantic and grammatical components of language occur when there are lesions to particular parts of this cerebral hemisphere. Monrad-Krohn (1947) noted long ago, however, that in addition to the semantic and grammatical aspects of language there is the component of *prosody*. This component is associated with the right hemisphere and refers to the distribution of stress and melodic contour in speech. Modulation of prosody imparts to speech affective coloration, and can be used to reflect nuances of meaning and to vary the emphasis in verbal communication (Weintraub, Mesulam & Kramer, 1981). Six types of prosody disturbance, generally referred to as *aprosodias*, have been described and

linked to damage to specific parts of the right cerebral hemisphere
(Ross, 1981); these include a motor or expressive aprosodia, which
renders the individual's speech affectless and monotone, and a receptive aprosodia, which prevents the individual from appreciating the
affective colouring of other's speech. Individuals with aprosodias may
also have problems making appropriate gestures and facial expressions
of emotion (Ross, 1985). But even when patients with aprosodias
show an absence of emotional gesturing and speech that lacks affective
colouring, their non-cognitive ability to either experience emotions
inwardly or display extreme emotional behaviours (such as laughing,
crying, anger, or depression) remains relatively intact, unless there is
associated damage to temporal–limbic or hypothalamic structures
(Mueller, 1983; Ross et al., 1994).

There is evidence that the right hemisphere plays a special role also in
the cognitive processing of facial expressions of emotions (see, for
example, Mandal & Singh, 1990). Studies of patients with right
hemisphere lesions have often revealed deficits in the perception of
facial expressions of emotion (Borod et al., 1993; Bowers et al., 1985;
Voeller, Hanson & Wendt, 1988). In addition, when stimuli are
presented separately to the left and right visual fields of neurologically
intact subjects, the left visual field (linked with the right hemisphere)
shows an advantage over the right visual field in discriminating facial
emotional expressions (Bradshaw, 1989; Young, 1986). This right
hemisphere advantage is found regardless of whether realistic photographs of facial expressions are used or abstract cartoon drawings
(Bradshaw, 1989; Ley & Bryden, 1979).

Laterality research has shown that the right hemisphere is superior to
the left hemisphere not only in recognizing facial emotional expressions, but also in recognizing the emotional characteristics of other
types of information (Silberman & Weingartner, 1986). For example,
dichotic advantages for the left ear (right hemisphere) have been found
for the recognition of emotional sounds (e.g. crying and laughter), and
for emotionally toned sentences (Bradshaw, 1989). Similarly, a right
hemisphere superiority has been found when neurologically intact
individuals have been asked to make discriminations between emotional and non-emotional pictures presented either to the left or right
visual field (Silberman & Weingartner, 1986).

Along with research on the perception of emotional stimuli, a
sizeable body of work has examined the roles played by the two
cerebral hemispheres in the regulation of mood and affect. In a recent
review, Gainotti, Caltagirone and Zoccolotti (1993) refer to a number
of early studies with brain-damaged individuals that found a differential pattern of emotional reactions when the left or right cerebral

hemisphere was damaged. Left-hemisphere lesions produce depressive (negative) emotional reactions in patients, while right-hemisphere lesions produce either euphoric (positive) emotional reactions or indifference reactions. Gainotti and colleagues described a similar pattern of results in studies in which sodium amytal was injected into the left or right carotid arteries of neurologically intact individuals to temporarily inactivate one of the cerebral hemispheres.

Several recent reviews note that two different hypotheses have been proposed in the cerebral laterality literature to account for the differential pattern of results that have been found in various brain-damage and sodium amytal studies (Camras, Holland & Patterson, 1993; Gainotti *et al.*, 1993; Ross *et al.*, 1994). The *right hemisphere hypothesis* argues that the right cerebral hemisphere is not only superior for the perception of emotional stimuli, but that it also plays the dominant role in the processing and regulation of all primary emotions, regardless of valence. The *valence hypothesis*, on the other hand, views the right hemisphere as involved in the processing of negative emotions, whereas positive emotions are mediated by the left hemisphere.

In an attempt to reconcile the valence and right hemisphere hypotheses, Fox and Davidson (1984; Davidson & Fox, 1988) proposed an *approach–withdrawal hypothesis* that stresses the contribution of both cerebral hemispheres and takes into account anatomical development. According to this hypothesis, in early childhood, when interhemispheric connections have not yet fully matured, basic emotions (such as distress or pleasure) are mediated solely by the right hemisphere. As the child grows and the corpus callosum and other brain structures become fully myelinated, the left hemisphere becomes involved in the processing and regulation of social approach (positive valence) emotions. The right hemisphere, however, is viewed as continuing to play a dominant role in the processing and regulation of withdrawal (negative valence) emotions.

Evidence that different normal emotional states are associated with activation in different brain regions was provided by a recent report of changes in regional cerebral blood flow measured by the radioactive tracer $H_2^{15}O$ and positron emission tomography in a group of healthy women who induced sadness, happiness, or neutral emotion by recalling affect-laden or neutral memories while looking at sad, happy, or neutral faces (George *et al.*, 1995). Although different anatomical structures were associated with happiness and sadness, the study did not demonstrate hemispheric predominance in the mediation of positive or negative emotion. In evaluating the role of the cerebral hemispheres in emotional processing, however, Davidson (1993) has made the important comment that the neural substrates of perceiving emotional information are likely to be different from those involved in the experience and expression of emotion. He points out that the data upon which the right hemisphere hypothesis is based have 'come largely from studies of the perception of emotional information (e.g. facial expressions), where the weight of the evidence does indeed suggest that the right *posterior* region is specialized for the perception of emotion, regardless of valence' (p. 145). However, studies in which emotions were elicited and measured, with simultaneous recording of brain electrical activity, have yielded evidence that it is the *anterior* regions of the two cerebral hemispheres (frontal and anterior temporal) that are differentially involved in the positive and negative emotions associated with approach and withdrawal behaviours (Davidson, 1993; Davidson *et al.*, 1990).

Several other emotion theorists also have adopted a broader perspective that gives the two cerebral hemispheres complementary roles in emotional behaviour. Ross *et al.* (1994), for example, argue that certain types of emotion, which are derived biologically from attachment, should be categorized as 'social' emotions, and distinguished from primary emotions. Social emotions include pride, shame, guilt, joy, envy, and scorn. Although both social emotions and primary emotions have positive and negative valences, 'primary emotions . . . have a predominantly negative bias' (Ross *et al.*, 1994, p. 2). As part of a research study designed to assess prosody, patients were asked to recall an emotionally charged life event before, during, and after an injection of sodium amytal into their right carotid artery. Besides a distinct loss of spontaneous and affective prosody during the procedure, 'almost all of the patients dramatically altered their affective recall of the life event by denying, minimizing, or decathecting the primary emotion and, in many instances, substituting a social emotion ' (p. 3). On the basis of this unexpected experimental finding, Ross and colleagues proposed that the right hemisphere is associated with both positive and negative primary emotions, and the left hemisphere with social emotions.

Gainotti *et al.* (1993) proposed a more complex model, which attempts to integrate specialized functions of the two cerebral hemispheres with subcortical mechanisms in the processing of emotional behaviour. On the basis of anatomical considerations, as well as a variety of research findings, these theorists suggest that the right hemisphere is involved preferentially in functions of emotional arousal, especially the autonomic response to emotional stimuli, and that the left hemisphere is more involved in the inhibition and control of emotional expression.

Thus, rather than focusing on cerebral asymmetries, current emotion theorists and researchers are promoting the view that affect regulation involves an integration of specialized functions provided by the two cerebral hemispheres, as well as interactions between cortical and subcortical levels of brain organization.

**Cerebral laterality and imaginal processes**

In Chapter 1, we described how fantasy, dreams, and other imaginal activities play an important role in affect regulation. As with other aspects of emotional processing, recent thinking about the contributions of the cerebral hemispheres to imaginal activity has shifted from an exclusive emphasis on cerebral asymmetry to an appreciation for the close cooperation that occurs between the two hemispheres in normal individuals (Brown, 1991).

The early cerebral laterality literature had proposed that fantasy and dreaming were associated with a predominance of right hemispheric activation (Bakan, 1978; Cartwright, 1977; Galin, 1974; Ley, 1979). Support for this view came from reports that some patients with damage to parts of the right hemisphere claimed that they no longer dreamed (Humphrey & Zangwill, 1951), and from EEG studies that demonstrated greater activation in the right hemisphere (decreased amplitude on the EEG) during rapid eye movement (REM) sleep, the phase of the sleep cycle from which most dreams are reported, and during self-generated visual imagery (Goldstein, 1984; Goldstein, Stoltzfus & Gardocki, 1972). An association between frequent daydreaming and a predominance of right hemisphere activity was demonstrated also by Singer (1966), who used the technique of observing conjugate lateral eye movements as an index of hemispheric activation. [We will discuss this technique later in the chapter.] In addition, highly susceptible hypnotic subjects, who are generally more open to fantasy and other experiences (Lynn & Rhue, 1988; Tellegen & Atkinson, 1974), were reported to show a greater tendency to left lateral eye movements, suggesting right hemispheric preference during usual consciousness (Bakan, 1969). However, not all of these studies controlled for moderating variables, such as gender and handedness of the subjects, and the subjects in Goldstein *et al.*'s (1972) EEG study were not awakened during REM sleep to check for dream mentation.

More recent neurophysiological research, which has employed improved methodologies to explore the relationship between dream mentation and activation in both cerebral hemispheres, has yielded evidence that both cerebral hemispheres play important roles in dream mentation (for reviews, see Antrobus, 1987; Gabel, 1988). Whereas the right hemisphere plays a role in the prosodic or affective components of dreams and in generating some of the visual imagery, the left hemisphere is involved in the verbal organization and narrative structure of dreams (Antrobus, 1987; Greenberg & Farah, 1986). Dream mentation would appear to be the result of an integration of the different information-processing styles of the two hemispheres.

There is recent evidence also that despite the co-occurrence of the more bizzare and self-involving narrative type of dreams with REM sleep, the dream process is regulated by forebrain structures rather than by neurones in the pontine part of the brainstem, as has been asserted chiefly by Hobson and McCarley (1977). In a study of a large sample of neurological and neurosurgical patients, Solms (1995) found that patients with damage to the brainstem-core reported preservation of dreaming, whereas patients with lesions in the inferior parietal lobule of either cerebral hemisphere, and patients with bilateral frontal damage, reported global cessation of dreaming. Those patients with inferior parietal lesions also showed disturbances in symbolic and spatial thought, and those with bilateral frontal damage manifested impulsivity, disinhibition, and problems with affect regulation. A few patients with lesions involving the medial occipito-temporal region of the hemispheres reported a loss of visual dream imagery, but they continued to dream in sensations or words; these patients also manifested deficits in waking visual imagery. Patients who reported completely normal dreaming had lesions in the dorsolateral frontal lobes, the part of the brain 'thought to be the highest executive end of the motor system, essential for the planning, regulation, and verification of all voluntary activity' (Solms, 1995, p. 58).

In considering these findings, Solms (1995) not only called into question prevailing theories of the relationship between dreaming and REM sleep, but also identified the neuropsychological mechanisms involved in dream mentation:

> Those parts of the brain which are *most* essential to the dream process (which, when damaged, produce a total *cessation* of dreaming) are responsible for *symbolic operations, spatial thought, and impulse control*. On the other hand, the part of the brain that is *least* essential to the dream process (which, when damaged, has *no effect* on dreaming) is responsible for *goal-directed thought and action* (p. 58).

The evolution of research on the neuropsychology of mental imagery parallels the work done on dream mentation. More systematic studies, using both neurologically intact and brain-damaged individuals, have not supported an exclusively right hemisphere specialization for mental imagery (Ehrlichman & Barrett, 1983; Farah, 1984). Whereas the right hemisphere has an advantage in processing simple imagery tasks, there is evidence now that the left hemisphere also plays a significant role (Bakan & Glackman, 1981; Farah *et al.*, 1985). As summarized by Brown (1991), 'elementary organization of visual imagery is a role for the right hemisphere, but its organization into a complex whole and the interpretation of its significance seem to be tasks involving predominantly the left hemisphere' (p. 101).

One of the weaknesses of the early research was that it treated mental imagery as a single, unitary process. As Kosslyn (1987) has noted, mental imagery represents a variety of mental phenomena. For example, imagery may be used to activate stored visual information in memory, or to perform mental simulations of possible outcomes. Instead of proposing that one processing system is responsible for all types of imagery, Kosslyn (1987) suggests that mental imagery is better conceptualized as a function of a variety of processing subsystems. Although some subsystems appear to be linked to the right cerebral hemisphere and others to the left hemisphere, mental imagery requires activation and close collaborative integration of both hemispheres.

A capacity to integrate or rapidly alternate between left and right hemispheric activities appears to be important also during hypnosis. Whereas several studies have shown right hemisphere lateralization in highly susceptible hypnotic subjects and during hypnosis, other studies have failed to replicate these findings (Brown, 1991; Gabel, 1988). However, studies that have examined shifts of cortical activation between hemispheres before or during hypnosis have demonstrated that highly hypnotizable subjects show more dramatic shifts between hemispheres and more specific lateralization, depending on the nature of the task (verbal versus imagery), than do low hypnotizable subjects (Brown, 1991).

Given the strong association between imaginative ability and hypnotizability (and the negative relationship between alexithymia and the openness to experience dimension of personality that was discussed in Chapter 4), one would expect alexithymic individuals to show low hypnotic responsivity. Preliminary support for such a relationship was provided by a study with patients referred for treatment of anxiety; there was a significantly higher percentage of alexithymic patients among those who rated low on measures of hypnotizability, and a significantly higher percentage of non-alexithymic patients among those who rated high for hypnotizability (Frankel *et al.*, 1977). Further studies are needed, however, as alexithymia was assessed with the BIQ and interrater reliability was not determined.

An important requirement for imaginative activity is the ability to shift from concrete to abstract thinking and to use language creatively as a transitional phenomenon (Deri, 1984; Weich, 1978). Although speech and the semantic and grammatical aspects of language are lateralized to the dominant left hemisphere, this is not true for the highest aspects of language. Studies of brain-damaged individuals have shown that metaphor, humour, proverb interpretation, and creativity are more affected by lesions in the right hemisphere than in the left hemisphere (Bihrle, Brownell & Gardner, 1988; Cutting, 1992; Gardner et al., 1983). The absence of these aspects of language contributes to the externally orientated cognitive style of alexithymic individuals (Hoppe, 1988).

Notwithstanding the mounting evidence that most cognitive tasks normally require a varying amount of interhemispheric cooperation, so that the two hemispheres function as a unified system, it should be emphasized that many individuals show a trait-like preference or tendency to rely on the processing style of one hemisphere over the other (Crossman & Polich, 1989), a tendency that has been termed hemisphericity. The left hemisphere displays an advantage for verbal and analytical thinking, while the right hemisphere is at an advantage for a non-verbal spatial and holistic mode of processing. It has been suggested that individual preferences for one hemisphere over an another might be relevant for understanding individual differences in personality. For instance, some studies have found that introverted individuals, and those with an obsessive–compulsive personality style, demonstrate left hemisphericity in contrast to extraverted individuals, and those with an hysterical personality style, who show right hemisphericity (Charman, 1979; Crossman & Polich, 1989; Smokler & Shevrin, 1979). However, there is evidence also that some individuals show a greater capacity for interhemispheric integration than do others (Christman, 1994; Hellige, 1993). Christman (1995), for example, has found that left-handed individuals display a relatively greater ability to integrate left and right hemisphere processing than right-handed individuals. The anatomical substrate of this difference might be the larger corpus callosum found in non-right-handers (Witelson, 1995).

There is evidence also of gender differences in functional brain asymmetry. Dichotic listening, tachistoscopic, and brain lesion studies have found that women show less hemispheric specialization than men (Bradshaw, 1989; McGlone, 1978; Rybash & Hoyer, 1992). This might be the result of a sex difference in the distribution of androgen receptors in the fetal brain, which would alter androgen-mediated neurohumoral interactions and thereby affect brain development differentially (Witelson, 1995).

Cultural factors might also influence the functional organization of the human brain. In discussing Tadanobu Tsunoda's research on the Japanese brain, Racle (1980, 1986) reported that Japanese people process both linguistic sounds and non-linguistic sounds (e.g. animal sounds, emotional utterances, singing of insects, and traditional Japanese instrumental music) predominantly with the left hemisphere, in contrast to people in Western countries who generally process non-linguistic sounds with the right hemisphere. This does not appear to be an hereditary phenomenon, as Japanese people raised in countries where Western languages are spoken do not show the typical Japanese pattern. Given the predominance of left hemisphere processing in Japanese people, one might expect a greater prevalence of alexithymia than among people in Western countries.

## The neurobiology of alexithymia

Interest in the neurobiology of alexithymia began initially with observations of alexithymic characteristics in epileptic patients who had undergone complete or partial cerebral commissurotomies (Hoppe & Bogen, 1977), as well as in individuals with agenesis of the corpus callosum (Buchanan, Waterhouse & West, 1980), and later from reports of similar characteristics among children, adolescents, and adults with evidence of lesions or other deficits in the right cerebral hemisphere (Fricchione & Howanitz, 1985; Voeller, 1986; Voeller et al., 1988; Weintraub & Mesulam, 1983). These observations generated two preliminary neurobiological hypotheses to account for alexithymia: (i) that alexithymia might be a result of a deficit in interhemispheric communication; and (ii) that alexithymia might be a result of a dysfunction in the right cerebral hemisphere.

Although the right hemisphere dysfunction hypothesis and the interhemispheric communication deficit hypothesis are sometimes presented as competing neurobiological explanations for alexithymia (e.g. Dewaraja & Sasaki, 1990), it needs to be emphasized that there are still many unanswered questions concerning the unique and integrated roles of the two cerebral hemispheres in emotional processing. It is possible that evidence that has been used to support either hypothesis may result from the same underlying neurobiological factors. Thus, while alexithymia may be associated with right cerebral hemisphere dysfunction, it is unclear whether the emotional processes being affected are a direct result of a deficit in a particular part of the right hemisphere, or a result of subsequent factors. It is possible, for example, that right hemisphere dysfunction affects the normal communication between the two cerebral hemispheres, and that alexithymia is a consequence of a deficiency in interhemispheric communication and poor coordination of the functions performed by the two hemispheres. It is possible also that a dysfunction in the right hemisphere causes an over-activation of the left hemisphere, with a subsequent disruption in the normal process of interhemispheric communication and integration.

**Interhemispheric transfer deficits and alexithymia**

In their study of 12 patients who had undergone complete cerebral commissurotomies, Hoppe and Bogen (1977) found an impoverishment of dreams and fantasies, and difficulty in describing feelings, as well as a pronounced operative style of thinking – core features of the alexithymia construct. In a case study of a 37-year-old man with agenesis of the corpus callosum, Buchanan et al. (1980) reported a cluster of alexithymic features, similar to those described by Hoppe and Bogen (1977), including an inability to recall dreams despite a normal amount of REM activity. On the basis of his findings with split-brain patients, Hoppe (1977) postulated that alexithymia may involve an interruption of the normal flow of information between the two cerebral hemispheres; he referred to this as a 'functional commissurotomy'. A few years earlier, Galin (1974) had proposed that a similar inhibition of neuronal transmission across the corpus callosum and other cerebral commissures might be the neurophysiological mechanism for at least some instances of repression.

Support for the interhemispheric communication deficit hypothesis has come from experimental research with both split-brain patients and neurologically intact individuals. Using a complex method of content analysis to assess emotional expressiveness and the quality of fantasy and symbolization, TenHouten et al. (1986) compared the spoken and written responses of eight patients who had had cerebral commissurotomies (six complete and two partial) with those of eight neurologically intact control subjects to a film that was aimed at evoking emotions and fantasies by symbolically representing death and loss. The results showed that the commissurotomized patients were more alexithymic than the control subjects.

Zeitlin et al. (1989) tested the hypothesis that alexithymia reflects a functional disconnection between the left and right cerebral hemispheres in a group of neurologically intact adults. The efficiency of interhemispheric communication was assessed with a tactile finger localization task in 25 male combat veterans with posttraumatic stress disorder (PTSD) and 10 normal adult male control subjects.

Alexithymia was assessed with the TAS, and the pre-established upper and lower cutoff scores were used to compose groups of combat veterans with and without alexithymia. The investigators found that alexithymic PTSD subjects (N = 15) had a significant bidirectional deficit in the interhemispheric transfer of sensorimotor information when compared with non-alexithymic PTSD subjects (N = 7) and normal control subjects. Zeitlin and her colleagues also tested the hypothesis that alexithymia may be linked with either left or right hemisphere dysfunction. Using only alexithymic PTSD subjects, they compared left-hand with right-hand performance in the uncrossed conditions on the tactile finger localization task; this procedure allowed the processing speed of each hemisphere to be assessed. There was no significant difference in the processing speed of either hemisphere, leading the investigators to conclude from their overall results that 'the deficit in alexithymic individuals is specific to interhemispheric transfer and is not due to a dysfunction in either hemisphere' (p. 1437).

In an extension of the study with combat veterans, Dewaraja and Sasaki (1990) examined the relationship between interhemispheric transfer and alexithymia using both linguistic and non-linguistic symbolic stimuli. Alexithymic (N = 27) and non-alexithymic (N = 26) right-handed undergraduate students were given a series of lateralized visual matching tasks (using a tachistoscope) that involved presenting either linguistic or non-linguistic material. Although alexithymia was measured with the SSPS, which has certain psychometric limitations (see Chapter 3), Dewaraja and Sasaki used only subjects scoring at a very extreme range on the measure (the top 3% and the bottom 3% from a large undergraduate student sample). Differences in left- and right-hand reaction times were used to indicate speed of callosal transfer. Although the alexithymic and non-alexithymic groups did not differ in the speed of callosal transfer for linguistic information, there was a significant difference for non-linguistic information. Consistent with the results reported by Zeitlin et al. (1989), no difference was found in the processing speeds of the two hemispheres, thereby allowing the investigators to relate their findings to the callosal transfer process. Whereas Zeitlin et al. (1989) found a bidirectional relationship between alexithymia and the callosal transfer process, Dewaraja and Sasaki (1990) found a unidirectional (right to left) relationship. The significance of the right to left relationship for alexithymia is unclear at this time. A recent meta-analysis of 16 studies examining interhemispheric transfer time found that transfer from the right hemisphere to the left hemisphere is usually faster than transfer from the left hemisphere to the right hemisphere (Marzi, Bisiacchi & Nicoletti, 1991).

Though the results from the two studies with neurologically intact individuals support the interhemispheric deficit hypothesis, the use of combat veterans with PTSD in Zeitlin et al.'s (1989) study raises uncertainties concerning the generalizability of the findings to other populations, and the study by Dewaraja and Sasaki (1990) is limited by the use of the SSPS to measure alexithymia. Replication studies are needed using diverse populations and psychometrically sound measures of the alexithymia construct.

**Right hemisphere dysfunction and alexithymia**

As mentioned earlier, several researchers have noted that some of the salient features of the alexithymia construct can be observed in individuals with right hemisphere damage or lesions. Fricchione and Howanitz (1985), for example, reported motor aprosodia and a reduced ability to fantasize and describe feelings in an adult patient who had suffered damage to the right frontotemporal–parietal area. Voeller (1986), and Weintraub and Mesulam (1983), reported expressive aprosodias and alexithymic-like difficulties in the identification and communication of affects among children and adolescents with right cerebral hemisphere deficits. Indeed, the disturbance of affective communication observed in children, and reports of similar difficulties in other members of their families, has led to the suggestion that alexithymia might represent an inherited dystrophy of the right hemisphere analogous to the dyslexia associated with developmental abnormalities of the left hemisphere (Bear, 1983; Weintraub & Mesulam, 1983). Furthermore, as with alexithymia, right hemisphere developmental learning disabilities seem to create a range of interpersonal difficulties as well as a vulnerability for later disorders of affect regulation, including major depression and substance use disorders (Grace & Malloy, 1992; Rourke, Young & Leenaars, 1989).

In experimental research with neurologically intact subjects, alexithymia has been found to be associated with emotional processes linked predominantly to the right cerebral hemisphere. Several studies have found alexithymia to be related to poor performance on tasks that require subjects to interpret emotion-relevant information. For example, in a study with undergraduate students (Parker et al., 1993c), we found alexithymia to be associated with a diminished ability to recognize posed facial expressions of basic emotions as depicted in a set of photographs selected by Izard (1971). A similar finding was reported recently by Mann et al. (1994), who had adult volunteers label posed facial expressions of emotion. Lane et al. (1995) examined the relationship between alexithymia and four different emotion labelling tasks in a large community based sample. The different verbal and non-verbal tasks required subjects (a) to match emotion words with sentences depicting specific emotions that did not include emotion words, and with photographs of facial emotional expressions, and (b) to match facial expressions with sentences depicting emotions, and with photographs of scenes depicting an emotion without human faces. Alexithymia was found to be associated with decreased accuracy rates on all of the labelling tasks.

Cole and Bakan (1985) examined the hypothesis that alexithymia is associated with a right hemisphere dysfunction by using conjugate lateral eye movements (CLEMs) as an index of hemispheric activation. Individuals demonstrating a predominance of left CLEMs (left movers) during ongoing cognitive processing are assumed to rely more on the right cerebral hemisphere, while those showing a predominance of right CLEMs (right movers) are thought to rely more on their left hemisphere (Bakan, 1969; Gur, 1975). Reliance on a particular hemisphere implies that the other hemisphere is under-utilized (possibly because of a dysfunction). Although Cole and Bakan (1985) expected alexithymia to be positively associated with right CLEMs (indicating left cerebral lateralization), the opposite result was found in a sample of right-handed undergraduate students. However, the magnitude of the correlation between alexithymia and left CLEMs was low, which is especially problematic as alexithymia was assessed with the SSPS, a measure with questionable internal reliability.

In an effort to better understand the relationship between alexithymia and CLEMs, we conducted a similar experiment, also with right-handed undergraduate students, but used the TAS as well as the SSPS to measure alexithymia (Parker, Taylor & Bagby, 1992). A significant and higher magnitude positive relationship was found between the TAS and right CLEMs, but the association between the SSPS and CLEMs was not significant. Though these findings offered some support for the hypothesis that alexithymia is associated with right hemisphere dysfunction, there is controversy over the validity of CLEMs as an index of hemispheric activation. There is evidence, for example, that the direction of CLEMs can be influenced by the experimental situation (e.g. the distance between the subject and the examiner), and by the type of questions asked (verbal vs. spatial in nature); in addition, the relationship between CLEMs and hemispheric functioning may be moderated by gender and handedness (Dunn et al., 1989; Ehrlichman & Weinberger, 1978).

In another study examining the right hemisphere dysfunction hypothesis, Berenbaum and Prince (1994) used a free-vision chimeric face task to assess hemispatial bias in a sample of undergraduate students. The rationale for this measure of hemispatial bias is that 'the degree to which an individual's right hemisphere is more active than his or her left hemisphere will be associated with the degree to which attention is paid to the right and left halves of visual space, and hence to the likelihood of considering faces with smiles in the left half of visual space to be happier than faces with smiles in the right half of visual space' (p. 234). Consistent with the results of our CLEMs study, Berenbaum and Prince (1994) found that high levels of alexithymia were associated with diminished right hemisphere activity.

Overall, the findings from research exploring the neurobiology of alexithymia suggest that the trait is associated, at the very least, with a variation in brain organization. It remains unclear, however, whether this variation represents a dysfunction of the right hemisphere, an interhemispheric transfer deficit, an inhibition of the right hemisphere by a highly activated left hemisphere, or merely a preferred hemispheric mode. Before the neurobiology of alexithymia can be better understood, however, researchers must learn more about the mechanisms and means by which the hemispheres coordinate their activities and work as a unified entity (Banich, 1995). Given the increasing realization that emotional processing, imaginal activity, and other cognitive functions involve the participation of both hemispheres, it seems likely that future research will demonstrate that alexithymia reflects a deficiency in how the two hemispheres coordinate their respective operations.

# [6] Somatoform disorders

To demonstrate the clinical usefulness of conceptualizing certain medical and psychiatric illnesses as disorders of affect regulation, we begin with the extremely common but poorly understood problem of patients who seek medical care with persistent somatic symptoms and little or no identifiable disease. Such patients typically present initially to primary care physicians, and are believed to account for as many as 10% to 30% of all visits to family doctors (Kellner, 1990). They are often misunderstood and unnecessarily referred to multiple medical and surgical specialists, which leads to over-investigation and excessive costs to the health care system (Bacon *et al.*, 1994; Bass & Murphy, 1990; Shaw & Creed, 1991; Wickramasekera, 1989). Indeed, their use of inpatient and outpatient services is as much as nine times greater than that of the general population (Smith, Monson & Ray, 1986). When it becomes evident that no adequate medical diagnosis can be made for these patients, the persistent and puzzling somatic symptoms are usually attributed to *somatization* and described as 'functional' with the implication of an underlying psychiatric disorder.

Several studies have shown that many somatizing patients do in fact meet criteria for an anxiety disorder or a major depressive disorder (Bridges & Goldberg, 1985; Kirmayer & Robbins, 1991a); we will discuss this category of somatizing patients in Chapter 7. The present chapter will focus on those patients who are less easily diagnosed (Kaplan, Lipkin & Gordon, 1988; Robbins & Kirmayer, 1991) and who are sometimes pejoratively labeled 'chronic somatizers', 'hypochondriacs', 'medical care abusers', or 'medical crocks', especially when they fail to respond to standard medical and psychiatric treatments (Bass & Murphy, 1990). The therapeutic impasse leaves this group of patients dissatisfied with their medical care and prone to increasing impairment of social and occupational functioning as their symptoms become chronic. As Tyrer (1973) aptly observed, '[they] occupy the hinterland between psychiatry and medicine, seeking help from both specialties but finding haven in neither' (p. 915).

Historically, patients with medically unexplainable somatic symptoms were given diagnoses of hysteria, hypochondriasis, neurasthenia, or melancholia (Lipowski, 1988); nowadays, however, such patients are classified among one of the somatoform disorders unless they fulfil criteria for an anxiety or depressive disorder. The DSM-III-R (American Psychiatric Association, 1987) describes five somatoform disorders (body dysmorphic disorder, conversion disorder, somatization disorder, hypochondriasis, and somatoform pain disorder) and two residual categories (undifferentiated somatoform disorder, and somatoform disorder not otherwise specified) for patients who do not meet full criteria for any of the distinct disorders. The DSM-IV (American Psychiatric Association, 1994) has retained these categories but modified slightly the criteria for some of the disorders.

Although the DSM classification has stimulated much-needed research in the hazy borderland between psychiatry and medicine, several clinicians and researchers have noted that 'it does not entirely correspond to clinical realities' (Kirmayer, Robbins & Paris, 1994, p. 125). In particular, the DSM criteria may be too restrictive, the various disorders overlap in clinical practice, and patients with undifferentiated or not otherwise specified somatoform disorders are far more common than those with distinct disorders (Fink, 1993; Kirmayer et al., 1994; Lipowski, 1988). In addition, the requirement that the symptoms of the somatoform disorders have 'no demonstrable organic findings or known physiologic mechanisms' creates the impression that they occur 'as it were in a physiological vacuum' (Lipowski, 1987, p. 164), and has led also to confusion over the classification of functional physiological disorders, such as irritable bowel syndrome and fibromyalgia, which are thought to be influenced by emotional states (Kellner, 1991, 1994; Kirmayer & Robbins, 1991b).

Although there is some empirical support for classifying functional physiological disorders and some of the somatoform disorders as discrete entities (Kirmayer & Robbins, 1991b), we believe, as do Sensky (1994) and Kirmayer and Robbins (1991c), that attention should focus less on classification and phenomenology and more on trying to understand the pathological processes that underly functional somatic distress. We therefore will attempt to show how the concept of affect dysregulation, and the construct of alexithymia, can contribute to a better understanding of somatization that may aid in developing more effective treatments for many patients with somatoform disorders. Although the closely related functional physiological disorders also involve regulatory disturbances, we will discuss them in Chapter 10 along with several other medical illnesses and diseases. We are aware that the presence of a medical disease with structural tissue changes does not exclude the possibility of coexisting functional somatic symptoms.

## Background

Much of the difficulty in understanding the pathogenesis of the somatoform disorders can be traced to ambiguity of the term somatization, which has been used to denote a *process* as well as a symptom or disorder. The term somatization was coined by the Viennese psychoanalyst Wilhelm Stekel (1925) to refer to a process whereby a deep-seated neurosis could be expressed through a physical disorder. Stekel regarded somatization as equivalent to the concept of conversion, which was introduced by Breuer and Freud (1895) to explain the development of motor or sensory symptoms in hysteria. Like conversion, somatization represented a defense mechanism for keeping conflicts over drive-related wishes and associated dysphoric affects unconscious, yet at the same time permitting their partial expression and gratification through bodily symptoms.

As summarized by Barsky and Klerman (1983), somatization and hypochondriasis provided ways of deflecting sexual, aggressive, or oral drives as well as defenses against guilt or low self-esteem. Vaillant (1977) and Brown and Vaillant (1981), for example, emphasized the transformation of aggressive and hostile impulses into hypochondriacal complaints; these impulses were presumed to stem from past disappointments, but achieved partial expression through the patients' complaining and reproaching other people for their suffering. Other psychoanalytic theorists conceptualized somatic symptoms and hypochondriacal complaints as an expression of pregenital wishes for caring, nurturance, attention, sympathy, and physical contact. Somatic symptoms were also thought to defend a person against becoming aware of certain personality deficiencies, and to serve as atonement and punishment for past wrongdoings and a sense of inner badness. That is, like psychoneurotic symptoms, functional somatic symptoms were considered to have motivational as well as defensive functions, and to provide both primary and secondary gains.

In constructing these formulations of functional somatic symptoms, most psychoanalytic theorists adopted Freud's (1917) conception of the psychogenesis of hysterical conversion symptoms, and overlooked the important distinction he made in 1898 when he contrasted the *psychoneuroses* with the *actual neuroses* and proposed different etiological mechanisms. Whereas Freud (1895a, 1898) regarded the psychoneuroses (including hysteria) as originating in psychic conflict over unconscious impulses and fantasies from childhood, he believed that the actual neuroses were *somatic* in origin and therefore without primary psychological meaning. Freud (1914) classified anxiety neurosis and neurasthenia as actual neuroses and added hypochondriasis to the list more than a decade later.[1]

Although most contemporary theorists view somatization as a type of abnormal illness behaviour, rather than a type of unconscious defense, their attempts to redefine the construct have failed to transcend the mind–body interactionist view that medically unexplained somatic symptoms result from underlying *psychological* distress. Lipowski (1987), for example, who was perhaps the first to pursue this issue, defined somatization as 'a tendency to experience and communicate psychological distress in the form of physical symptoms, and to seek medical help for them' (p. 161). Similarly, Swartz *et al.* (1989) defined somatization as 'a bodily or somatic expression of psychic distress' (p. 44). Even the DSM-III-R description of the essential features of the somatoform disorders includes 'positive evidence, or a strong presumption, that the symptoms are linked to psychological factors or conflicts' (American Psychiatric Association, 1987, p. 255).

This presumption about mechanism or cause is not far from earlier psychogenic theories of somatization, and is promulgated further by Wickramasekera (1989), who defines somatizers as 'people who transduce *psychosocial conflicts* into somatic complaints and disorders such as chronic muscular and vascular headaches, irritable bowel, and chronic low back pain' (p. 105, our italics). Such misconceptions are found also in a book by the medical historian Shorter (1992) who, as was noted in a review of the book (Taylor, 1993a), ignores the important distinction between the mechanisms of conversion and somatization.

British psychiatry also has, in general, not fully disavowed earlier psychoanalytic conceptions, as evidenced in the work of Bridges and Goldberg (1985) who view somatization as 'a common and important *psychological* mechanism' (p. 653, our italics); in their operational definition of somatization, these researchers require evidence of a psychiatric disorder as well as the presentation of somatic complaints.

---

1. Freud's (1895a) description of actual anxiety neurosis corresponds partly to the DSM-III-R and DSM-IV diagnosis of panic disorder, which is discussed in Chapter 7. Although neurasthenia is classified among the neuroses in the 10th revision of the *International classification of diseases* (World Health Organization, 1992), as it was also in DSM-II, it was viewed as a mood disorder (dysthymia) in DSM-III and DSM-III-R, and is classified as an undifferentiated somatoform disorder in DSM-IV.

As another British psychiatrist correctly notes, such definitions fail to include 'the large number of patients who present in primary care with medically unexplained somatic symptoms which are not accompanied by an overt psychological symptom' (Mayou, 1993, p. 70). Moreover, there is evidence that many somatizing patients are not only without concurrent anxiety or depression, but also have a lifetime history free from anxiety and depressive disorders (Kirmayer & Robbins, 1991a).

Recognizing the inappropriate theoretical implications of most definitions of somatization, some researchers recommend avoiding any use of the term, or choosing a definition that encompasses only the presence of one or more somatic complaints without demonstrable organic disease or in excess of what one would expect on the grounds of objective medical findings (Kellner, 1990; Mayou, 1993). Lipowski (1988) also modified his definition of somatization after realizing that 'somatizers actually experience and communicate primarily somatic, not psychological, distress and that this feature characterizes them' (p. 1359).

Thus, in their efforts to formulate an atheoretical and purely descriptive definition of somatization, contemporary theorists have inadvertently resurrected Freud's concept of the actual neuroses in which somatic symptoms are not given a psychological origin. Though Freud (1898) was incorrect in attributing the actual neuroses to an excessive accumulation or marked depletion of libido (resulting respectively in anxiety neurosis and neurasthenia), or to a shift of libido from objects in the external world to a bodily organ (as in hypochondriasis), implicit in his theory, as Grotstein (1986) first pointed out, is the concept of *disorders of self-regulation*. The simplistic idea that poorly regulated libido causes symptoms has long been abandoned, but the concept of unregulated affect offers a new perspective on somatization that was glimpsed by MacAlpine (1952) over four decades ago when she described somatization as a variant of the actual neuroses that could be attributed to rudimentary and partly expressed emotions.

**Somatization and deficits in the cognitive processing of emotions**

The concept of actual neurosis and Lipowski's (1988) revised definition of somatization shift attention to the much-neglected physiological basis of functional somatic symptoms and to the often-forgotten fact that emotions are primarily biological events, subjective feelings being a secondarily developed component, as we outlined in earlier chapters.

It is part of normal experience, therefore, for individuals to perceive somatic sensations that accompany states of emotional arousal, and also to experience brief episodes of bodily discomfort associated with normal physiological functioning (e.g., borborygmi produced by intestinal peristalsis, and aches and pains from increased muscle tension). While most people give little attention to these bodily experiences, some individuals become preoccupied with the sensations, misinterpret them as symptoms of disease, and continually seek medical care despite reassurance that no serious medical disease exists (Barsky & Klerman, 1983). Tyrer (1973) proposed an explanation for these differences, which is based on a modified version of the James–Lange theory of emotion:

> In normal emotion the subject recognizes the provoking stimulus, usually an external one, which gives rise to the emotion. He experiences the somatic feelings of physiological arousal, but as he has already detected the source of arousal he regards these as secondary phenomena. In morbid emotion the subject may or may not recognize the provoking stimulus. He is particularly prone to ignorance if the stimulus is an internal psychic one. If he fails to recognize it, the bodily feelings that he experiences are not understood. He is therefore likely to look upon these as primary phenomena and deny the psychic aspects of his condition. Further exposure to the stimulus tends to reinforce the initial interpretation of the feelings experienced (p. 916).

This proposal reflects a cognitive (information) processing model of emotion, and obviously borders on the alexithymia construct and Krystal's (1990) observation that alexithymic individuals fail to use emotions as signals in information processing, but instead may focus on the physiological sensations as entities in themselves. Although later we will elaborate and slightly modify Tyrer's formulation, he clearly links functional somatic symptoms to the activating aspects of emotions and to deficits in the cognitive processing of emotions.

Kellner (1985, 1987, 1990) also attributes the majority of functional somatic symptoms to the physiological changes that accompany emotions. He emphasizes that the symptoms are not conversions or replacements for emotions, and may even reinforce emotions; for example, somatic symptoms that induce anxiety may lead to more somatic symptoms as a consequence of autonomic arousal (Kellner, 1986). We concur fully with Kellner's (1985, 1990) view that conversion disorders are different phenomena, and believe that they are still best understood within the traditional psychoanalytic framework for conceptualizing psychoneurotic symptom formation. Some patients present with a combination of conversion and somatization symptoms, just as Freud (1898) described patients with admixtures of psychoneurotic and actual neurotic symptoms.

Kellner (1985, 1987) and Sharpe and Bass (1992) are among the few theorists and researchers who have highlighted some of the physiological mechanisms associated with emotional arousal (especially anxiety states) that may produce somatic sensations or symptoms in the absence of medical disease. These include increased activity of the sympathetic nervous system (resulting in tachycardia, sweating, smooth muscle contractions), increased tension in voluntary muscle (producing tension headaches, local muscle pain, and fatigue) and hyperventilation (resulting in hypocapnia, hyperirritability of peripheral nerves associated with alkalosis, and chest pain from spasm of intercostal muscles). Indeed, based on observations of patients attending his general medical practice, Zalidis (1994) has compiled an extensive list of somatic symptoms resulting from hyperventilation, which he has come to view as 'one of the commonest causes of functional symptoms' (p. 1). Zalidis conceptualizes the hyperventilation syndrome as a consequence of a maladaptive way of handling affects, and reports examples of patients who responded favourably to a treatment approach that combines behavioural and psychotherapeutic interventions aimed at elevating emotions from a primitive sensorimotor level of experience to a verbal representational level.

Consistent with the theoretical link between alexithymia and somatization, several studies have yielded preliminary evidence that alexithymic individuals show higher tonic levels of sympathetic arousal than non-alexithymic individuals, and a decoupling of the autonomic and cognitive responses to stressors (Martin & Pihl, 1986; Papciak, Feuerstein & Spiegel, 1985; Rabavilas, 1987). There is some evidence also that facial affective expression is correlated inversely with the level of physiological activation in response to stressors (Notarius & Levenson, 1979; Traue et al., 1985). Conversely, verbal communication of affective distress (which is limited in alexithymic individuals) reduces autonomic arousal and appears to protect against somatic symptom formation (Anderson, 1981; Berry & Pennebaker, 1993; Pennebaker, 1985; Pennebaker & Susman, 1988).

### Somatization and dimensions of personality

One necessary refinement to Tyrer's (1973) modified version of the James–Lange theory of emotion is removal of the implication that people can be categorized into those who somatize and those who do not. Recognizing that there is wide individual variation in the experiencing and reporting of functional somatic symptoms, several researchers have recommended conceptualizing somatization as a dimensional construct, with the relatively rare DSM-III-R somatization disorder (also referred to as Briquet's syndrome) at one extreme, and the majority of somatizing patients who present to primary care physicians manifesting a subsyndromal form with fewer symptoms (Escobar *et al.*, 1991; Katon *et al.*, 1991; Kirmayer *et al.*, 1994; Swartz *et al.*, 1991). Milder and transient forms of somatization would also fall on this spectrum and are often simply a type of adjustment reaction shown by some people to stressful situations (Katon *et al.*, 1991). Kirmayer *et al.* (1994) propose three distinct dimensional constructs of somatization that reflect their finding that somatizing patients can be categorized into a 'functional' subgroup (the tendency to experience and report functional symptoms), a 'hypochondriacal' subgroup (the tendency to worry or be convinced that one is sick), or a 'presenting' subgroup (individuals with anxiety or depressive disorders who present clinically with predominantly somatic symptoms).

Given these dispositional tendencies and the chronic and enduring nature of the somatoform disorders, several researchers have suggested that somatization and hypochondriasis should be viewed as personality traits; some even propose reclassifying the somatoform disorders as personality disorders (Bass & Murphy, 1995; Escobar, 1987; Pennebaker & Watson, 1991). Tyrer and colleagues (1990), for example, recently made a case for regarding hypochondriacal personality disorder as a diagnosis in its own right in addition to retaining hypochondriasis as an Axis I psychiatric mental state diagnosis.

Such proposals raise questions concerning the relationships that hypochondriasis and somatization might have with other dimensional constructs and personality traits, including the alexithymia construct. Most of the research to date has centred on neuroticism (N) or the closely-related construct negative affectivity (NA) which, as outlined in Chapter 4, reflect the tendency to experience both emotional and somatic distress (Costa & McCrae, 1992; Eysenck & Eysenck, 1975; Watson & Clark, 1984). Measures of N and NA have been found to correlate highly with measures of somatic symptom reporting (Costa & McCrae, 1987*b*), even in studies in which high and low NA individuals did not differ on objective markers of health (Pennebaker & Watson, 1991). As Kirmayer *et al.* (1994) suggest, this may be because neurotic individuals experience more physical sensations as a result of their autonomic lability (Eysenck, 1963; Eysenck & Eysenck, 1985) and also because they focus more attention on their bodies.

Given that imagination and receptiveness to inner feelings likely influence the meanings that individuals ascribe to somatic sensations, one would expect the broad Openness to Experience (O) dimension of personality and the narrower absorption trait (which is related to hypnotic susceptibility) also to be related to somatization. To date, empirical findings are limited and inconsistent. Whereas McCrae (1991) found a negative correlation between O and the Somatization Scale of the Millon Clinical Multi-Axial Inventory, Watson (1991) and Vassend (1987) found positive correlations between absorption and measures of somatic complaints. Wickramasekera (1986, 1995), however, has found that both high and low hypnotizability may contribute to somatic distress; interestingly, somatizing patients with low hypnotic ability were found to complain the least of psychological symptoms. Certainly 'inner-directness', which is the converse of an externally orientated cognitive style (Loiselle & Dawson, 1988), is associated negatively with self-reported somatic symptoms (Vassend, 1987).

As outlined in Chapter 4, alexithymia is related positively to N and NA, and negatively to O. Several studies that used dimensional measures have shown that alexithymia is associated positively also with somatization. In samples of university students, for example, low, but significant, positive correlations were found between the TAS and several different measures of functional somatic complaints including the hypochondriasis subscale of the Basic Personality Inventory, the SUNYA revision of the Psychosomatic Symptom Checklist, the somatization subscale of the SCL-90R, the Pennebaker Inventory of Limbic Languidness (a checklist of 54 common physical symptoms and bodily sensations), and the somatic complaints subscale of the Cornell Index (Bagby et al., 1988a,b; Bagby et al., 1986b; Parker et al., 1989a). Similar or slightly higher magnitude correlations have been obtained between the TAS-20 and several of these measures of somatic complaints in university student samples, although it is important to note that the measures do not distinguish between functional symptoms and symptoms from actual disease.

A positive association between alexithymia and somatization was demonstrated also in a community sample of 2243 middle-aged Finnish men who completed a translated version of the TAS and the hypochondriasis scale of the MMPI (Kauhanen, Julkunen & Salonen, 1991). A slightly larger sample of the men also completed a frequency checklist of symptoms, which included 26 common complaints. The alexithymia score, adjusted for age, smoking, and socioeconomic status, was associated positively with the MMPI hypochondriasis scale and also showed a graded and statistically significant relationship with recent (12-month) symptoms. Indeed, in a stepwise multiple regression analysis, the TAS was found to be a stronger predictor of recent symptoms than either age or smoking. Men in the upper quartile of

TAS scores (N = 451) also reported worse perceived level of health than men in the lower quartile of TAS scores (N = 508). Collectively, the results of studies examining the relationships between somatization and other personality constructs indicate that the tendency to develop medically unexplained somatic symptoms is associated with a proneness to, and limited ability to, modulate negative affects. Such findings refute the early psychoanalytic view of somatization as a defense against distressing affects, but are consistent with our proposal that the somatoform disorders (with the exception of conversion disorder) be reconceptualized as disorders of affect regulation.[1]

Several researchers have used the findings of a positive association between somatization and NA to challenge the view that many somatizing individuals are alexithymic. Simon and VonKorff (1991), for example, rejected the concept of alexithymia after analyzing data from the NIMH Epidemiologic Catchment Area (ECA) Study which showed that an increasing number of functional somatic symptoms was associated with reported psychological distress (especially sadness, depression, fear, or anxiety). Oxman et al. (1985) also rejected the concept of alexithymia after demonstrating through speech content analysis a similar high level of reported emotional distress in patients with somatization disorder and patients with major depression. However, these and many other investigators mistakenly have taken the term alexithymia literally, as meaning 'no words for feelings', and misconstrued the construct as a defense against distressing affects, as though it were equivalent to earlier notions of somatization.

As we outlined in earlier chapters, alexithymia is conceptualized primarily as a deficit and not as a defense, and does not imply an absence of affect or an inability to report any emotional distress. Indeed, the definition of the construct emphasizes *difficulty* (not inability) in identifying and describing feelings (Taylor et al., 1991). This cognitive difficulty might have been detected in the ECA and speech content analysis studies if the investigators had measured the range of affective vocabulary in their subjects, as well as the subjects' abilities to elaborate spontaneously used words (such as sad, anxious, and depressed) and to link reported emotions to internal or external events. As Nemiah and colleagues (1976) described, 'many alexithymic individuals will spontaneously use words such as "sad", "nervous" and

---

1. Although distressing affects may underly conversion symptoms, these are associated with unconscious drive-related conflicts and fantasies, which are defended against and represented symbolically through the somatic symptoms.

"frightened"; it is necessary to ask them specifically to state what it "feels like" to be sad or angry or nervous; only then will it become apparent that they have little or no vocabulary available to describe these affects' (p. 431).

Although Kirmayer and Robbins (1991c) have made substantial contributions to the understanding of somatization, they too partly misrepresent the alexithymia construct by claiming that 'Some accounts of alexithymia . . . imply that if strong emotions cannot be symbolically transformed and given verbal expression, they are "discharged" along autonomic pathways, causing physiological disorders' (p. 4). This assertion presumably stems from speculations in an early paper by MacLean (1949), which reflect the outmoded view that affects are derived from drives and the economic notion that affects accumulate and need to be discharged (Karush, 1989). Emotions are certainly not 'discharged' along autonomic pathways; nor are they 'transformed' by symbolic mental representations and verbal expression. Heightened autonomic activity is a normal correlate of emotional arousal that may contribute to functional somatic symptoms, as outlined earlier, or produce conditions conducive to the development of somatic disease if the activity is prolonged and not adequately regulated (see Chapter 10). The mental representation of emotions aids in modulating the intensity and duration of distressing emotional states by allowing individuals to evaluate and reflect on their emotional responses to both internal and external stimuli, and also intentionally to communicate emotions verbally to others who may provide additional aid in regulating stress (Dodge & Garber, 1991). Indeed, there is evidence that patients with hypochondriasis tend not to confide in others about distressing personal experiences, thereby reducing the opportunity for interactional regulation of affect (Barsky et al., 1994).

These ideas are evident in modern psychoanalytic theories which now emphasize the signal, integrative, and communicative functions of affects as well as the cognitive mechanisms involved in their regulation and modulation (Basch, 1976; Krystal, 1988; Lichtenberg, 1983; Spezzano, 1993). These functions and mechanisms appear to be deficient in alexithymic individuals leaving them vulnerable to states of affect dysregulation that may produce psychological distress as well as somatic distress; the former may be reported verbally, though with a limited emotional vocabulary. The externally orientated cognitive style of alexithymic individuals, in contrast to the inner-directed or introspective style of non-alexithymic individuals, leads to further somatic distress and dysregulation as attention is focused on the puzzling somatic sensations, which may be amplified and/or misinterpreted, thereby triggering further anxiety and hypochondriacal concerns. A vicious circle may develop (Kellner, 1990).

This tendency to amplify and misinterpret bodily sensations is captured also in the concept of *somatosensory amplification*, which was introduced by Barsky (1992) and Barsky and Klerman (1983) as a possible factor in the pathogenesis of somatization and hypochondriasis. To explore this concept, Barsky et al. (1988; Barsky & Wyshak, 1990; Barsky, Wyshak & Klerman, 1990) developed a self-report Somatosensory Amplification Scale (SSAS) which demonstrated adequate psychometric properties and correlated positively with measures of both general dysphoria and functional somatic symptoms. Wise and Mann (1994) recently examined the relationship between alexithymia and somatosensory amplification by administering the TAS and SSAS to a group of psychiatric outpatients, most of whom manifested an anxious or depressed mood. Although partial correlations controlling for depression revealed a significant relationship between the two constructs, when examined by gender the partial correlation remained significant only for females. However, previous research has shown that amplification is stronger in women than in men (Barsky & Wyshak, 1990), and that women are more prone to somatization (Cloninger et al., 1986). Although further research is needed to evaluate the validity of the amplification construct, findings from experimental studies strongly suggest that somatic amplification is due to expectancy and selective attention to bodily sensations (Farthing, Venturino & Brown, 1984; Pauli et al., 1993; Schmidt et al., 1994). There are also very preliminary findings from studies of brain function, which suggest that patients with somatization disorder have more difficulty than normal subjects in dividing their attention efficiently between relevant and irrelevant sensory input (James et al., 1987).

## Clinical illustrations

The following vignettes illustrate some of the clinical manifestations of somatizing patients that were described in the preceding sections, as well as the dimensional nature of the somatization construct and its association with alexithymia.

### Case 1

Peter had suffered from multiple somatic symptoms for 8 years. Initially, at age 31, he experienced pain in the epigastric region; this had spread gradually to other parts of his abdomen and later was accompanied by unpleasant sensations throughout his entire body. On one occasion, he had developed melaena and a duodenal ulcer was identified and treated. When his abdominal pains continued, he was given a diagnosis of irritable bowel syndrome. In addition to abdominal symptoms, Peter complained of dizziness, aching eyes, ringing in his ears, and a constant feeling of pressure in his head. Affected by unpleasant and widespread bodily symptoms every day, Peter had developed a hypochondriacal preoccupation with the idea that he had a more serious physical illness. He had consulted many physicians and surgeons and undergone numerous investigations, but eventually was told that his problem was 'psychological' and that he should seek psychiatric treatment.

In a psychiatric interview, Peter manifested a rather wooden, largely expressionless face, had difficulty identifying and elaborating his feelings, and indicated that he rarely fantasized and had no recall of dreams. When asked about upsetting life events, he acknowledged feeling depressed and having difficulty sleeping over the past year following his wife's death from cancer. He emphasized, however, that his somatic symptoms predated the onset of his wife's illness by several years. In response to further questions about his mood, Peter merely indicated that he liked listening to loud music.

Although this patient did not meet full DSM-III-R or DSM-IV criteria for a diagnosis of somatization disorder, the pattern and chronic nature of his symptoms, and his high use of medical services, indicated a subsyndromal form of the disorder. Consistent with an absence of vegetative symptoms other than a sleep disturbance, he showed only a mild to moderate level of depression on the Beck Depression Inventory (BDI). On the TAS-20, however, he obtained a score of 80, which confirmed the clinical impression of marked alexithymia.

## Case 2

Nick, a 28-year-old musician, sought psychiatric treatment for three major symptoms: obsessional doubting of his competency as a musician, a preoccupation with his physical appearance, and a preoccupation with the fear of having a serious disease. For several years he had struggled with intrusive and persistent thoughts that there was something wrong with the sound of his cello playing; he often spent several hours daily evaluating and re-evaluating tape-recordings of his playing, wondering whether he was truly perceiving a serious defect or merely imagining one. In addition, Nick was excessively concerned with his facial appearance; he constantly checked himself in the mirror, compared himself with other men, and concluded that he was physically unattractive and therefore unappealing to women. Nick's third complaint was a preoccupation with bodily sensations and physical symptoms, and a concern that he must have a serious disease that his physicians had not yet detected. Prior to developing obsessional doubts about his cello playing, he had been preoccupied with a fear that he had multiple sclerosis. Over a period of 2 or 3 years, Nick had complained of weakness in his arms and fingers, consulted numerous neurologists and other physicians, and undergone many medical investigations. Despite negative findings, he could not be reassured that he did not have a neurological disease. His symptoms of muscle weakness and preoccupation with multiple sclerosis eventually were replaced by several other bodily symptoms including nausea, abdominal or pelvic pain, chronic headaches, chest pain, and frequency of urination. He invariably responded to these symptoms with the fear that he had cancer or heart disease, and immediately sought medical attention from his family physician or by going to the emergency department of a local hospital. On several occasions these visits led to additional and sometimes extensive medical investigations; despite repeated negative findings, Nick could not be reassured.

This patient's obsessional, hypochondriacal, and functional somatic sympto-matology reflects the not uncommon overlap among anxiety and somatoform disorders. Nick met DSM-IV diagnostic criteria for somatization disorder, obsessive–compulsive disorder, body dysmorphic disorder (dysmorphophobia), and hypochondriasis. His physicians also made a diagnosis of irritable bowel syndrome. Although the onset of these disorders occurred soon after his mother's death from heart disease, Nick recalled being somewhat hypo-chondriacal even during childhood and adolescence, and how he had regularly sought reassurance from his mother who was a physician.

In psychiatric interviews, Nick was able to report some psychological distress, especially of an acute and intense type, which he experienced when he thought music he had just played 'sounded bad' or when a woman he admired showed no special interest in him. However, much of this distress was expressed behaviourally by pounding his head with his fists or precipitating arguments with his father or friends. Certain everyday experiences, such as brief separations or minor criticisms, were often followed by the recurrence of a somatic symptom and the seeking of medical attention. Nick also showed a striking lack of an inner fantasy life, an inability to recall dreams, and a marked tendency to become preoccupied with communi-cating the details of physical symptoms or obsessional concerns. It became evident that he focused attention on the somatic accompaniments of emotional states, which were then amplified and misinterpreted as signs of disease. Consistent with these clinical observations, Nick scored in the alexithymic range on the TAS-20, and in the very high range on a measure of neuroticism; he showed a moderate degree of depression on the BDI. Treatment with selective serotonin reuptake inhibitor drugs reduced only partially his obsessional and somatic symptoms and concerns, but there was progressive improvement when these were combined with modified psychotherapeutic interventions, which are described in Chapter 11.

## Empirical studies of alexithymia and somatization

One of the earliest empirical studies of alexithymia and somatization in a clinical population was conducted by Shipko (1982), who administered the Schalling–Sifneos Personality Scale (SSPS) to a group of 12 somatizing patients (4 of whom had a concurrent classical psychosomatic disease) and a control group of 27 healthy subjects, as well as to a group of 15 subjects who had a history of one or more of the seven classical psychosomatic diseases. Whereas the mean SSPS scores of the control group and the psychosomatic disease group did not significantly differ, the somatizing patient group was significantly more alexithymic than both other groups. Although these findings provided some preliminary support for an association between alexithymia and somatization, the study was limited by the poor psychometric properties of the SSPS (see Chapter 3), by a failure to match the three subject groups on sociodemographic variables, and by a possible sample selection bias.

Extending our own research with the TAS to a clinical population, we investigated the relationship between alexithymia and somatic complaints in an ethnically heterogeneous group of 118 patients referred to the psychiatric outpatient department of a large metropolitan general hospital in Honolulu, Hawaii (Taylor et al., 1992b). The majority of patients suffered from anxiety, depressive, or adjustment disorders; no patient received a diagnosis of somatoform disorder. Almost 40% of the group scored in the alexithymic range on the TAS. Compared with the non-alexithymic patients, the alexithymic patients manifested significantly more somatic complaints, as measured by the following MMPI scales – the Hypochondriasis Scale, the Somatic Complaints Harris Subscale, the Physical-Somatic Concerns Subscale, the Poor Health Scale, and the Organic Symptoms and Poor Health Wiggins Content Scales. These MMPI scales collectively measure a diverse and extensive range of somatic symptoms and bodily concerns (Graham, 1987). In addition, the alexithymic patients had significantly higher levels of anxiety, depression, and general psychological turmoil. Consistent with the construct, the alexithymic patients also had significantly less ego strength than the non-alexithymic patients, and were more dependent and more likely to engage in impulsive and acting out behaviours.

Although the cross-sectional design of this study prevents any determination of whether alexithymia is an actual cause of somatic complaints or a consequence of more extreme levels of anxiety, depression, or other psychopathology, the overall pattern of results is consistent with the view that alexithymic individuals are prone to both functional somatic symptoms and symptoms of emotional turmoil because they lack the necessary psychological capacities for modulating emotions. Similar findings were obtained in an earlier study in which newly abstinent male substance abusers with alexithymia had significantly less ego strength than their non-alexithymic counterparts, and significantly higher levels of somatic complaints and general dysphoria (Taylor, Parker & Bagby, 1990b).

Surprisingly, in a recent study of 45 psychiatric inpatients in Austria, Bach et al. (1994) found that alexithymic patients and non-alexithymic patients did not significantly differ in scores on the somatization subscale of the SCL-90R nor in their current or lifetime history of somatoform disorders. However, all of the patients in this study met criteria for an anxiety disorder and, consistent with the construct, the alexithymic patients showed higher levels of psychological turmoil and overall psychopathology. Furthermore, in a subsequent follow-up study of 30 of the patients, alexithymia was found to be a significant predictor of persistent somatization and poor treatment outcome, independent of other types of psychopathology, severity of illness, and sociodemographic variables (Bach & Bach, 1995).

It is possible also that a relationship between alexithymia and somatization may be demonstrated more strongly in clinical populations by avoiding the somatoform diagnostic categories and alexithymia cutoff scores and instead viewing both somatization and alexithymia as dimensional constructs, as was done in the studies with university student and community samples that were reviewed earlier. Indeed, in a separate study with psychiatric inpatients, Bach et al. (1996) obtained a statistically significant positive correlation between the TAS-20 and the somatization subscale of the SCL-90R. In another recent clinical study, Cohen et al. (1994) found no significant differences in alexithymia scores among groups of somatizing patients, psychiatric patients, and dental patients; however, in a multiple regression analysis, alexithymia (as measured by the TAS) was significantly predicted by several measures of the tendency to experience and report somatic symptoms.

## Somatization and chronic pain

Pain for which no adequate organic cause has been found is one of the commonest symptoms of somatizing patients. When pain is the predominant focus of the clinical presentation and has been present for at least six months, a diagnosis of somatoform pain disorder is usually made. This DSM-III-R category of somatoform disorder replaced the diagnosis of 'psychogenic pain disorder' in DSM-III, which required evidence that psychological factors played an etiological role.[1] Indeed, for many years, the conceptualization of medically unexplained chronic pain was influenced by Engel's (1959) view that pain-prone patients struggle with unconscious guilt and conflicts over intense

1. To encompass acute as well as chronic pain, DSM-IV has replaced somatoform pain disorder with the new diagnostic category of 'pain disorder' with four subtypes and a role for psychological factors in the onset, severity, exacerbation, or maintenance of the pain.

aggressive and forbidden sexual impulses. Engel attributed these conflicts to deficiencies in the childhood home including an ill parent and the trauma of emotional, verbal, or physical abuse. Though the presence or absence of conflicts was not evaluated, subsequent research yielded some empirical support for an association between psychogenic pain disorder and a history of traumatic childhood experiences (Adler et al., 1989).

Although clinical experience confirms that intrapsychic conflicts may lead to chronic pain through the mechanism of conversion (i.e. psychogenic pain), pain might also be a direct manifestation of unregulated emotion and thus a symptom of somatization. Many studies have shown a high incidence of anxiety and depression, as well as somatization symptoms, in chronic pain populations (Bacon et al., 1994; Iezzi et al., 1994), but there is considerable controversy as to whether the affective component is a consequence of the impact of chronic pain on a person's mood or a predisposing factor in the development of chronic pain (Gaskin et al., 1992; Turk & Salovey, 1984). For example, Blumer and Heilbronn (1982) regard chronic pain as a specific variant of depressive illness and recommend treatment with antidepressant drugs. Other researchers, however, note that many chronic pain patients do not respond to antidepressant drugs (Merskey, 1982; Roy, Thomas, & Matas, 1984), and that when depression is present it has more likely occurred after the onset of pain (Bacon et al., 1994).

A possible solution to the controversy is found in Swanson's (1984) hypothesis that chronic pain is a third pathologic emotion that is separate from, but interfaces closely with, anxiety and depression. Recognizing that modern pain theorists view pain as an abnormal affective state and not as a primary perceptual experience, Swanson suggests that chronic pain, like anxiety and depressive states, has its own neurochemical correlates in the integrative centers of the brain. Extending Swanson's hypothesis, we would argue that acute pain can be viewed as a signal affect serving a protective function that is comparable to the functions of signal anxiety and signal depression, which will be described in the next chapter.

Whether chronic pain be viewed as a third pathologic emotion, as a variant of depression, or as a cause of negative affective states, we believe it qualifies for inclusion in our general category of disorders of affect regulation. Circular feedback systems are involved, with anxiety and depression provoking pain by increasing pain sensitivity and by lowering pain tolerance thresholds, and pain serving as a stressor that evokes anxiety and depression (Beutler et al., 1986; Gaskin et al., 1992). This dysregulation may be suspected when the patient is alexithymic and anhedonic which, in the experience of some clinicians (e.g.

Blumer & Heilbronn, 1982), can be observed commonly among chronic pain patients.

### Clinical example

Richard, a junior accountant, was referred for psychiatric consultation after extensive medical investigations failed to find an organic basis for his complaint of 'pain in the head'. The patient reported that he had experienced this pain every day for 15 years and that it was aggravated by shaving, combing his hair, taking a shower, or other ordinary daily activities. Apart from this pain and an attack of migraine headache approximately once a year, Richard claimed to be in good physical health. He was reluctant to take any medication for his symptom.

In response to questioning, Richard denied being depressed, but admitted to a mild feeling of sadness which he believed was a result of the chronic discomfort in his head. At the time of onset of his head pain, he was achieving in high school and had imagined himself doing something 'great' in his life; the development of his chronic symptom, however, had prevented the fulfilment of this wish. Richard stated that he thought he might have brain damage because of a cold sensation he experienced in his nose when breathing.

The patient manifested considerable difficulty identifying and describing his feelings. He was aware of dreaming, but was unable to recall any dream content other than a vague memory of other people being in his dreams. Although he had a strong desire to have a girlfriend, and claimed to become aroused when he had sexual fantasies, Richard reported that he had never masturbated and that his sexual fantasies were not accompanied by penile erections. This suggested a decoupling of cognitive and imaginal processes from peripheral physiological activity similar to the decoupling that has been reported in experimental studies of alexithymia (Martin & Pihl, 1986; Papciak et al., 1985).

Consistent with the clinical impression that he was alexithymic and only mildly depressed, Richard scored in the alexithymic range on the TAS-20 and obtained a score of only 10 on the BDI.

### Empirical studies of alexithymia and chronic pain

Findings from early investigations of the relationship between alexithymia and chronic pain are of questionable validity because of the measures used as well as a failure to adequately define the criteria for diagnosing the patient samples, which are well known for being heterogeneous. For example, Mendelson (1982) and Papciak et al. (1986/87) reported relatively high rates of alexithymia among chronic pain patients but measured alexithymia with the MMPI-A, a scale that lacks reliability and validity.

Postone (1986) used the interviewer-rated BIQ as well as the MMPI-A to compare the rates of alexithymia among 18 inpatients with chronic pain, 9 of their spouses who were in good health, and 19 outpatients who were being treated with psychotherapy and who did not have physical symptoms. Both alexithymia measures showed the pain patients to be significantly more alexithymic than the psychoneurotic control subjects, but not more alexithymic than their healthy spouses. Based on the criterion score of 6 on the BIQ, alexithymia was identified in 33% of the pain group, 50% of the spouse group, and 16% of the psychotherapy group.

Other researchers used the $SAT_9$ to assess alexithymia in a sample of 30 chronic pain patients and reported evidence of an impaired capacity for fantasy and symbolic activity in all of the patients (Catchlove et al., 1985). Despite the limitations of the $SAT_9$ as a measure of alexithymia, most of the pain patients also scored in the alexithymic range on the BIQ which, as noted in Chapter 3, correlated significantly with the $SAT_9$ (Demers-Desrosiers et al., 1983).

Following the introduction of the TAS, Sriram et al. (1987a) validated an Indian dialect (Kannada) translation, which they used together with the BIQ to assess 30 patients fulfilling DSM-III criteria for psychogenic pain disorder who were attending a psychiatric outpatient clinic. The patients were not dependent on alcohol or drugs, and their pain symptoms were of at least six months duration. Alexithymia was assessed also in a sociodemographically matched control group of 30 healthy individuals who were recruited from the hospital staff and friends and relatives of patients. The TAS and BIQ correlated significantly, and the pain patients scored significantly higher than the control subjects on both alexithymia measures. Alexithymia was identified in 27.1% of the pain patients compared with 9.5% of the control subjects.

In contrast, in a study conducted in New Zealand, James and Large (1991) found no difference between a group of chronic pain patients and a group of normal control subjects on the TAS nor on the BIQ and $SAT_9$. One wonders, however, whether these negative results were influenced by a sample selection bias and by the investigators lack of experience in using the alexithymia measures. From a random selection of patients attending the outpatient pain clinic, only one-third agreed to participate in the study and 38.8% of this group were not experiencing pain at the time of the study. Furthermore, despite the significant correlation between the TAS and BIQ in the Indian study (and in several other studies; see Chapter 3), these two measures failed to correlate significantly in the New Zealand study; the $SAT_9$ also failed to correlate with the BIQ. Although James and Large (1991) obtained adequate inter-rater reliability for the $SAT_9$, ratings of the BIQ appear to have been made by only one investigator as inter-rater reliability for this measure was not reported.

In another study, Millard and Kinsler (1992) investigated a group of 195 patients with chronic non-malignant pain who were consecutive referrals to an outpatient pain centre in the United States. Although the patients were not required to meet DSM-III-R criteria for a diagnosis of somatoform pain disorder, they had all suffered from pain for at least 4 months, the mean duration being 60 months; back pain, headache, or pain in the limbs were the most frequent primary complaints. More than one-third of the patients were receiving a financial compensation package in association with their pain complaint. The mean TAS scores of men and women were not significantly different, and were independent of age, education, and financial compensation status. Based on the TAS cutoff score, 34.4% of the pain patients were categorized as alexithymic. Alexithymia scores were associated with affective distress, but were unrelated to pain intensity and to global reports of functional disability.

Similar findings were reported by Zayfert, McCracken and Gross (1992) in a study of 142 patients with chronic non-malignant pain who were consecutive referrals to a multidisciplinary pain clinic located also in the United States. The majority of patients complained of back pain; the remainder complained of pain in their torso, extremities, face, or head. The median duration of pain was 18.5 months. Based on the same TAS cutoff score, alexithymia was found in 36% of the sample. TAS scores were again associated with measures of affective distress, and unrelated to measures of the intensity of pain and only weakly related to perceived level of disability.

While the rates of alexithymia reported in the two American studies are similar to rates that have been found in heterogeneous samples of psychiatric outpatients (Taylor et al., 1992b; Todarello et al., 1995; Wise & Mann, 1994), a somewhat higher rate of 53% was reported recently by Cox et al. (1994), who used the TAS-20 to investigate alexithymia in 55 motor vehicle accident survivors (19 males, 36 females) in Canada. The subjects in this study had complained of chronic pain for at least two years and met the DSM-III-R criteria for a diagnosis of somatoform pain disorder.

In studies evaluating the Rorschach alexithymia indices, Acklin and Bernat (1987) initially compared a group of 33 patients with chronic low back pain with reference data for non-patients, depressed inpatients, and patients with mixed personality disorders, who were randomly selected from the protocol pool established by Exner (1986) at the Rorschach Research Foundation. The low back pain patients scored in the predicted direction on all of the Rorschach alexithymia indices and showed greater similarity to the personality disorder patients than to either depressed patients or non-patients. In a later study, Acklin and Alexander (1988) compared the same group of low back pain patients with three groups of patients suffering from gastrointestinal disorders, skin disorders, or migraine headaches. Though all four patient groups were found to be highly distinguishable from a non-patient reference group on all or most of the seven Rorschach alexithymia indices, there was considerable variability among the somatically ill groups with the back pain patients being the most alexithymic. The differences between the back pain and migraine headache patients were due largely to greater impairments in affect management and perceptual processing in the back pain group. Acklin and Alexander (1988) considered these findings preliminary, however, as the groups were not matched on demographic variables.

The Rorschach was used also by Julkunen, Hurri and Kankainen (1988) in an exploratory study examining the role of alexithymia and other psychological factors in the outcome of chronic low back pain. The subjects were female employees of a large, cooperative commercial enterprise in Finland. Alexithymic characteristics were assessed by the number of human movement responses (with the content of play or other pleasurable activity) on the Rorschach, and by an index of affective words on a modified Sentence Completion Test. Whereas subjects who showed spontaneous recovery were found to be relatively outgoing and expressive of their feelings, those who showed increasing disability at a one-year follow-up were characterized by alexithymic features. Further outcome studies are obviously needed using the more clearly defined set of Rorschach alexithymia indices and other better validated measures of the alexithymia construct.

**Somatization, dissociation, and trauma**

Consistent with Krystal's (1978b, 1988, 1997) clinical impression that problems in affect regulation often stem from early trauma, several studies have demonstrated an association between somatoform disorders and recalled histories of childhood trauma (Loewenstein, 1990). Pribor and Dinwiddie (1992), for example, found a greatly elevated prevalence of somatization disorder (13.5%) (together with elevated rates of most other psychiatric disorders) in adult survivors of childhood incest. Morrison (1989) found a significantly higher rate of sexual molestation during childhood among women with somatization disorder than among women with affective disorder. In a study of primary care patients, Craig et al. (1993) found that acute somatization was associated with a history of early parental neglect, indifference, and abuse. Walker et al. (1988) found that women with chronic pelvic pain reported a significantly higher prevalence of histories of childhood and adult sexual abuse than did women with specific gynaecological disease. The chronic pain patients also had a significantly greater prevalence of major depression and substance abuse, and reported significantly more somatic symptoms. The rate of childhood sexual abuse was 64%, which is double the rate found in a general population survey. More recently, Barsky et al. (1994) compared a group of patients with DSM-III-R hypochondriasis with a group of non-hypochondriacal patients attending the same general medical outpatient clinic. The hypochondriacal group reported significantly more traumatic sexual contact, victimization by physical violence, and major parental upheaval before age 17.

In a further investigation of women with chronic pelvic pain, Walker et al. (1992) also found high rates of dissociation among the women with histories of sexual abuse. This is not surprising in that dissociation is a common response to severe trauma and studies have demonstrated positive correlations between the Dissociative Experiences Scale (DES) and scores on child abuse and trauma questionnaires (Sanders & Giolas, 1991). There is evidence also of a strong association between dissociation and somatization (Loewenstein, 1990). Saxe et al. (1994), for example, found that 64% of a group of inpatients with dissociative disorders also met DSM-III criteria for somatization disorder and reported an average of 12.4 somatic symptoms. Furthermore, the finding of a significant correlation between the scores on the DES and the number of reported somatic symptoms, suggests that the more a patient dissociates, the more somatic symptoms he or she will experience. A comparison group of age and gender matched inpatients, who scored very low on the DES, reported an average of only 3.1 somatic symptoms, and none of these patients met criteria for somatization disorder. In another study, almost two-thirds of a group of patients with multiple personality disorder also met the DSM-III-R criteria for somatization disorder (Ross et al., 1989). Pribor et al. (1993) found an association between dissociative symptoms and somatization disorder in a group of female psychiatric outpatients, as well as a strong association with histories of sexual abuse as a child or as an adult and/or physical or emotional abuse as a child. While empirical evidence of a strong association between alexithymia and posttraumatic stress disorder will be presented in Chapter 7, we remind the reader of the study by Berenbaum and James (1994), which found a positive association between alexithymia and dissociation.

The finding of a strong association between somatization and dissociation should not be surprising since, as several authors have commented (Loewenstein, 1990; Nemiah, 1991; Saxe *et al.*, 1994), the two phenomena were linked historically as prominent features of hysteria. Briquet (1859) related hysteria to a variety of traumatic experiences including sexual abuse. Freud (1896; Breuer & Freud, 1893) also, in his early papers on hysteria, attributed the physical symptoms to childhood sexual traumas. He subsequently relinquished this theory, however, after deciding that his patients' reports of childhood seduction were largely the product of fantasies. Although the association between somatization and dissociation was buried within DSM-III as hysteria evolved into the diagnostic category of somatoform disorders, the separation of hysteria from dissociative disorders helped clarify the distinction between somatization and conversion, which we outlined earlier.

The associations between somatization, dissociation, alexithymia, and trauma, have led to the suggestion that dissociation (rather than somatization) acts as a defense against emotionally distressing memories, and that the functional somatic symptoms are direct manifestations of the emotions and sensations associated with the traumatic event (Nemiah, 1991; Saxe *et al.*, 1994). This idea was considered more than 100 years ago by Janet (1889), who proposed that memories of traumatic experiences might be stored outside of conscious awareness and expressed in somatic symptoms. Furthermore, as Krystal (1978*a,b*, 1988) and van der Kolk and van der Hart (1989) have indicated, intense emotions evoked by trauma interfere with the cognitive processing of experience so that the affects are encoded on a sensorimotor, enactive level rather than in a semantic and linguistic way. This alexithymic deficit prevents the individual from making a conscious link between the somatic symptoms and the original traumatic experience. As one patient in Saxe *et al.*'s (1994) study stated, 'My mind may not remember, but my body keeps the score' (p. 1333).

Not all somatizing patients have associated dissociative symptoms, and dissociation is not the only defense that people might use in their attempts to cope with traumatic experiences. As we outlined in Chapter 2, Freud's (1915*a*) concept of primal repression also can account for an arrest in the formation of verbal representations of traumatic experiences and associated affects, which then 'exist as pathological memory forms, protosymbolically organized' (Dorpat, 1985, p. 102), and compulsively enacted through abnormal illness behaviour and the experiencing of somatic symptoms and hypochondriacal worries. This latter conceptualization leads us to a further elaboration of Tyrer's (1973, p. 916) proposal that people who somatize 'deny the psychic aspects of [their] condition'. The denial employed is primitive in nature and corresponds to primal repression, which involves a constriction and arrest in cognitive functioning and does not respond in the usual way to interpretation of defenses (Dorpat, 1985; Krystal, 1988). Though traditionally referred to as defenses, dissociation, primal repression, and primitive denial also signify deficits in the cognitive processing of distressing affects and a failure to assimilate the totality of traumatic events. It is the 'unmentalized' and unregulated emotions, rather than the events themselves, that underly the somatic symptoms (van der Kolk & van der Hart, 1989). The therapeutic implications of these concepts will be elaborated in Chapter 11.

# [7] Anxiety and depressive disorders and a note on personality disorders

Numerous studies of primary care populations have found that many somatizing patients have diagnosable anxiety or depressive disorders that are commonly undetected by general practitioners. In a study of two family medicine clinics in Canada, for example, Kirmayer and Robbins (1991a) found that 11% of patients met DSM-III criteria for major depression and/or anxiety disorder, and almost three-quarters of these patients had presented with exclusively somatic symptoms. Similarly, in a survey of 15 primary care practices in the Greater Manchester area of England, Bridges and Goldberg (1985) found anxiety and depressive disorders that were unrelated to physical disease in almost 25% of patients, with more than three-quarters of the patients seeking medical help for somatic symptoms; although general practitioners detected the majority of psychiatric disorders in patients who sought help for psychological symptoms, only half of the psychiatric disorders were detected when somatization was present. An American study found clinical depression in 12% of ambulatory medical patients in a prepaid health program, and demonstrated a failure of primary care physicians to diagnose the depression in 50% of cases (Nielson & Williams, 1980). Studies of patients with somatization disorders referred to psychiatrists by primary care physicians have also demonstrated high rates of comorbidity with other psychiatric disorders, especially major depression, panic disorder, and generalized anxiety disorder (Brown, Golding & Smith, 1990; Liskow et al., 1986).

The failure to recognize anxiety and depressive disorders in somatizing patients results in unnecessary consultations and investigations, and leads to increased rates of alcohol abuse and suicide when these psychiatric disorders remain untreated (Haddad, 1994; Weissman et al., 1989). The burden placed on the health care system is compounded by other costs to society as patients become functionally impaired and dependent on disability payments or welfare (Leon, Portera & Weissman, 1995; Rice & Miller, 1995). These costs could be reduced if detection and treatment of anxiety and depressive disorders in somatizing patients were improved. To enhance detection and to implement successful treatments, however, more needs to be known about why some patients focus predominantly on the somatic components of anxiety and depression. This chapter shows how the alexithymia construct can help explain the somatic presentation of certain anxiety and depressive disorders. Also included in this chapter is a discussion of alexithymia and affect dysregulation in borderline and other primitive personality disorders, which may overlap with subsyndromal forms of these Axis I disorders.

### Anxiety and depression as signal affects

Before discussing specific anxiety and depressive disorders, and commenting on primitive personality disorders, it is important to re-emphasize that the affects of anxiety and depression provide essential functions in normal mental life. In the course of development, as outlined in Chapter 1, anxiety and depression (like other primary affects) come to be experienced not merely as emotional reactions to internal and external situations, but also as types of information generated by the ego about its relative degree of safety and possible need for mobilizing defenses against the emergence of a more intense level of unpleasant affect. This *signal function* of anxiety was described first by Freud (1926) when he relinquished his initial theory that anxiety was merely transformed libido and reconceptualized anxiety as a signal that alerts the ego to danger, in particular, danger arising from the emergence of forbidden impulses and unconscious fantasies. Whereas in his first theory, Freud (1895a) regarded anxiety as entirely somatic in origin, resulting from repressed libido, in his second theory he viewed anxiety as a psychological phenomenon that motivates the operation of repression and other ego defenses and leads to intrapsychic conflict (Nemiah, 1988).

Freud (1926) broadened his second theory to include, along with anxiety, pain and mourning (i.e. depression) as signal affects that may also elicit defensive activity. But whereas anxiety was viewed as a signal that something unpleasant is about to happen, depression was seen as a signal that some calamity has already occurred, namely that one has lost the tie to a loved and need-gratifying person (object loss). Subsequent psychoanalytic theorists have also emphasized the signal function of both anxiety and depression and extended the anticipated dangers, or calamities that have already occurred, to include loss of self-esteem, loss of the object's love, and the fantasy of castration (Bibring, 1953; Brenner, 1975, 1991; Hoffman, 1992; Jacobson, 1994; Rangell, 1968; Sandler & Joffe, 1965; Spezzano, 1993).

Rangell, and more recently Jacobson, regard the signal sequence of affects as the quintessential psychobiological event:

> The affects, with their biological grounding . . . are sampled *experientially*, setting in motion psychological processes that are experienced as dangers, motives, and purposes . . . (Jacobson, 1994, p. 21).

From this perspective, one can see that an individual's capacity to use affects as signals and to mobilize effective defenses plays an important role both in normal affect regulation and in the formation of psychoneurotic symptoms. In simple phobias, for example, anxiety elicited by the danger of the threatened loss of control over forbidden unconscious impulses or wishes is successfully bound through its displacement onto an object or situation that can be avoided; intense anxiety or panic is then experienced only when the phobic object is approached. Similarly, as conceptualized within the framework of classical psychoanalytic theory, the symptoms of obsessive compulsive disorder reflect the binding of anxiety through the defenses of reaction formation, isolation, intellectualization, and undoing (Fenichel, 1945; Nemiah, 1988).

Under certain circumstances, however, an individual may be unable to use affects as signals or mobilize adequate defenses, and will then experience affective flooding of the unmodulated signal (Jacobson, 1994). This is especially evident in panic disorder, posttraumatic stress disorder (PTSD), and borderline personality disorder, which are conceptualized in this chapter as disorders involving major deficits in the cognitive processing and regulation of affects. Although advances in biological psychiatry have led to the realization that most depressive disorders and many of the anxiety disorders probably involve constitutional-inherited or acquired disturbances in the regulation of neurotransmitter systems that mediate affects (Gorman *et al.*, 1989; Kolb, 1987; Siever & Davis, 1985; van der Kolk & Greenberg, 1987), we consider it useful to identify those disorders in which there appears also to be a failure in the information-processing or signal function of affects. In addition to panic disorder and PTSD, we will discuss somatic presentations of depression, and some of the personality disorders that appear to be associated with temperamental affective dysregulations.

## Panic disorder

Panic disorder is characterized by recurrent, unexpected panic attacks. Although panic attacks can occur in other anxiety disorders, they are more likely to be situationally bound, as in social and simple (specific) phobias, or evoked by stimuli associated with a severe stressor, as in PTSD. The diagnosis of panic disorder, according to DSM-III-R and DSM-IV (American Psychiatric Association, 1987, 1994), requires the presence of unexpected (spontaneous) panic attacks, although some patients also have situationally bound attacks or a predisposition to attacks during or after exposure to situational triggers.

The essential feature of a panic attack is a discrete period of intense fear or discomfort that is accompanied by a variety of somatic symptoms that are associated with autonomic overactivity. In addition, there may be symptoms of derealization or depersonalization, as well as cognitive symptoms such as a fear of dying or a fear of going crazy and losing control (American Psychiatric Association, 1994). After experiencing a succession of panic attacks, some patients develop an anticipatory anxiety that may progress to avoidant behaviour and agoraphobia as they become concerned about having a recurrence of panic in situations where previously they have experienced an attack. Other patients may become hypochondriacal as a result of focusing on normal bodily sensations or mild physical symptoms, and misinterpreting these as indicators of serious illness.

A panic attack is a clear example of a failure in the signal function of affects. While such failures might happen occasionally to any person, some individuals, especially patients with panic disorder, seem to 'possess a psychological organization that does not permit the typical development of signal anxiety' (Baumbacher, 1989, p. 75). Instead of perceiving warning signs of developing anxiety, these patients experience sudden overwhelming floods of undifferentiated affect. In Krystal's (1992) view, what they experience 'is not a true panic, but an "attack" of mixed physiological elements of dysphoric affects' (p. 407). Krystal considers this 'a perfect example of regression in affects to their infantile, somatic, undifferentiated form' (p. 407).

Like Freud's (1915b, p. 121) concept of instincts, panic arises 'on the frontier between the mental and the somatic' and has yet to be organized and differentiated into cognitive schemata that allow affects to be used as signals by the ego and provide a structure for the internal processing of emotions (Baumbacher, 1989; Isenstadt, 1980; Lane & Schwartz, 1987). Indeed, recognizing that panic 'results from a direct translation of internal arousal into somatic pathways of discharge without any modification by higher order psychic processes', Nemiah

(1984, p. 134) suggests that one may view panic disorder as 'the prototypical psychosomatic disorder'. It may be more correct to apply Engel's (1962) term *somatopsychic–psychosomatic* to panic disorder, since the psychological symptoms (derealization/ depersonalization, fear of going crazy, etc.) during a panic attack reflect a state of psychic disorganization that is seemingly secondary to the experience of intense autonomic arousal, and further panic may be induced by the catastrophic misinterpretation of physiological sensations. Moreover, a psychological predisposition to panic disorder might be determined directly or indirectly through an interplay between a temperamental trait, such as 'behavioural inhibition', and the childhood environment (Rosenbaum et al., 1988). All of these ideas are encompassed by our conceptualization of panic as a disorder involving deficits in the cognitive processing and regulation of emotion.

Alarmed by the puzzling somatic symptoms produced by panic attacks, patients with panic disorder frequently present to hospital emergency departments and overutilize other medical services as well. According to Katon (1984), 6% to 10% of patients in primary care practice suffer from panic disorders, the majority presenting with somatic symptoms. He found that the three most common presentations are cardiologic, gastrointestinal, and neurologic symptoms. Misdiagnoses are common, especially when the physician focuses on only a part of the symptom complex (Sheehan, 1982).

Prior to DSM-III, which was published in 1980, panic disorder was not recognized as a separate diagnostic entity. Instead, unexpected panic attacks were grouped with more generalized forms of anxiety and given the diagnosis of anxiety neurosis. However, syndromes that closely resemble contemporary definitions of panic disorder have been reported in the medical literature since at least the late nineteenth century. Da Costa (1871), for example, described a condition of 'irritable heart' to refer to a cluster of symptoms resembling panic attacks that he had observed in some soldiers around the time of the American Civil War. Similar panic-like syndromes were reported subsequently by other cardiologists and given a variety of names including 'soldier's heart', 'neurocirculatory asthenia', 'effort syndrome', and 'cardiac neurosis' (Cohen & White, 1950; Oppenheim, 1918).

The diagnostic entity of anxiety neurosis was introduced by Freud (1895a) around the turn of the nineteenth century when he made an argument for detaching a certain cluster of anxiety symptoms from the broad syndrome of neurasthenia.[1] Freud described chronic anxiety

1. As noted in Chapter 6, anxiety neurosis and neurasthenia were classified by Freud (1898) as actual neuroses and contrasted with the psycho-neuroses, which he considered psychological in origin.

symptoms and acute anxiety or panic attacks, the latter bearing a remarkable similarity to the description of panic attacks given in DSM-III-R and DSM-IV. Equally striking is Freud's description of how anxiety could either remain 'free-floating' and produce a state of 'expectant anxiety' or become attached to a particular object or situation thereby leading to the development of a phobia. 'In the case of agoraphobia', he wrote, 'we often find *the recollection of an anxiety attack* and what the patient actually fears is the occurrence of such an attack under the special conditions in which he believes he cannot escape it' (Freud, 1895b, p. 81).

Although Freud eventually relinquished his initial theory that anxiety was somatic in origin (the result of an automatic and direct transformation of excess libido) and replaced it by his psychological theory, which viewed anxiety as a signal affect arising in the ego, he never entirely abandoned his concept of a type of anxiety that invades the ego involuntarily and is outside of its control. As Rangell (1968) and Nemiah (1988) have outlined, Freud's concept of 'actual' anxiety referred to a state of psychic helplessness in which the ego has been flooded by overwhelming instincts, tensions, and undifferentiated affects. Freud (1926) called this state a 'traumatic situation' and contrasted it with a minimal state of anxiety that has been brought about by the ego and under its control, and which moves the ego to erect psychological defenses that determine the form of specific psychoneurotic disorders. In other words, Freud preserved his concept of a contentless or automatic biological anxiety alongside his concept of signal anxiety which could become associated with specific ideational content (Frosch, 1990); he acknowledged also that some patients may show admixtures of actual neurotic and psychoneurotic symptoms (Freud, 1898).

Gediman (1984) has since elaborated the importance of actual neurotic states in psychoneurotic patients, and attributes these to a *'failure to dose and regulate stimuli, both internal and external'* (p. 192) because of a low stimulus barrier, determined either constitutionally or by chronic early trauma. Gediman notes that, because of secondary elaboration, such states do not remain devoid of mental content for very long and are quickly drawn into the orbit of neurotic conflict. This is evidenced in panic disorder patients by thoughts of dying or going crazy during panic attacks and by fantasies that subsequently may evolve. Like Schur (1955) and McDougall (1980b), Gediman (1984) views actual neurotic states as signifying 'a deficiency in the capacity to represent symbolically the related affective and tension states' (p. 197); that is, a deficit in the cognitive processing of emotion.

After Freud introduced his structural theory of the mind and elaborated his theory of signal anxiety, the distinction between 'actual' anxiety neurosis and neurotic anxiety as a reaction to forbidden impulses and fantasies was almost completely discarded, as most of his followers concluded that 'cases diagnosed as *Aktualneurose* in the early days would reveal themselves as genuine psychoneuroses if looked at with the more experienced diagnostic eye of a later day' (Waelder, 1967, p. 23). Consequently, the majority of psychoanalysts came to regard panic as a quantitative extension of ordinary anxiety, which was always traceable to intrapsychic conflicts; interpretive psychotherapies became the recommended treatment.[1]

Over the years, however, there has been increasing consensus that traditional psychoanalysis and psychodynamic psychotherapy for panic disorder and agoraphobia are generally ineffective (Nemiah, 1984; Roth, 1987). Psychological conflicts over drive-related wishes can certainly be detected in many patients with panic disorder, but these now appear to be only one of a variety of triggers rather than the direct cause of panic attacks (Aronson & Logue, 1988). Other factors that seem capable of triggering panic attacks in individuals with panic disorder include hyperventilation, separations, ingestion of caffeine or yohimbine, infusions of sodium lactate, and inhalation of carbon dioxide (Gorman et al., 1989). Some patients seem to panic because of faulty cognitions – they perceive and misinterpret as dangerous the normal bodily sensations of autonomic arousal (Clark, 1986), a phenomenon that is encompassed by the recently formulated construct of 'anxiety sensitivity' (S. Taylor, 1995). Furthermore, findings from pharmacological studies suggest strongly that panic is discontinuous and qualitatively different from ordinary anxiety and requires a different etiological explanation (Klein, 1981).

As researchers focused their attention on investigating specific mechanisms and testing the efficacy of different treatments, competing biological, cognitive/behavioural, and psychodynamic models of panic disorder and agoraphobia have emerged (Clark, 1986; Margraf, Ehlers & Roth, 1986; Marks, 1987; Michels, Frances & Shear, 1985; Sheehan, 1982; Shear et al., 1993). Several researchers have attempted to integrate these models (Busch et al., 1991; Gorman et al., 1989;

1. Although the term actual neurosis fell into disrepute, several authors have noted that actual neurotic states have been acknowledged all along within the field of psychoanalysis by other terms such as terror, traumatic neuroses, neurocirculatory asthenia, organ neuroses, somatization, and psychophysiological or psychosomatic disorders (Blau, 1952; Gediman, 1984; Rangell, 1968). These conditions correspond to several of the illnesses and diseases in this book that we have conceptualized as disorders of affect regulation.

Taylor, 1989), but the majority of panic patients still receive only pharmacologic and/or cognitive–behavioural treatments. These approaches fail to correct the underlying deficits in emotional processing which, in our view, account for the high rates of relapse and chronic, residual symptoms observed in follow-up studies of panic disorder patients (Faravelli & Albanesi, 1987; Katon et al., 1987; Noyes et al., 1993; Roy-Byrne & Cowley, 1994/1995). We will show how the overarching concept of panic as a disorder of affect regulation permits an integration of the salient features of the different etiological models.

Contemporary biological theorists have moved away from Freud's emphasis on the regulation of libidinal and aggressive instincts and taken a broader ethological perspective, thereby widening the range of biological regulatory systems that might become dysregulated and result in spontaneous panic attacks (Klein, 1994). Donald Klein (1981), for example, who is a leading proponent of the biological approach to panic, proposed that individuals prone to panic disorder might have a constitutionally determined lowered threshold in the neurobiological control mechanism underlying normal separation anxiety. Consequently, the mechanism may fire spontaneously or it may be activated by minimal triggers. Klein suggested that antidepressant medications may exert their beneficial effect on panic disorder by raising the threshold within this innate regulatory mechanism to a normal level.[1]

In developing this hypothesis, Klein was influenced strongly by Bowlby's (1969, 1973) theories of attachment and separation. The reader will recall that Bowlby's theories cast new light on the problem of separation anxiety by considering it a direct response to the loss, or threat of loss, of the mother, rather than a consequence of accumulated drive and need tensions. Bowlby linked anxiety disorders in adult life to the experience of long or repeated separations, or frequent threats of such, during childhood. Such a history is not uncommonly obtained from patients with panic disorder and has been found to be related to poor outcome (Noyes et al., 1993; Yeragani et al., 1989).

Klein's hypothesis is appealing in that it essentially conceptualizes

1. More recently, Klein (1994) shifted somewhat from his separation anxiety theory and suggested that panic is not fear, but stems from a malfunction of an innate 'suffocation alarm' system. This suggestion is consistent with the impression of the psychoanalyst Rangell (1984) that all pathological anxiety is ultimately 'a respiratory panic of the unavailability of the air to breathe' (p. 79). As Rangell points out, however, the snout or perioral region of the body, through which breathing occurs, is very much involved in attachment and separation, from the time of the infant's grasping, holding, and withdrawal from the maternal breast.

panic as a disorder of regulation involving a biological mechanism that normally is concerned with maintaining the infant's proximity to and contact with the mother. However, Klein's model resembles Freud's first theory of anxiety in giving no role to psychological mechanisms. As in actual neurosis, panic is seen as biological in origin, but now it is associated with an inherited tendency for a neurobiologic mechanism to become dysregulated rather than with an accumulation of 'toxic' libido.

Other biological models of panic disorder are very similar, and usually link panic to an increased firing of the brainstem noradrenergic center, the locus coeruleus; the hypersensitivity of this locus and/or other brainstem loci is believed to be inherited. As Gorman *et al.* (1989) point out, this hypothesis is supported by the observation that the symptoms of panic attacks are consistent with 'storms of autonomic nervous system activity', and by extensive experimental studies showing that panic attacks can be provoked in panic disorder patients by the various chemical agents that we listed earlier.

Although central neurotransmitter systems undoubtedly play an important role in regulating the activity of the biological mechanisms underlying separation anxiety, a person's close relationships, symbols, and inner psychological life might also play a significant role in modulating their activity. We know, for example, that disruptions in important interpersonal relationships can trigger the onset of panic disorder (Faravelli & Pallanti, 1989; Klein, 1964; Roy-Byrne, Geraci & Uhde, 1986), and patients with panic disorder often report experiencing less panic, anticipatory anxiety, and phobic avoidant behaviour when accompanied by persons with whom they feel safe (Rachman, 1984; Seligman & Binik, 1977); these 'safe people' would appear to function as external regulators of the level of their anxiety and thus compensate for deficits in their inner representational worlds (Hofer, 1984; Taylor, 1989). Indeed, in a recent experimental study with panic disorder patients, Carter *et al.* (1995) demonstrated that the presence of a safe person significantly reduced the physiological response to a $CO_2$ challenge, as well as the level of distress and number of catastrophic cognitions.

Klein seems to have overlooked completely Bowlby's (1969, 1973, 1988b) discussion of how the child organizes his knowledge of the external world by developing 'internal working models', including models of the dynamic attachment relationship between self and caregivers and of associated affects. As we outlined in Chapters 1 and 2, these working models (internal representations) reflect the quality of early social relationships and have the potential both for modulating anxiety and for evoking it.

Klein and other advocates of biological models of panic disorder have overlooked also important research in the field of developmental biology (Hofer, 1984, 1987; Pipp & Harmon, 1987; Reite & Field, 1985), which has shown that, hidden within the interactions between infant and mother, at least in lower animals, are a number of sensorimotor processes whereby the mother 'serves as an external regulator of the infant's behaviour, its autonomic physiology, and even the neurochemistry of its maturing brain' (Hofer, 1983, p. 199) until the infant's self-regulating mechanisms mature. These discoveries have led to important revisions to Bowlby's attachment theory and to a realization that the infant's responses to separation are due not simply to the breaking of an emotional bond with the mother, but also to withdrawal of the biological and behavioural regulation previously supplied by the mother (Field, 1985; Reite & Field, 1985; Hofer, 1984; Taylor, 1992b). Furthermore, as Weiner (1982, 1984) has suggested, the withdrawal of these 'hidden' regulatory processes in early life might affect the maturation and organization of homeostatic mechanisms in the brain and body and thereby alter susceptibility to medical and psychiatric disorders later in life. In other words, separation experiences in early life might modify the genetic expression of neurotransmitter systems regulating anxiety in humans and produce the lowered threshold or heightened sensitivity in brainstem loci postulated by Klein and his colleagues. These may be activated later in life by the stress of a real or threatened object loss.

The process of separating and individuating from the mother and internalizing her anxiety-regulating functions is facilitated in normal development by the child's attachment to a transitional object. As outlined in Chapter 1 and in an earlier contribution (Taylor, 1987a), transitional objects are initially 'sensation objects' that provide tactile and olfactory stimulation that has regulatory effects comparable to the 'hidden' regulatory processes that Hofer and others have discovered within animal infant–mother relationships. The subsequent endowment of the transitional object with symbolic meaning, and its evolution during childhood into interests and imaginative functioning, increase further the person's capacity to self-regulate affects. Alexithymic patients with panic disorder, however, are likely to show incomplete transitional object development, because of an impaired symbolizing capacity (Deri, 1984; Taylor, 1987a), and may still rely on sensation objects for self-regulation. For example, one of our patients, a 21-year-old woman with panic disorder, did not recall having a transitional object during childhood, but discovered that she could abort her panic attacks by inhaling the residual aroma from her husband that remained in the bedsheets after he had left for work.

Given that individuals with insecure childhood attachments and corresponding faulty internal representations often remain excessively dependent on others, it is not surprising that a high prevalence of dependent personality disorder or dependent personality traits has been reported among patients with panic disorder, especially among those with agoraphobia (Mavissakalian, 1990; Reich, Noyes & Troughton, 1987). Although the extent to which the dependency is an antecedent or a consequence of panic disorder and agoraphobia is not clearly established, it is our view that the dependency on a 'safe' person shown by some patients compensates for a failure to achieve the usual and proper level of self-regulation. Moreover, patients with high levels of dependent and other personality disorder traits have been found to respond less well to treatment (Mavissakalian, 1990).

In summary, our integrated model of panic disorder includes a role for disturbances in early object relationships, which might influence certain biological mechanisms involved in affect regulation, and also influence the internal representations (Bowlby's working model) of early experience that function as modulators of affect at a cognitive level. In addition, the model places importance on a predisposed person's current relationships, which might trigger dysregulation of brain stem loci through separations, or function as external regulators that help stabilize hypersensitive loci. The descending neural connections between brainstem, limbic system, and neocortex that we referred to in Chapter 5 (and are outlined also in a model proposed by Gorman et al. (1989)), provide pathways for mediating these effects. And while ascending connections from the brainstem and afferent input from the periphery convey to the neocortex information about states of arousal, descending connections provide a pathway for catastrophizing cognitions to further dysregulate brainstem mechanisms (Clark, 1986). We concur with Gorman and his colleagues that the limbic system is involved in anticipatory anxiety and the neocortex in the development of phobic avoidant behaviours.

### Clinical illustration

Mrs Jones, a 74-year-old widow, developed recurrent panic attacks soon after her husband died from a sudden heart attack. She had experienced panic attacks for several months during her teenage years, and had a recurrence of the disorder in her late thirties after emigrating. On the latter occasion, the patient's doctor made a diagnosis of 'homesickness' and sent Mrs Jones back to her mother for six months, which resulted in a complete remission of the disorder. She remained symptom-free during the rest of her adult life, but was markedly dependent on her husband, who was not only a good companion to Mrs Jones, but also functioned as an external psychic regulator, compensating for her shaky self-esteem and limited ability to make decisions and cope with solitude. During the few months before her husband's death, Mrs Jones had a premonition that something dreadful was about to happen and she became mildly agoraphobic. Although mildly depressed when she sought psychiatric treatment after her husband's death, Mrs Jones was not mourning this loss. Instead, she was overwhelmed by almost daily panic attacks which she related to her fear of being alone and helplessness when faced with the need to make decisions about her future. She had become extremely dependent on frequent telephone calls or visits from her daughter and friends, and she experienced further panic when these people could not be immediately available.

Mrs Jones was a markedly alexithymic person; she never recalled dreams and was unable to evoke mental images of her husband or remember their happy times together. Nor was she able to describe a range of feelings. She was mostly aware of sensing her husband's absence, which was 'like losing part of herself' and made her all the more anxious. Aside from her immediate family, the patient had no interests that she could become absorbed in or derive pleasure from. The focus in psychotherapy, therefore, was on the barrenness of the patient's inner world and on increasing her awareness of the solace that could be derived from memories and other transitional experiences. Mrs Jones discovered that she could reduce her level of anxiety by wearing one of her husband's pyjama jackets that had not been washed and still contained his body odour. Whereas a photograph of her husband provided little comfort, the tactile and olfactory sensations provided by the pyjama jacket evoked the illusion of his presence. Antipanic medication had previously been ineffective, but when combined with this direct sensory stimulation and the evolving regulatory psychotherapeutic relationship, Mrs Jones's panic attacks and fear of being alone gradually subsided.

## Empirical studies of alexithymia and panic disorder

Two empirical studies have yielded results that support our theoretical view that panic disorder is distinguishable from simple phobia and obsessive compulsive disorder as a disorder that is associated more strongly with deficits in the cognitive processing and regulation of affects.

In the first study, Zeitlin and McNally (1993) administered the Toronto Alexithymia Scale (TAS) and the Anxiety Sensitivity Index (ASI) to 27 patients with panic disorder and 31 patients with obsessive compulsive disorder, both groups being diagnosed by DSM-III-R criteria. The ASI measures the fear of anxiety-related sensations, which arises from the belief that these sensations have harmful consequences (Reiss et al., 1986; S. Taylor, 1995). The panic disorder patients scored significantly higher on the TAS than the patients with obsessive compulsive disorder. Based on the pre-established TAS cutoff score, 67% of the panic disorder patients were alexithymic compared with only 13% of the patients with obsessive compulsive disorder. Consistent with the view that alexithymic individuals tend to focus on and misinterpret the bodily sensations of emotional arousal, the panic disorder patients scored significantly higher on the ASI than the patients with obsessive compulsive disorder.

In the second study, we collaborated with Dr Marvin Acklin at the University of Hawaii who administered the TAS, the MMPI, and several other scales to 30 patients who met DSM-III-R criteria for panic disorder and 32 patients who met DSM-III-R criteria for simple phobia (Parker et al., 1993d). The two patient groups were compared on the alexithymia measure and selected MMPI scales by two-tailed t tests with the level of significance set at 0.007 for the Bonferroni correction. The panic disorder patients scored significantly higher on the TAS than the patients with simple phobia; based on the TAS cutoff score of $\geqslant 74$, 46.7% of the panic disorder patients were alexithymic compared with only 12.5% of the patients with simple phobia. Moreover, only 20% of the panic disorder patients scored 62 or lower on the TAS, compared with 65.6% of the patients with simple phobia; such extremely low scores indicate the absence of alexithymic characteristics.

Given the diagnostic criteria to select the two anxiety disorder groups in our study, the patients with panic disorder, not surprisingly, scored significantly higher on the manifest anxiety and somatic complaints scales of the MMPI than the patients with simple phobia. However, these indices of more intense symptoms of autonomic hyperarousal in the panic disorder patients were also consistent with their greater alexithymia and lesser ability to regulate affect. Although the two patient groups did not differ on the hysteria and repression scales of the MMPI, which suggests a similar use of denial and repressive defense mechanisms, the panic disorder patients scored significantly lower on the ego strength scale, indicating that they were less well-equipped psychologically to deal with problems and stresses than were the patients with simple phobia. The patients with panic disorder also scored significantly higher on the MMPI dependency scale, which was consistent with results of previous research comparing field dependence in patients with panic disorder and patients with simple phobia (Rock & Goldberger, 1978).

In a more recent study, Cox et al. (1995) used the TAS-20 to assess alexithymia in 100 patients with panic disorder and 46 patients with social phobia, as diagnosed by DSM-III-R criteria. Both patient groups also completed the ASI and several other questionnaires. A comparison of the two patient groups found no significant differences in the mean scores for the total TAS-20 and for its three factor scales. Based on the cutoff score of the TAS-20, which provides a more conservative estimate of alexithymia than the TAS, 34% of the patients with panic disorder and 28.3% of the patients with social phobia were alexithymic, a non-significant difference. Although a comparison of mean ASI scores for the two patient groups was not reported, the ASI correlated positively with all three factors of the TAS-20 in the panic disorder group, but the correlations were statistically significant only for Factors 1 and 2. This finding is consistent with the conceptualization that an alexithymic difficulty in distinguishing between feelings and the bodily sensations of emotional arousal would be associated with a fear and misinterpretation of bodily sensations, the latter being the essence of the anxiety sensitivity construct.

A major problem with Cox et al.'s (1995) study is the use of patients with social phobia as the comparison group. There is considerable overlap in the symptomatology of social phobia and panic disorder and also a substantial comorbidity of the two disorders. For example, Schneier et al. (1992) found in a large epidemiologic study that individuals with social phobia had more than a threefold increased risk of lifetime panic disorder when compared with individuals without social phobia. Argyle and Roth (1989) found in a study of patients who had both diagnoses that the social phobia invariably appeared first. Other investigators have found that patients who recover from an episode of panic disorder are sometimes left with residual symptoms of social phobia (Katon et al., 1987). Although Cox and his colleagues reported that none of the social phobic patients in their study had a concomitant diagnosis of panic disorder, they did not report whether these patients had a prior history of panic disorder; nor did they report whether the patients with panic disorder had any history of social phobia.

On theoretical grounds one would predict that patients with social phobias would resemble panic disorder patients in manifesting deficits in self-representation and in the cognitive processing of affects. Although patients with social phobia can control their panic attacks by avoiding the social situations in which they occur, this is a primitive defensive manoeuvre (comparable to the agoraphobia of some patients with panic disorder), which does not resolve the deficits in self-regulation that underly the socially phobic person's fear of being scrutinized and evaluated by others. Patients with simple phobia or obsessive compulsive disorder may also experience panic attacks but, as we outlined earlier, their ability to use anxiety as a signal and to mobilize higher-order defenses (such as displacement and undoing) permit the formation of more structured psychoneurotic symptoms that generally contain the anxiety (Nemiah, 1988).[1]

### Posttraumatic stress disorder

PTSD is another type of anxiety disorder in which the signal function of affects has been lost and the symptoms are related directly to unregulated emotions. The disorder develops following exposure to an extreme traumatic stressor which evoked intense fear, horror, or helplessness. As outlined in both DSM-III-R and DSM-IV, there are three clusters of symptoms in PTSD: (i) intrusive symptoms such as 'flashbacks' and distressing images, thoughts, perceptions, or dreams of the traumatic event; (ii) avoidance symptoms, including efforts to avoid thoughts, feelings, places, and people associated with the trauma or that evoke recollections of it, a feeling of detachment from others, and a restricted range of affect; and (iii) persistent symptoms of increased arousal, such as irritability and outbursts of anger, an exaggerated startle response, difficulty sleeping, and physiologic reactivity on exposure to internal or external cues that symbolize or resemble an aspect of the traumatic event.

Although DSM-III-R specified that the psychologically traumatic stressor is an event 'that is outside the range of usual human experience', this diagnostic criterion was changed in DSM-IV, which emphasizes events involving actual or threatened death or serious injury, or damage to physical integrity. In addition, DSM-IV requires both a 'persistent avoidance of stimuli associated with the trauma' and a 'numbing of general responsiveness' rather than one or the other, and it specifies acute and chronic subtypes of PTSD depending on the duration of the symptoms. We note these differences because all of the empirical studies on PTSD that we review in this chapter are based on DSM-III or DSM-III-R diagnostic criteria for PTSD.

PTSD was not formerly recognized as a distinct diagnostic entity until 1980, when it was included in DSM-III, partly in response to the need for describing severe stress syndromes observed in many Vietnam war veterans (Andreason, 1995). However, as noted by Tomb (1994), 'the symptoms of PTSD have been described since the inception of war [and] are well detailed . . . in Homer's *Iliad* and Cicero's *Letters to his friends*' (p. 237). During the American Civil War and the

---

1. This formulation of obsessive compulsive disorder does not exclude the accumulating evidence that there are also neurobiological abnormalities underlying the symptoms, including dysregulated serotonergic systems.

first and second World Wars, soldiers who developed PTSD symptoms received a variety of diagnostic labels including 'war neurosis', 'shell shock', 'soldier's heart', 'combat fatigue', 'gross stress reaction', and 'traumatic neurosis' (Choy & de Bosset, 1992). World War II also led to the identification of severe stress syndromes among individuals exposed to non-combat related traumas, including prisoner of war camps, concentration camps, and torture. By the time of DSM-III-R, it was clear that the stressors for PTSD included civilian-related events such as natural disasters, sexual assault, automobile accidents, chronic medical disorders, and even severe job stress (Andreason, 1995; Tomb, 1994).

In attempting to understand the etiology and nature of posttraumatic syndromes, most psychiatrists have described the presence of both psychological and physiological components to the trauma response along with an alternation between intrusive and avoidant symptoms. Kardiner (1941) referred to the traumatic syndrome resulting from war as a *physioneurosis* because of the irritability, heightened startle reaction, and outbursts of anger he observed. Although Freud (1919, 1920) minimized the role of external stressors in psychoneurotic pathology when he abandoned his seduction theory in favour of an intrapsychic conflict model, he did emphasize that in the war neuroses the ego had been overwhelmed by an external threat resulting in a disorganization and loss of ego functions. At the same time, Freud attributed the tendency to re-experience the trauma in dreams to a physical fixation to the trauma.

The consequences of massive psychic trauma on ego functions were elaborated subsequently by Krystal (1968, 1978b, 1981, 1988) on the basis of extensive observations of concentration camp survivors. Among the after-effects of trauma, Krystal described a disturbance of affectivity that corresponds to alexithymia, as we noted in Chapter 2. In addition to 'impairment in the verbalization of emotion and in the capacity for symbolic representation and fantasy formation', Krystal observed a lack of affect tolerance, anhedonia, a general psychic numbing, operative thinking, and a proneness to chronic anxiety and depression and physical illnesses. In Krystal's view, the mixed pattern of physiological responses experienced by trauma victims represents the physiological aspects of the emotions, which are no longer experienced as distinct subjective feelings. Both Krystal's (1981) long-term observations of Holocaust survivors and a study of prisoners-of-war survivors 35 years after the Korean conflict (Sutker et al., 1991) showed that the alexithymic difficulty in expressing feelings persists over time.

van der Kolk (1994) also regards a loss of affective modulation as a central feature of PTSD, and suggests that this may explain the inability of traumatized individuals to use affect states as signals:

In subjects with PTSD, feelings are not used as cues to attend to incoming information and arousal is likely to precipitate fight-or-flight
reactions. Thus they often go immediately from stimulus to response
without psychologically assessing the meaning of an event. This
makes them prone to freeze or, alternatively, to overreact and intimi-
date others in response to minor provocations (p. 254).

In his extensive writings on PTSD, van der Kolk (1987, 1993, 1994) has
repeatedly emphasized the psychobiological foundation of the disorder, in particular the failure to cognitively process the intense emotions
evoked by a traumatic event and the effects of a prolonged biological
stress response. He also considers the alternation between intrusive/
hyperactivity responses and numbing/avoidant responses as the two
primary dimensions of a person's response to any overwhelming and
uncontrollable traumatic experience.

Through a reappraisal of the work of Pierre Janet, van der Kolk and
van der Hart (1989) have helped also in clarifying some of the mechanisms that might underly the clinical features of PTSD. According to
Janet (1889), it is the 'vehement emotions' that accompany extreme
experiences that makes them traumatic; such emotions cause memories of the experience to be dissociated from consciousness and to be
stored instead as somatic sensations and visual images (van der Kolk,
1994). It is known now, as we indicated in Chapter 5, that intense
emotions interfere with the functioning of the hippocampus and hence
with the integration of the associated experience into existing memory
schemas; instead, the memories of the experience are organized on a
sensorimotor enactive or iconic level, which could explain the emergence of somatic symptoms, nightmares, flashbacks, or behavioural
re-enactments in individuals with PTSD (van der Kolk, 1993, 1994).
Consistent with our clinical experience of the types of dreams reported
by many alexithymic patients, van der Kolk et al. (1984) found that the
traumatic nightmares of combat veterans with PTSD tend to be exact
replicas of actual events, suggesting a failure to psychologically integrate their traumatic experiences.

There is growing evidence also that the somatosensory memories of
traumatic experiences may be activated by arousal of the autonomic
nervous system. As van der Kolk (1993) explains, this is a form of
state-dependent learning in which the memories were laid down under
conditions of similar arousal. Furthermore, some patients with chronic
PTSD display abnormal noradrenergic neuronal regulation. The noradrenergic system is more readily activated, especially by circumstances that resemble the original traumatic event; this results in
secretion of noradrenaline and abnormal elevations of blood pressure
and heart rate. A high percentage of patients with PTSD experience

panic attacks or flashbacks in response to an ingestion of yohimbine, and the disorder is often comorbid with panic disorder (Southwick *et al.*, 1993; Tomb, 1994). There is evidence of effects on other stress hormones in the hypothalamic–pituitary–adrenal axis as well, including persistent low cortisol levels in individuals with chronic PTSD (Yehuda *et al.*, 1995). And although still somewhat speculative, serotonin, dopamine, and endogenous opioids are also thought to play a role in the arousal and affective disturbances that characterize PTSD (Charney *et al.*, 1993; van der Kolk, 1994). Kolb (1987) and Charney *et al.* (1993) have proposed that the acute neurobiologic responses to a traumatic event may lead to persistent changes in synaptic transmission in brainstem, limbic, and cortical brain sites that have a negative effect on learning, extinction, and stimulus discrimination. Recent research has found evidence even of a decreased size of the right hippocampus in individuals with combat-related PTSD that was associated with deficits in short-term verbal memory (Bremner *et al.*, 1995).

It is important to emphasize that, like Janet, contemporary theorists attribute the symptoms of PTSD to the persistence of intense unregulated emotions and efforts to reduce their impact, and not to the repression of undesirable wishes or impulses. Hence our distinguishing PTSD from other anxiety disorders and categorizing it (along with panic disorder) as a disorder of affect regulation. This conceptualization does not exclude the possibility that premorbid personality characteristics and background experiences might render some individuals resilient and others vulnerable to developing PTSD. Indeed there is evidence that only about one-quarter of people exposed to catastrophic stress develop PTSD-like reactions (Breslau, Davis & Andreski, 1991).

Although the results of a recent 50-year prospective study of World War II veterans confirmed that 'severity of trauma is the best predictor of who is likely to develop PTSD' (Lee *et al.*, 1995, p. 521), other studies have found neuroticism, dysthymia, a history of childhood separations, maladaptive coping mechanisms, alcohol abuse, borderline personality disorder, and individual and family history of psychiatric disorder to be significant risk factors (Breslau *et al.*, 1991; Green *et al.*, 1990; Gunderson & Sabo, 1993; McFarlane, 1988). There is evidence also that persons who are less educated and have personality traits of neuroticism and extraversion are more likely to be exposed to traumatic events, and thus may be at greater risk for PTSD (Breslau, Davis & Andreski, 1995). Krystal (1978*b*) and Frosch (1990) point out that the specific meaning of a traumatic event for a person also influences the outcome. Childhood anxieties and early traumatic experiences may be reactivated and associatively connected with a current traumatic event, and injuries to specific parts of the body may be more likely to evoke a traumatic reaction.

### Clinical illustration

Morgan, a young factory worker, had received plastic surgery on two fingers of his right hand after the tips of the fingers had been severed when they became caught in a machine he was operating. He was referred for psychiatric consultation because of a failure to respond to a rehabilitation program aimed at returning him to work. The referring physician noted that the patient was depressed and also phobic about ever using the same machine again.

When seen in consultation, Morgan complained of pain and partial loss of sensation in the two injured fingers, and indicated also that he sometimes experienced a sensation that the two injured fingers were missing. Despite the absence of any neurological abnormality, he claimed that he was unable to perform many routine functions with his right hand, such as brushing his hair, typing, or writing with a pen. He indicated that he was depressed and sometimes suicidal, and described difficulty falling asleep and staying asleep, as well as recurrent vivid nightmares in which he was reliving the accident with the machine. He had lost interest in activities that had previously given him pleasure including playing sports, reading, watching television, and going to the movies. The patient also reported that he had become forgetful. Although he tried to avoid thinking about the accident, distressing thoughts and images of the traumatic event often intruded into his mind. He vowed that he would never go near the machine again, and was very angry that his boss had insisted he use it on an occasion when he had tried to return to work.

Morgan described being chronically irritable and having frequent outbursts of anger; because of this, he had lost his girlfriend and most of his other friends, and was becoming increasingly socially isolated. Although he reported being tearful and 'fed-up' with not feeling himself, he was unable to elaborate further on his feelings of depression other than to state that his whole life had changed and that he could see no hope for the future.

There was no opportunity to administer any psychological tests to this patient. In the clinical interview, however, he manifested typical alexithymic features including a limited affective vocabulary, a lack of psychological mindedness, and an externally-oriented mode of thinking. He had no dreams or fantasies other than the intrusive nightmares.

### Empirical studies of alexithymia and PTSD

Several investigators have explored the relationship between alexithymia and PTSD. In some of the studies, however, alexithymia was assessed either with measures that have poor psychometric properties or with measures whose validity has not yet been adequately established. Consequently, although significant results were reported, some of these must be interpreted cautiously.

One of the first studies to examine the relationship between alexithymia and PTSD was conducted by Shipko, Alvarez and Noviello (1983) who administered the Schalling–Sifneos Personality Scale (SSPS) to a sample of 22 Vietnam combat veterans diagnosed with PTSD according to DSM-III criteria. Of these subjects, 41% scored in the alexithymia range of the SSPS; this rate was considered five times greater than the rate of alexithymia found in normal samples. In another study, Hyer et al. (1990) assessed alexithymia with the MMPI alexithymia scale (MMPI-A) and found that a group of Vietnam veterans with PTSD scored more alexithymic than a diagnostically heterogeneous group of psychiatric patients but were no more alexithymic than a group of alcohol abuse patients.

In addition to the self-report SSPS and MMPI-A, Krystal et al. (1986) used the observer-rated Alexithymia Provoked Response Questionnaire (APRQ) and Beth Israel Hospital Psychosomatic Questionnaire (BIQ) to assess alexithymia in separate groups of Vietnam veteran inpatients and outpatients with PTSD, a group of medical inpatients with somatic diseases traditionally regarded as 'psychosomatic', and a comparison group of psychiatric inpatients with a diagnosis of affective disorder. Consistent with the prediction that PTSD and 'psychosomatic diseases' are disorders involving deficits in emotional processing, the PTSD inpatients and the medical inpatients were found to be significantly more alexithymic on both the BIQ and the APRQ than the inpatients with affective disorders. There were no significant differences among the groups on the SSPS and MMPI-A; nor were there any significant differences between the PTSD outpatients and the affective disorder inpatients on any of the alexithymia measures. It is important to note that the BIQ, which is the most reliable and valid of the four measures, found group differences in the predicted direction.

The finding that the PTSD outpatients were no more alexithymic than the inpatients with affective disorders might be explained by the severity of the PTSD symptoms. Zeitlin et al. (1989), for example, reported that severity of PTSD predicted 22% of the variance in TAS scores in a sample of 25 male Vietnam combat veterans. These results suggest that the more severe the disorder the more likely there are to be disturbances in the cognitive processing and regulation of affects. In the study by Zeitlin and her colleagues, it is possible to calculate from the TAS cutoff score that 60% of the men with PTSD were alexithymic.

In a later study of victims of sexual assault, Zeitlin, McNally and Cassiday (1993) compared scores on the TAS of 12 rape victims with PTSD, 12 rape victims without PTSD, and 12 non-traumatized comparison individuals who were matched sociodemographically with the rape victims. Both groups of rape victims scored more alexithymic than the non-traumatized comparison group, but the mean TAS scores of rape victims with PTSD and those without PTSD were not significantly different. However, persons who had experienced multiple assaults were more alexithymic than persons who had experienced a single assault. The mean TAS score for the subjects who had experienced multiple assaults was above the cutoff score of 74 for alexithymia.

The chronicity of physical injury following a traumatic event has also been found to be associated with more severe disturbances in affect regulation. In a study assessing the relationship between alexithymia and trauma, Fukunishi, Chishima and Anze (1994) administered a Japanese translation of the TAS to 24 patients with burn injuries and a control group of 24 healthy persons matched for age and gender. Based on the time since the burn, 10 patients were considered to be in the acute phase (less than 4 months after the burn), and the remaining 14 patients were in the chronic phase (greater than 10 months after burn). The latter subgroup of patients scored significantly higher on the TAS than both the healthy controls and the burn patients in the acute phase. No significant difference was found between the healthy controls and the burn patients in the acute phase. Fukunishi and his colleagues also reported that, among the 14 burn patients in the chronic phase, 8 patients met DSM-III-R criteria for a diagnosis of PTSD and these patients were significantly more alexithymic than the 6 patients in the chronic phase without PTSD.

Overall, the results of empirical studies indicate a strong association between alexithymia and PTSD; in addition, the data suggest that alexithymia is influenced by the severity of the precipitating trauma, the intensity of the PTSD symptoms, and the chronicity of any physical injury caused by the traumatic event. The most obvious and immediate interpretation of these findings is that alexithymia is a state reaction to trauma, presumably a consequence of affect regression and a breakdown in affect regulating functions in an overwhelmed ego, as Krystal (1988) has suggested (see Chapter 2). Because of cross-sectional designs, however, none of the empirical studies addresses directly the question of whether alexithymia is a risk factor for PTSD or merely a consequence of severe psychological trauma. Zeitlin et al. (1993) found that repeated sexual assaults result in higher alexithymia scores, but they did not speculate as to why some of the victims of sexual assault in their study did not develop PTSD. Moreover, of the 12 rape victims who did not have PTSD, 8 had previously met the criteria for this diagnosis; this is a confound that further compromises interpretation of the results. None the less, the findings that not all sexual assault victims and victims of burn injuries develop PTSD support the idea of predisposing dispositions.

To date, there is only one published investigation of the influence of alexithymia on treatment outcome of patients with PTSD. Kosten *et al.* (1992) administered the APRQ and the Impact of Events Scale (IES) to 57 outpatient Vietnam combat veterans who met DSM-III criteria for PTSD. The IES is divided into two subscales that assess avoidance type and intrusive type symptoms associated with PTSD. The patients were entered into a randomized, 8 week pharmacotherapy trial of either placebo, desipramine, or phenelzine under double-blind conditions. All patients also received once weekly psychotherapy, medication monitoring, and symptom assessments with the IES. At the end of the treatment trial, 72% of the patients were reassessed with the APRQ. The results indicated that alexithymia was a significant predictor of treatment outcome, especially in the placebo group, but was associated only with changes in avoidance symptoms. A finding of no significant change in mean APRQ scores across the 8-week trial suggested that alexithymia was a stable trait in these patients.

## Somatic depressions

The criteria for a diagnosis of major depression in DSM-III-R and DSM-IV include vegetative symptoms as well as a depressed mood, a loss of interest or pleasure, and a preoccupation with thoughts of worthlessness and guilt. While an altered mood and negative cognitions are commonly present and are considered the main criteria for making the diagnosis, there has been repeated reference in the clinical literature to a type of depression with a primarily somatic presentation (Lesse, 1983; Lopez Ibor, 1972; Pinard, 1987). Over the years this type of depression has been given a variety of labels including 'depressio sine depressione', 'depressive equivalent', 'affective equivalent', 'hidden depression', 'somatic depression' and, most commonly, 'masked depression'.

Although the majority of primary care patients with major depression present to their physician with exclusively somatic symptoms, less than 10% deny any relationship between their symptoms and their emotions and fit a strict definition of masked depression (Kirmayer *et al.*, 1993; Kirmayer, Robbins, & Paris, 1994). The somatic complaints presented by this latter group are usually chronic, are sometimes described rather vaguely, and lead frequently to overinvestigation by physicians and to hypochondriacal concerns in patients (Katon, Kleinman & Rosen, 1982; Lipowski, 1990). Some of these patients present with headache, atypical facial pain, or some other chronic pain as their chief complaint, and others have symptoms involving multiple organ systems (Blumer & Heilbronn, 1982; Lesse, 1983). If they admit to experiencing anxiety or depression, they blame it mostly or entirely on their somatic discomfort and related concerns about their physical health (Lipowski, 1990).

While the affective component of depression is generally known to patients through the cognitive processes of perceiving, labeling, and giving meaning to subjective feelings, some non-Western cultures traditionally discourage and suppress the expression of emotional distress, and in others there are few words for describing internal emotional states (Katon et al., 1982; Lipowski, 1990). Leighton et al. (1963), for example, claimed that the Yoruba of Nigeria had no word for the feeling of depression and no concept of depressive disorder;[1] similar observations have been reported among Chinese people, who also may use words that function to keep emotions undifferentiated (Katon et al., 1982; Leff, 1973). In a study of 'neurasthenic' patients attending a psychiatric outpatient clinic in China, Kleinman (1986) found the majority had a major depressive disorder and all had presented with physical symptoms. Even in Western cultures, some families discourage the experience and expression of feelings, and some encourage minimization or denial as a way of coping with emotional distress (Katon et al., 1982).

Although some patients may be aware of a depressed mood and choose not to communicate it, and others may be limited by their language or cultural background, Katon et al. (1982) conclude that there is a group of patients who present with somatic depressions who seem simply to lack the capacity to perceive and label internal emotional states. Such patients are likely to be alexithymic and to selectively focus on the somatic symptoms of depression. Although there have been no empirical studies to date exploring the relationship between alexithymia and somatic presentations of depression, we report two clinical vignettes, one from the literature and one from our own clinical practice.

1. In recent years this claim has been challenged by Oyebode and Oyebode (1990), who note that the Yoruba language has several words both for anxiety and for depression, as well as different words for qualitatively distinct experiences of sadness.

## Clinical illustrations

Fisch (1989) reported the case of a 58-year-old woman with a masked depression and history of multiple losses, who scored in the alexithymic range of the BIQ. The patient had been referred for psychiatric evaluation after extensive medical investigations had failed to find an organic explanation for her three-year history of gastrointestinal and other somatic symptoms. Psychiatric assessment revealed that the patient had grown up in Europe, but at age 12, shortly before the outbreak of World War II, her mother had a sudden heart attack and died instantly in the patient's presence. During the war, she had to hide and was in constant danger of being found and deported to a concentration camp. Her sister was sent to a camp and died, as did most of the patient's other relatives and acquaintances. The patient emigrated to Israel after the war and had then been able to function normally because, as she stated during the psychiatric consultation, she had 'built a partition between [her] mother's death and [her]self' and later repressed the Holocaust completely and did not even dream about it.

This patient's somatic symptoms began many years later, shortly after the death of her severely handicapped and retarded grandchild and the subsequent departure of her daughter and son-in-law from Israel. Although she denied being depressed or emotionally distressed, she obtained a score of 23 on the Hamilton Rating Scale for Depression, indicating a moderately severe major depression. In clinical interviews, she showed 'a complete lack of emotional expression, both verbal and non-verbal', and a restricted ability to describe fantasies, claimed to have no dreams, and failed to see any connection between emotions and her somatic symptoms. According to Fisch (1989), 'her world was strictly cognitive and somatic, with no place for emotions' (p. 709). The patient was treated with antidepressant medication and had a favourable response; she became free of her somatic symptoms and even regained a capacity for emotional expression; however, her paucity of fantasies and dreams continued.

We describe another patient with somatic depression who presented in our own clinical practice:

Rod, a married man of 40, sought psychiatric consultation for a variety of somatic symptoms that his physicians were unable to explain despite exhaustive medical investigations. The symptoms had been present for over one year and included abdominal discomfort, pain in his left ear, an intolerance of noise, excessive sweating, a feeling of unsteadiness, parasthesiae on both sides of his face, a pulling sensation in his left eye, dizziness, diffuse muscle pains, fatigue, and a sense that there was something loose in his head. Rod feared that he had an undetected cancer. Although his father had suffered several heart attacks in recent years and died just one month before the patient was seen in psychiatric consultation, Rod claimed that he was not distressed by the loss as he had not been close to his father for several years. When questioned further, he acknowledged that he was sleeping poorly, had been occasionally impotent, and was mildly depressed, but he denied any change in appetite or sexual desire. Despite numerous stresses related to his mother and teenage children, Rod expressed little affect and admitted only to a 'shivering' sensation if he heard of someone dying. He did not recall dreams and rarely had fantasies.

Rod participated in one of our research studies and was rated as alexithymic on the BIQ by three experienced clinicians. He scored in the alexithymic range on the TAS, and had elevated scores also on the depression and somatic anxiety subscales of the Crown-Crisp Experiential Index. He was treated with antidepressant medication and supportive psychotherapy for over one year and gradually lost most of his somatic symptoms. His alexithymia did not change; indeed, it appeared to be a stable trait, as he had been known to one of us in a non-professional capacity 15 years earlier and was remembered well for his marked lack of psychological mindedness and rather boring communicative style that focused only on the details of external events.

## Affect dysregulation in primitive personality disorders

Over the past decade there has been an increasing interest in the genetic and biological substrates of personality along with research suggesting that the phenomenology of borderline and other so-called 'primitive' personality disorders is determined not only by personality characteristics linked to traumatic childhood experiences, but also by temperamental differences in affect and impulse regulation (Rothbart & Ahadi, 1994; Siever & Davis, 1991; Zuckerman, 1991). These temperamental dysregulations are thought to explain the affective instability and episodic impulsive–aggressive behaviours that are so typical of severe personality disorders, particularly borderline personality disorder, and that result in unstable relationships as well as self-destructive, sensation-seeking, and antisocial behaviours (Akiskal, 1994; Siever & Davis, 1991).

Evidence of a high comorbidity of borderline personality disorder and affective disorders led Akiskal (1992, 1994) to propose that a substantial proportion of borderline personality disorders are best conceptualized as 'subaffective depressions' with different types of temperament (dysthymic, irritable, cyclothymic, and anxious–sensitive) corresponding to different types of affective disorder. Stone (1988, 1993) also acknowledges a significant overlap between borderline personality disorder and affective disorders, but suggests that *hyperirritability* is the basic temperamental substrate for most borderline patients. While he refers to this disposition as the 'neurophysiological red thread' running through the borderline, and considers it a precursor of outbursts of inordinate rage and other impulsive behaviours, Stone (1988) includes early traumata among the factors that could dysregulate neural mechanisms and cause this hyperirritability. He notes a similar chronic irritability of the nervous system in PTSD, and reminds us of Kolb's (1987) proposal that excessive stimulation of the central nervous system caused by a traumatic event sets off reverberating circuits and lasting dysregulation of arousal.

Several other authors have explored the conceptual and phenomenological interface between borderline personality disorder and PTSD. Although the two disorders can be distinguished on the basis of clinical, longitudinal, and developmental histories, Gunderson and Sabo (1993) and Herman and van der Kolk (1987) point out that the disorders share major disturbances in affect regulation, impulse control, interpersonal relationships, and self-integration, as well as a propensity to states of dissociation. Gunderson and Sabo (1993) review a series of studies in which a large percentage of patients with borderline personality disorder reported histories of sexual and/or physical abuse during childhood; they note also that as many as one-third of borderline patients meet criteria for a concurrent diagnosis of PTSD. Even after allowing for inaccurate memories of childhood due to cognitive distortions, Paris (1995) concludes that 'the weight of the research evidence supports the hypothesis that abuse during childhood is an important risk factor for borderline personality disorder' (p. 15).

Thus, while there is increasing evidence that biological factors play a role in the etiology of borderline personality disorder, the histories of abusive experiences during childhood, which were reported originally by Stern (1938), but ignored for a long time by most psychoanalysts, indicate that developmental and intrapsychic factors also play an important role. Indeed, as Soloff (1994) recently suggested, 'there may be complex interrelationships between biologic and psychosocial traits, including possible "cause and effect" relationships' (p. 50). This view was advanced originally by Grotstein (1987), who regards borderline personality disorder as a disorder of self-regulation, and conceives of reciprocal influences between biological and psychological variables. Grotstein indicates that in addition to inherited variants of endogenous affective disorders, borderline patients exhibit psychic developmental deficits that may be due to faulty nurturing caregivers, a faulty inherent temperament, a lack of 'goodness-of-fit' in the bonding between infant and parent, and/or family psychopathology. The intense affective displays of borderline patients, their difficulty being alone, and their pattern of tumultuous relationships, suggest an anxious/ambivalent attachment style, which, as described in Chapter 1, is associated in childhood with unpredictability of maternal responsiveness; divorced from cognition, affective displays become a way of coercing others into making desired responses that will help modulate distressing affective states (Crittenden, 1994). Indeed, there is some empirical evidence that borderline personality disorder is associated with features of anxious attachment, but it appears that repeated frustration also gives rise to angry withdrawal behaviour (West & Sheldon-Keller, 1994).

In elaborating upon his view of the borderline as a disorder of self-regulation, Grotstein (1987) notes how such patients, 'failing in their capacity for normal self-soothing and soothing through object relations, must resort to drugs, food, or other devices to regulate psychic states' (p. 352). In a similar way, van der Kolk *et al.* (1994) propose that self-mutilation, which is very common in borderline patients, may 'be a way of regulating the psychological and biological equilibrium for patients in whom ordinary means of self-regulation were disturbed by early trauma' (p. 719). As will be described in later chapters, borderline personality disorder has a high comorbidity with substance use disorders and eating disorders, which we conceptualize also as disorders of affect regulation.

Though Grotstein (1986, 1987) refers to alexithymia as one of the developmental deficits underlying the regulatory disturbances in borderline personality disorder, there has as yet been no systematic empirical research exploring this relationship. In a sample of overweight women, Bach *et al.* (1994*b*) found in a series of stepwise multiple regression analyses that dimensional measures of schizotypal, dependent, and avoidant personality features, and a lack of histrionic features (i.e. negative $\beta$ value), emerged as significant predictors of alexithymia, as measured by the TAS. Future studies need to assess alexithymia in samples of patients who meet DSM-IV diagnostic criteria for borderline personality disorder.

Despite their proneness to chronic dysphoria and intense affect storms, borderline patients are capable of genuine affective experience and expression (Brown, 1993); one therefore might not expect them to manifest alexithymic characteristics in clinical interviews or to show a high rate of alexithymia in empirical studies. In the course of working psychotherapeutically with such patients, however, it soon becomes evident that there are fundamental deficits in affect tolerance as well as severe impairments in the signal function of affects and in the capacity to modulate emotions through the employment of neurotic defenses and mature coping behaviours. Indeed, on the basis of extensive clinical observations, Robbins (1989) has concluded that the phenomenology of primitive personalities should be understood 'in terms of arrested and pathological cognitive and affective development . . . rather than in terms of conflict and defense ' (p. 454). Among the fundamental characteristics of borderline and other primitive personalities, Robbins emphasizes an inability to form and sustain mental representations of affects, and a persistence of a preconceptual organization of emotions, the latter corresponding to the lower levels of functioning in Lane and Schwartz's (1987) hierarchical model of affect development. Robbins also elaborates upon the associated immature style of object relations in borderline patients, in particular the symbiotic attachments they attempt to form and how these are employed adaptively to stimulate more positive affects and to provide a sense of completeness.

Fonagy (1991), also writing from a psychoanalytic perspective, attributes the borderline patient's impaired mental representation of affects to childhood traumatic interactions with an abusive parent that led the child to defensively disregard perceptions related to the thoughts and feelings of the parent.[1] This strategy, which is a form of primitive denial corresponding to primal repression (Dorpat, 1985), protects the child from unbearable thoughts about the parent's wish to harm him or her. However, the disavowal of the mentalizing capacity results in a proneness to experiences of undifferentiated and poorly regulated affects, as well as to states of meaningless, chaos, and nameless dread, as the person is unable to reflect upon and think about his or her own feelings or the feelings of others. Emotions, uncontained by representations, demand immediate discharge through action; and thoughts and words may generate terror as they are experienced 'not [as] vehicles for encoding and communicating meaning, but [as] concrete implements of seduction, assault, manipulation and control' (Robbins, 1989, p. 446). Without a conception and the experience of a mind of one's own, and a mind in others, that thinks about desires, thoughts, wishes, and fantasies, the boundaries between self and other remain poorly developed and the borderline person experiences terrifying threats of fusion, abandonment, and loss of identity (Fonagy, 1991). As with other disorders of affect regulation, psychotherapy of patients with borderline personality disorders should focus primarily on the deficits in cognition and affect. Pharmacotherapy is likely to be a useful adjunct in managing the affective dysregulation of some patients (Soloff, 1994).

1. As noted in Chapter 2, Krystal (1978b, 1988) also attributes arrests in affect development to early psychic trauma.

# [8] Substance use disorders

Alcoholism and drug abuse are major public health problems in many countries. In the United States, for example, it is estimated that 8–10% of men and 3–5% of women abuse or are dependent on alcohol, and that 5% of senior high school students consume alcohol on a daily basis (Bukstein, Brent & Kaminer, 1989; Group for the Advancement of Psychiatry, 1991; Schuckit, 1986). In 1985 there were over 500000 known heroin addicts in the United States, 5 million people were using cocaine, and at least 7 million were regularly using prescription drugs, mostly addictive ones, without medical supervision (Barchas et al., 1985).

The economic, social, and health consequences of psychoactive substance abuse are enormous. More than a decade ago, the estimated annual cost of alcohol and drug abuse to the economy of the United States was $177.4 billion (Group for the Advancement of Psychiatry, 1991). Substance abusers have high levels of morbidity and mortality from accidents and diseases, and also high prevalence rates of psychiatric disorders. In addition, the violent or other pathological behaviour of many substance dependent individuals frequently has adverse effects on the mental health of their spouses or children. Added to these sequelae in recent years is the rapid spread of HIV infection among intravenous drug users. Consequently, there is renewed interest in the treatment and prevention of substance use disorders with much of the current research focused on elucidating factors that increase peoples' risk for developing these disorders.

The etiology of alcoholism and other substance use disorders is undoubtedly multifactorial involving hereditary or constitutional factors, as well as personality and sociocultural factors (Donovan, 1986). Exploration of all of these factors is beyond the scope of this chapter and we limit ourselves to the personality factors; in particular, we focus on personality characteristics that can be integrated into a conceptual model in which deficits in affect regulation are considered a central aspect of substance use disorders. Ultimately, however, a comprehensive theory of substance dependence must also integrate genetic and sociocultural factors and account for their interaction with deficits in the ability to regulate affects.


## Background

The idea of conceptualizing substance use disorders as disorders of affect regulation emerged gradually as empirical research failed to identify a personality profile specifically associated with alcoholism (Bell & Khantzian, 1991; Graham & Strenger, 1988; Schuckit et al., 1994). Although there have been numerous studies searching for a link between personality and alcohol and drug abuse, the only consistent finding is that antisocial behaviour beginning in childhood and adolescence is a predictor of alcoholism (Nathan, 1988; Vaillant, 1983). The finding that alcoholics tend to have elevated scores on the Psychopathic Deviate Scale of the MMPI that are quite stable over time (Graham & Strenger, 1988), as well as reports of a high comorbidity between alcoholism and antisocial personality disorder (Regier et al., 1990), also suggest that alcoholics are antisocial and manifest the traits of aggressiveness and impulsivity. However, a large number of substance abusers have never demonstrated antisocial behaviours in childhood, and many antisocial or conduct-disordered children never develop alcohol or drug-related problems as adults (Nathan, 1988). Furthermore, as Schuckit et al. (1994) point out, individuals with antisocial personality disorder are not very common and 85% of alcoholics do not meet the DSM-III-R criteria for this diagnosis. In a recent 10-year prospective study of 223 young men, which excluded individuals with antisocial personality disorder or any other severe personality disorder, Schuckit et al. (1994) found no differences on a range of personality tests between men who went on to develop alcohol abuse or dependence and those men who did not develop alcoholism.

Depression is also a trait or symptom that frequently accompanies alcohol and drug dependence. This is a complex association which we discuss further later in the chapter; evidence suggests, however, that depression is often a consequence of alcoholism and that antecedent depression is probably a separate disorder (Donovan, 1986; Nathan, 1988; Schuckit, 1986; Vaillant, 1993). None the less, in cross-sectional studies alcoholics and drug addicts generally score high on measures of neuroticism or negative emotionality, and presumably are more prone to both anxiety and affective disturbances; their initial motivation to abuse psychoactive substances may be to find symptom relief (Lodhi & Thakur, 1993; Martin & Sher, 1994; Sher & Trull, 1994; Tarter, 1988).

Based on Freudian instinct theory, the early psychoanalytic view of alcohol and drug addiction emphasized regressive wishes and the pleasurable aspects of psychoactive substance use. A deeper understanding of the personality and motivation of substance dependent individuals may be found in the contributions of Glover (1932), Rado (1933), and Fenichel (1945). Focusing on psychic structure rather than personality traits, these psychoanalysts proposed that compulsive drug use is an attempt to relieve dysphoric affects or states of inner tension that reflect deficits in the ego or the self. As Donovan (1986) has noted, however, psychoanalysis was slow to pursue further understanding of substance abusing patients, perhaps because of its lack of commitment to treating preoedipal pathology. Consequently, treatment with traditional psychodynamic psychotherapy, with its usual emphasis on interpreting drive-related conflicts and regressive longings, was generally unhelpful to alcoholic and drug dependent individuals (Bell & Khantzian, 1991; Frosch, 1970).

Since the late 1960s several psychoanalysts have made further important contributions to the understanding and treatment of individuals with substance use disorders. An important feature of the contemporary psychoanalytic approach is its emphasis on the addictive process rather than on specific symptoms or diagnoses (Goodman, 1993). Accordingly, it is assumed that there is a common psychopathologic process underlying substance use disorders and other compulsive or habitual behaviours such as gambling, anorexia/bulimia, compulsive running, and even compulsive sexual behaviour. In addition to compulsivity, these behaviours are characterized by craving and withdrawal, and by a seeming inability to control them (Bell & Khantzian, 1991; Khantzian, 1993).

The renewed psychoanalytic interest in the addictive process may be attributed to advances in psychoanalytic theory, in particular to the conceptualizations of ego psychology, object relations theory, and self psychology, which have made it more possible to use psychoanalytic therapies to treat individuals with preoedipal pathology (Levin, 1987). Informed by these contemporary psychoanalytic theories, and also by advances in the understanding of affect development, observations made during patient interviews and in-depth psychotherapy have provided clinical evidence that the addictive process originates in a disorder of the self-regulation system, with impairment in affect regulation and related difficulties in object relations as the most salient components (Goodman, 1993; Khantzian, 1993).

## Affect regulation failures in substance use disorders

In Chapters 1 and 2, we noted the important contributions of Krystal (1974, 1975, 1978b, 1988) to our understanding of affect development and how early psychological trauma, or deficiencies in early childhood relationships, can result in primary deficits in affect regulation that predispose an individual to substance use disorders or to other disorders of affect regulation. Even before the term 'alexithymia' was coined, Krystal and Raskin (1970) had described cognitive and affective characteristics among drug dependent and alcoholic patients that were very similar to the characteristics described by Nemiah and Sifneos (1970) in patients with classical psychosomatic diseases. Krystal and Raskin observed that drug addicts experienced their affects mainly in an undifferentiated, global, primarily somatic way, and that they had great difficulty tolerating painful affects. The addicts reported their subjective states in a vague and unspecific manner as though they were experiencing an undifferentiated form of common affect precursors, so that separate feelings of anxiety and depression could not be described (Krystal, 1962). The experiencing of emotions in a primitive sensorimotor form seemed to amplify the pain of withdrawal from a psychoactive drug, creating a dread of being overwhelmed by negative emotions and by an insatiable craving for the drug. Unable to verbalize affects adequately or use affects as signals to themselves, the drug addicts tended to become preoccupied in a hypochondriacal way with the bodily sensations that accompany emotional arousal and with a compulsive need to block them through taking the drug (Krystal, 1982). Krystal points out that without the cognitive aspect of the emotion (i.e. the meaning of the affect and some indication of the 'story behind it'), as well as the expressive component and a capacity for self-reflection, alexithymic drug addicts are unable to recognize that they are experiencing feelings and also are unable to identify them.

In addition to failures in affect regulation, Krystal and Raskin (1970) identified impairments in self-care and in the capacity for self-solacing among their substance dependent patients. Rather than viewing these impairments as deficits, however, Krystal (1978a) concluded that they stem from 'the "walling-off" of the *maternal* object representation, and within it the self-helping and comforting modes' (p. 224). This inability to exercise comforting, mothering functions contributes to the apparent need of substance dependent individuals to use drugs to obtain relief from distressing affects. It also explains the insecure but extreme dependence that many of these individuals have on other people, as well as their fear of exploitative intrusion by others.

In Krystal's (1978a) opinion, the 'walling-off' of the maternal object representation is a defensive manoeuvre against extreme aggressive impulses toward it. Associated with this defense is an idealization of an external object with which substance dependent patients yearn to be united, while at the same time dread being fused with. This psychodynamic is enacted in the addictive behaviour during which the brief period of comfort or pleasure after taking a drug is followed rapidly by dysphoria. As Krystal explains, the drug is used both as a pharmacological means to manipulate the individual's affective states and as a placebo to permit a temporary regaining of the self-caring parts of the self that have been split-off and attributed to the object representation. The eventual confrontation of the underlying aggression during psychodynamic psychotherapy is fraught with difficulties and requires special care and caution so that the patient is not overwhelmed by his murderous rage or by guilt.[1]

Other important contributions to understanding the association between affect dysregulation and substance abuse have been offered by Wurmser (1974, 1978, 1984), who described a breakdown of affect defense in narcotic addicts as well as *hyposymbolization*. This latter term encompasses a cluster of characteristics that are virtually identical to those comprising the alexithymia construct, namely, an inability to articulate feelings, the experiencing of emotions as somatic sensations (such as craving and physical discomfort), a constricted fantasy life, and a tendency to externalize. In Wurmser's (1984) view, individuals prone to substance use disorders have given up the ability to experience their own affective world as well as the ability to empathize with the affects of others. He suggests that 'they "learned" from their parents how and why not to use "empathy into feelings", not to accept emotions and conflicts, and how to cover them up' (p. 44).[2] Wurmser (1974) attributes the onset of compulsive drug use to an acute crisis, typically first occurring during adolescence, in which powerful underlying narcissistic conflicts are mobilized along with a flood of intense emotions like disillusionment, rage, shame, loneliness, anxiety, and depression. Because of a breakdown of affect defense and an associated hyposymbolization, such emotions are experienced as 'overwhelming, global, archaic, physically felt, [and] cannot be articulated in

1. One of us (Taylor, 1993b) has provided clinical evidence of such aggression and described some psychotherapeutic strategies in a detailed case report of a male patient who abused alcohol and manifested an encapsulated alexithymic sector in his personality.
2. As noted in Chapter 2, there are some preliminary empirical data supporting this view that the development of alexithymic characteristics is influenced by childhood environment, in particular by reduced family expressiveness (Berenbaum & James, 1994).

words' (Wurmser, 1978, p. 109). Wurmser (1974) proposes that this massive emotional disruption leads to a search for drugs, which are then used as an artificial or surrogate defense against the overwhelming affects. In his view, the states of craving described by drug addicts stem from the upsurge of archaic and disturbing emotions. At other times, drugs are taken to alleviate vague discomfort and tension, which is only dimly perceived as an affect and more usually attributed to something wrong either in the body or in the environment.

Dodes (1990) and Levin (1987) have also drawn attention to the narcissistic vulnerability of individuals prone to addictive behaviour. Dodes suggests that the initiation of, or relapse to, alcohol or drug abuse, in many instances, serves to ward off a sense of helplessness or powerlessness via controlling and regulating one's affective state. In his view, the drive behind addictive behaviour is narcissistic rage, the rage being a response to feeling powerless to control one's affective states, as well as an aid in restoring an internal state of mastery. Levin (1987) similarly relates addictive behaviour to a disorder of self- and affect regulation, including a need for power and control, which are sought through fusion with an idealized selfobject – alcohol or drugs – to which the addict has attributed omnipotent powers. Recognizing that addicts need to relinquish their grandiosity, Dodes (1990) and Levin (1987) note that the toleration of powerlessness and helplessness, and modification of the underlying pathological narcissism, are an appropriate central focus of the Twelve-Step recovery program of Alcoholics Anonymous and Narcotics Anonymous.

Based on his extensive experience treating narcotic addicts, Khantzian (1990, 1993; Bell & Khantzian, 1991) also has concluded that self-regulation deficits and a need for control are the core issues in patients with substance use disorders. Like the other psychoanalysts working in this field, Khantzian (1982) observed that addicts become dependent on drugs because of enormous difficulties in modulating, regulating, and expressing affects and drives. Addicts, he writes:

. . . suffer in extremes, their feelings being either intense, unbearable, and overwhelming or diffuse, confusing, or absent. Most of all, addicts suffer because their feelings are out of control, and they believe a drug or alcohol 'solution' to this state of affairs provides relief even at the same time as it perpetuates their suffering (Khantzian, 1993, p. 261).

These ideas are consistent with Wurmser's (1974) observation that it is both intense and painful affects and those that are diffuse, nameless, and elusive that are hard for the addict to tolerate. There is a paradox, however, in that while drugs and alcohol are used to relieve these states, the calming effects are generally short-lived with the outcome usually being an exacerbation and perpetuation of psychological distress (Bell & Khantzian, 1991). As Khantzian (1982) explains, the addiction–withdrawal cycle, especially with short-acting opiates, has a powerful regressive and disorganizing influence on mental functions; he suggests that this may be why methadone works better as it has a longer sustained action than heroin. Despite the paradoxical effect, however, addictive behaviour has adaptive value as it allows these individuals to 'substitute dysphoria and a relationship with suffering they do not understand or control for one's they do understand and control' (Khantzian, 1993, p. 269).

Like Krystal, Khantzian (1978, 1990, 1993) attributes problems in affect regulation to dysfunctional relationships during childhood development that have led either to an arrest in affect development or to regression to a more primitive mode of functioning in which affective experiences are not fully encoded in words. He emphasizes also the lack of self-care in substance dependent individuals, noting that they generally show an apparent disregard to a whole range of real or possible dangers to their well-being, including the situations associated with their alcohol or drug abuse. Paralleling Bruch's (1962) ideas about patients with eating disorders (which we discuss in Chapter 9), Khantzian (1978) challenges the traditional assumption that the lack of self-care shown by patients with substance use disorders is consciously or unconsciously motivated. In his view, self-care is a complex function involving several component ego functions including signal anxiety, reality testing, judgement, control, and synthesis (Khantzian, 1978). He proposes that these ego functions are impaired, deficient, or absent in substance dependent individuals. This proposal is supported by empirical evidence that certain ego functions are significantly impaired in addicts when compared with normal individuals (Bellak, Hurvich & Gediman, 1973; Blatt et al., 1984; Treece, 1984).

Whereas Krystal (1978a) employs psychoanalytic object relations theory in attributing the substance-dependent individual's lack of self-care to a 'walling-off' of the object representation, Khantzian (1978, 1993) links the deficits in ego functions to a failure to internalize them from caring parents during early and subsequent phases of development. In this conceptualization, he employs self psychology theory, in particular Kohut's (1971) view that psychostructural weakness in the addiction-prone individual stems from traumatic disappointments with the mother who,

> because of her defective empathy with the child's needs (or for other reasons), did not appropriately fulfil the functions (as a stimulus barrier; as an optimal provider of needed stimuli; as a supplier of tension-relieving gratification, etc.) which the mature psychic apparatus should later be able to perform (or initiate) predominantly on its own (p. 46).

Recognizing the narcissistic and borderline features in the personalities of many people with addictive behaviour, Rinsley (1988) also refers to a deficiency of soothing object representations that ordinarily enable people to monitor, modulate, and regulate the emotional vicissitudes to which they are subject from time to time.[1]

Whether it is primarily a failure to internalize self-regulatory functions, or a failure to locate these functions within the self-representation through identification with a 'good-enough' primary caregiver (or a mixture of both), psychotherapy with substance dependent patients provides clinical evidence that the attainment of narcissistic and emotional equilibrium may be facilitated through the establishment of regulatory selfobject relationships, and by confronting and gradually modifying the pathologic introjects that tend to destabilize this equilibrium. Certainly the success of the Twelve-Step program of Alcoholics Anonymous, as Bell and Khantzian (1991) comment, 'seems to be its capacity to provide a kind of new edition of selfobject experience . . . that allows the acquisition of tension-regulating functions through its unconditional acceptance, affirmation, mirroring, and opportunities for idealization' (p. 279). It is helpful to remember Grotstein's (1983) qualifying point, however, that 'what we internalize are experiences with objects, not objects *per se*' (p. 177).

The following case illustrates a pattern of substance abuse and style of object relating that is employed adaptively by many addicts to compensate for deficits in self- and affect regulation.

### Clinical example

Henry, a married man of 43, began abusing alcohol in his early teens and eventually became alcohol dependent. He also habitually smoked marijuana between ages 20 and 34, after which he regularly abused cocaine until 36 when he was successfully treated for his addictions at a drug and alcohol treatment centre. Although he had remained abstinent for over six years, Henry continued to regulate his affective states by an addiction to nicotine and by a pattern of engaging in multiple affairs with women. He declared that he does not fall in love with any of the women and that the affairs are

1. Consistent with these formulations of dysfunctional childhood relationships and defective object representations, researchers have found that substance use disorders are associated strongly with a history of childhood trauma including loss and separation, physical and sexual abuse, witnessing of intrafamilial violence, and emotional neglect (Triffleman *et al.*, 1995).

primarily sexual and usually of short duration. Despite claiming to have a desire to experience emotional intimacy, this was absent in his marriage and in all of his extra-marital affairs. In a consultation interview, Henry indicated that his father had been an alcoholic as well as a chronic gambler; he described his mother as a woman who never expressed emotion. The trait of alexithymia was suggested by Henry's acknowledgment that he generally had difficulty describing his feelings and that he rarely used his imagination or recalled dreams. These difficulties had been brought to his attention by his group therapist and by other patients in the group, as they reacted to his bland inner life and unemotional way of reporting current and past events in his life. Henry was able to indicate, however, that he was prone to feelings of shame and mild depression, and that he frequently lost his temper.

On the Beck Depression Inventory (BDI), Henry obtained a score of 20, which was consistent with mild depression. He obtained a score of 74 on the TAS-20, which is well above the cutoff score for alexithymia. In addition, the patient scored low on the fantasy subscale of the Openness to Experience dimension on the Revised NEO Personality Inventory, and very low on the subscale assessing receptivity to his own feelings. Also consistent with the concept of failures in affect regulation, (as well as the empirical research reported in Chapter 4), Henry obtained elevated scores on Neuroticism and the subscales assessing proneness to anxiety, depression, self-consciousness, and vulnerability to stress, and very low scores on the warmth and positive emotions subscales of Extraversion.

These psychological test findings confirmed the clinical impression that Henry was alexithymic, and had a disorder of affect regulation as well as a limited ability to establish intimate relationships. As McDougall (1974) observed in many of her alexithymic patients, the women in Henry's life were interchangeable and, along with the various psychoactive substances, functioned as external (selfobject) regulators apparently compensating for an absent or unavailable inner symbolic dimension. Such attempts to compensate fail to modify the structural deficits in self- and affect regulation, as Kohut (1977) also has commented:

> It is the structural void in the self that the addict tries to fill – whether by sexual activity or by oral ingestion. And the structural void cannot be filled any better by oral ingestion than by any other forms of addictive behaviour (p. 197).

## A self-medication hypothesis

Further support for a model that conceptualizes substance use disorders as disorders of affect regulation comes from the observations of Khantzian (1985) and several other clinicians and researchers (e.g. Milkman & Frosch, 1973; Pervin, 1988; Wieder & Kaplan, 1969; Wurmser, 1978) that the drugs that addicts select are not chosen randomly. Although addicts usually experiment with multiple psychoactive substances, the majority show preference for a particular class of drugs, suggesting that the specific pharmacological actions of the different classes of drugs interact with the dominant affects with which the person struggles.

In his early work with narcotic addicts, for example, Khantzian (1978, 1982) observed how dysphoric affects associated with restlessness, anger, and rage were relieved by heroin and other opiates. He began to suspect that opiates might be craved not for a euphoric effect, but more because of a direct anti-aggression action. On the basis of his subsequent experience, Khantzian (1990) concluded that the problem with aggression in opiate addicts 'is a function of an excess of this intense affect – partly constitutional and partly environmental in origin – which interacts with ego and self structures that are underdeveloped or deficient and thus fail to contain this affect' (p. 265). Such individuals are usually distressed, however, by the feelings of aggression and rage that often prompt them to engage in violent behaviour; they experience opiates as having a calming effect on these emotions (Khantzian, 1993).

While Khantzian was impressed by the anti-aggression and anti-rage action of opiates for certain individuals, other investigators had observed that opiates may be used to counter feelings of shame and loneliness as well as rage (Wurmser, 1974). The use of other psychoactive drugs also appeared to be associated with attempts either to counteract specific intense affects or to evoke certain pleasurable affective states. Stimulants, for example, such as amphetamines and cocaine, seemed to relieve states of boredom and emptiness, as well as the anergia associated with depression; in high-energy individuals, they provide a sense of aggressive mastery and grandeur, and in hyperactive individuals they have a paradoxical calming effect (Khantzian, 1990; Milkman & Frosch, 1973; Wieder & Kaplan, 1969; Wurmser, 1974). As one of our young alexithymic female patients stated:

> If I could have it my way, I would be stoned on amphetamines all the time. This is because I am then able to do things; I can write, gather my thoughts together, overcome my inertia, and no longer fret and experience the doubts to which I am generally so prone.

Psychedelic drugs, such as lysergic acid diethylamide (LSD), seem to 'counteract the emotional state of emptiness, boredom, and meaninglessness' and to create an 'illusion that the self is mystically boundless and grandiose' (Wurmser, 1974, p. 834). In addition to using amphetamines, our young female patient occasionally abused large amounts of psilocybin; this drug enabled her to transcend her depression and chronic sense of futility about her life by inducing an altered but pleasurable perception of her immediate environment.

In contrast to the modulating action of opiates, alcohol and sedative drugs (including barbiturates and benzodiazepines) have a disinhibiting or releasing effect on emotions, thereby permitting neurotically inhibited individuals to briefly overcome their social and emotional constriction (Khantzian, 1990). In Khantzian's (1993) experience, however, 'the majority of individuals who have become and remained dependent on alcohol or sedatives have struggled with more severe inhibitions and restrictive personality structures involving rigid and unstable defenses against narcissistic longings and aggressive impulses' (p. 264). For some individuals, alcohol allows feelings of closeness and love to be experienced briefly and therefore 'safely'; such experiences are normally prevented by the rigid defenses against aggression.

On the basis of published reports and his own observations that addicts tend to select a particular class of drugs, plus a small amount of supporting empirical data, Khantzian (1985) proposed a *self-medication hypothesis* that individuals are compelled to overuse and depend on alcohol or other drugs to manage painful affective states and related psychiatric disorders. He emphasized that individuals vary, however, in the degree to which their emotions are differentiated (Khantzian, 1993). While some addicts may be aware of feelings such as depression or rage and use drugs primarily to self-medicate their suffering, other addicts may experience their feelings as vague or diffuse and use the painful effects or after-effects of drugs to counter their confusion by introducing an interpretable and understandable form of suffering. Khantzian (1993) has observed that most addicts experience an admixture of painful affective states and confusion, and thus feel overwhelmed and out of control. As noted earlier, they cope with this threat by adopting a pattern of addictive behaviour with alternating states of emotional distress and relief of distress, which they can understand and control.

Further support for the self-medication hypothesis was provided by a study of drug abusers receiving treatment who were asked to generate a set of situations from their daily lives in which they used or wanted to use drugs and also a list of affects they might experience in association with these situations (Pervin, 1988). Results of a statistical analysis of the data from this study were consistent with the view that people use drugs to modulate distressing affects, that some drugs are generally associated with relief from specific affects, and that individuals establish a pattern of preferred drugs to manage unique constellations of distressing affects.

### Relationships between substance abuse and depressive and anxiety disorders

Our proposal that substance use disorders be conceptualized as disorders of affect regulation is supported by a consistent finding that, in addition to high levels of emotional distress, alcoholics and drug addicts show a high lifetime and current prevalence of other DSM Axis I psychiatric disorders, especially depressive disorders and anxiety disorders (Brady et al., 1993; Bukstein, Brent & Kaminer, 1989; Hesselbrock, Meyer & Keener, 1985; Khantzian & Treece, 1985; Sonne, Brady & Morton, 1994). What is controversial, however, is whether substance abuse is a cause or a consequence of these other disorders. Those who favour the former alternative, namely that associated psychopathology is caused by the use of alcohol or drugs, marshall empirical evidence to refute or minimize the self-medication hypothesis advanced by Khantzian (see, for example, Vaillant, 1993). Bell and Khantzian (1991) have responded by drawing attention to empirical evidence that supports both possibilities.

In attempting to resolve the controversy as to whether anxiety and depressive syndromes precede or follow substance abuse, some researchers emphasize the need to distinguish between the general dysphoria that usually accompanies alcohol and heroin abuse, and the presence of psychiatric symptoms of sufficient severity to meet DSM-III-R or DSM-IV criteria for diagnosing a coexisting major anxiety or depressive disorder (Schuckit, 1986; Schuckit & Hesselbrock, 1994). It is well established, for instance, that alcohol has a biphasic effect on mood. After a few drinks of alcohol people generally feel stimulated and happy, but these emotions tend to change to sadness and irritability as the blood level of alcohol is falling (Schuckit, 1986). During prolonged bouts of drinking many alcoholics develop clinically significant depression that can look identical to an episode of major depressive disorder, but the symptoms usually disappear within days or weeks of abstinence.

Studies of alcoholic patients and depressed patients also demonstrate that the association between substance use disorders and depressive disorders is complex and that the chronology of the disorders is sometimes difficult to determine. According to Schuckit (1986), 20% to 30% of severely depressed patients increase their alcohol intake, but only 5% to 10% of depressed patients with primary affective disorders meet the criteria for secondary alcoholism. In a study of 321 hospitalized alcoholics, however, Hesselbrock, Meyer and Keener (1985) found a current or lifetime prevalence of major depression in 32% of the men and 52% of the women; moreover, 41% of the male alcoholics and 65% of the female alcoholics reported their first major depressive episode as having occurred prior to the onset of alcohol abuse and/or dependence. Comorbidity rates may vary depending on the population studied, as well as on the family history of alcoholism and affective disorder. The general consensus, however, is that alcoholism and major depression are independent disorders and that reports of a high comorbidity merely reflect the high prevalence of both disorders in the general population. It is likely that substance use disorders and affective disorders are significant risk factors for each other, as well as manifestations of underlying disturbances in affect regulation.

The same conclusion may apply to the comorbidity between substance use disorders and anxiety disorders (Kushner, Sher & Beitman, 1990; Schuckit & Hesselbrock, 1994). It is well known that individuals who are withdrawing from alcohol develop an acute abstinence syndrome characterized by tremors, feelings of tension, restlessness and insomnia; this often is followed by a more protracted state of anxiety and emotional instability that sometimes includes phobic symptomatology or panic attacks (Schuckit & Monteiro, 1988). Such symptoms generally subside as the period of abstinence continues. There are several studies, however, that have reported high rates of substance abuse in patients with primary anxiety disorders including generalized anxiety disorder, panic disorder, agoraphobia, and social phobia (Bibb & Chambless, 1986; Chambless et al., 1987; Johannessen et al., 1989; Kushner & Sher, 1993; Quitkin et al., 1972; Weiss & Rosenberg, 1985). Although Schuckit and Monteiro (1988) attribute this association to the high rate of alcoholism in the general population, Hesselbrock et al. (1985) found that symptoms of phobias and panic disorder preceded the onset of alcohol abuse in the majority of alcoholics with these conditions. The hypothesis that individuals are motivated to use alcohol or drugs to seek relief from anxiety or undifferentiated emotional distress is supported also by a study in which 41% of American senior high school students completing a self-report questionnaire about drug use cited 'to relax or relieve tension' as a reason for their alcohol and drug use (Johnston & O'Malley, 1986). Moreover, in a survey of coping behaviour in over 1000 adults in the United Kingdom, 27% reported that they used alcohol and cigarettes when faced with an emotional problem or personal difficulty (Barker *et al.*, 1990). This is despite empirical evidence that physiological measures of tension and subjective feelings of anxiety are increased, rather than decreased, by even modest doses of alcohol (Schuckit & Monteiro, 1988).

Although there is some empirical support for the hypothesis that many individuals abuse psychoactive substances in an attempt to relieve dysphoric affects, the major support comes from patient interviews and individual psychotherapy. This is illustrated by the following clinical vignette.

### Clinical example

Robert, a 39-year-old married pharmacist, sought psychiatric consultation for symptoms that met DSM-IV criteria for a diagnosis of major depressive disorder. He had been treated for an episode of major depression five years previously, and his father and three siblings had been treated on various occasions also for recurrent affective disorders. During the year prior to seeking psychiatric consultation, Robert had become tense and anxious and somewhat depressed, and, in an attempt to relieve his symptoms, he began abusing alcohol on a daily basis and also self-medicating with increasing doses of diazepam. One of his siblings had a history of alcohol abuse in addition to affective disorder.

On psychological testing, Robert obtained a score of 29 on the BDI, as well as high scores on Spielberger's trait and state anxiety scales. A score of 89 on the TAS, as well as restricted affective responses and a paucity of human movement responses on the Rorschach test, indicated that he was markedly alexithymic.

Robert was offered outpatient treatment and advised to discontinue his use of alcohol. He was weaned from diazepam and treated with a combination of psychotherapy and a tricyclic antidepressant that led gradually to a resolution of his anxiety and depressive symptoms. Four months after commencing treatment, he was retested and obtained a score of only 1 on the BDI. Although his score on the TAS had decreased to 74, this score, as well as observations made during the subsequent course of psychotherapy, indicated that alexithymia was a stable personality trait of Robert that reflected a limited ability to cognitively process emotions and instinctual drives.

As has been reported in other alexithymic patients (Levitan, 1989; Taylor, 1987a), Robert's dreams revealed impairments in the symbolizing and defensive functions of his ego as it struggled to contain threatening affective and instinctual material. For example, several of the dreams he reported in the early months of psychotherapy included menacing images of Adolf Hitler and Joseph Stalin, as well as a vulture that was threatening to attack and already had human flesh in its beak and claws. The careful analysis of these and similar dreams, together with a modified psychotherapeutic approach to reduce Robert's alexithymia (see Chapter 11), led gradually to a higher level of mental representation of his own primitive rage and to an ability to imagine and tolerate fantasies involving the expression of murderous impulses toward a colleague who had exploited and offended him. Although the experience with the colleague, and other experiences that also had invoked narcissistic injuries, created inner conflicts for Robert, his alexithymic trait intensified the inner tensions associated with these conflicts and limited his ability to reflect and find satisfactory resolutions.

### Comorbidity with personality disorders

Although decades of research have failed to identify a single personality type that is characteristic of individuals who develop substance abuse or substance dependence disorders, investigators acknowledge that many addicts have one or more coexisting personality disorders. In a recent study of 178 alcoholics and 86 polydrug users, for example, DeJong et al. (1993) used structured interviews and found that 78% of the alcoholics and 91% of the drug addicts met DSM-III criteria for at least one personality disorder. The average number of personality disorders was 1.8 per patient in the alcoholic group, and 4.0 per patient in the polydrug group.

The most common types of co-occurring personality disorder depend on other characteristics of the patient sample being assessed, including whether the subjects were referred for long-term psychotherapy or hospitalized only for detoxification. Most studies of alcoholics and narcotic addicts report high rates of coexisting antisocial personality disorder, borderline personality disorder, and dependent personality disorder (Brady et al., 1993; Khantzian & Treece, 1985). In the study conducted by DeJong et al. (1993), however, a much lower rate of antisocial personality disorder was found among the alcoholic patients, which could be explained (as the investigators suggested) either by the sample being selected from patients referred for long-term psychotherapy, or by a short history of addiction, which provided less time to develop a pattern of antisocial behaviour.

The temporal sequences and causal relations between substance use disorders and personality disorders are complex and not yet fully understood (DeJong *et al.*, 1993; Gerstley *et al.*, 1990). Substance abuse itself leads not only to many antisocial behaviours, but also to disruptions of personality organization. Furthermore, as with the substance use disorders, there is a high rate of co-occurrence between some of the DSM-III-R and DSM-IV Axis II personality disorders and the Axis I anxiety and affective disorders. Indeed, it has been suggested that antisocial behaviour sometimes may be an expression of an affective disorder (Akiskal, Hirschfeld & Yerevanian, 1983). And, as outlined in Chapter 7, the behaviour of some individuals with borderline personality disorders may be an expression of, and/or an attempt to cope with, a temperament that produces intolerable affective states. The cyclothymic temperament, for example, is characterised by instability of mood and a high association with substance abuse, especially an alternating pattern of stimulant and sedative abuse (Akiskal, Khani & Scott-Strauss, 1979; Mirin *et al.*, 1991). This association is evident also in the adolescent cyclothymic offspring and juvenile kin of adults with manic-depressive disorder, who have been found to have a greater rate of polysubstance abuse than their counterparts with full-blown manic and depressive presentations (Akiskal *et al.*, 1985). These findings, as Akiskal (1992) has emphasized, support the self-medication hypothesis, in that individuals with cyclothymic temperaments appear to use drugs in an attempt to self-treat subsyndromal shifts in affect, energy, and drive.

The high rate of personality disorders found among alcoholics and drug addicts has led some investigators to question 'the validity and usefulness of the distinction between Axis I and Axis II disorders in patients with substance use disorders' (DeJong *et al.*, 1993, p. 92). Noting that 'the effects of the drugs used and the emotional and defensive states of the user become inextricably intertwined, each affecting the other in turn', Khantzian and Treece (1985, p. 1071) view the characterological problems as evolving concurrently with the substance dependency. These investigators consider difficulties in regulating dysphoric affects as 'a central causative feature' of personality disorders as well as substance use disorders, with the disorders themselves exacerbating the dysphoric affects.

When substance abuse is successfully controlled, patients may still show evidence of an associated personality disorder as well as compulsive behaviours that attempt to compensate for their alexithymic deficit in affect regulation. This is illustrated by the following clinical vignette.

## Clinical example

A homosexual man of 40, was referred for consultation by his psychiatrist, who had observed that the patient seemed to lack a language for describing feelings and to become confused by individual psychodynamic psychotherapy. Tony, as we shall call him, had a long history of alcohol abuse, but had been abstinent for two years as a result of regular attendance at meetings of Alcoholics Anonymous. He had also recently commenced therapy in a group for patients with borderline personality disorders.

Information obtained from the consultation interview strongly suggested that Tony was alexithymic and had difficulty in regulating distressing affective states. His emotional vocabulary was extremely limited, and he reported rarely having fantasies or recalling dreams. The few dreams he had in recent years involved mutilation of parts of his body, and had awakened him. Tony was able to indicate, however, that he was prone to depression and also to becoming enraged like his father. The usual outlet for his anger was to have a temper tantrum and to break something. When he was depressed, he engaged in compulsive homosexual activity, or alternatively he would masturbate compulsively, as he had done since childhood to console himself. He stated that he was 'addicted to sex'. Consistent with the diagnosis of borderline personality disorder, Tony described an instability of his own identity – for example, even in his longstanding homosexual relationships, he was often dissociated and confused as to whether he had become the other man.

Psychological testing yielded a score of 84 on the TAS, thus confirming the clinical impression that Tony was alexithymic. A score of 5 on the BDI and low scores on measures of state anxiety indicated that he was not currently anxious or depressed.

### Comorbidity with eating disorders

Consistent with our conceptualization of both substance use disorders and eating disorders as disorders of affect regulation, the literature contains numerous reports of substance abuse in eating disordered women as well as eating disorders in women classified as substance abusers (Holderness, Brooks-Gunn & Warren, 1994). The associations are much stronger in patients with bulimic behaviours than in those with anorexia nervosa of the restricter type. The high comorbidity is discussed further in the next chapter.

## Assessment of regulatory disturbances in substance use disorders

One approach that has been used to investigate affect regulating and other self-regulating capacities in patients with substance use disorders has been to assess their ego functioning using an Ego Function Assessment (EFA) procedure developed by Bellak (1984) and his colleagues (Bellak *et al.*, 1973). Guided by psychoanalytic ego psychology, these researchers defined twelve ego functions in operational terms and developed scales that are rated on the basis of information obtained from a semistructured clinical interview. Two of the scales are of particular relevance to studies with substance use disorder patients – Regulation and Control of Drives, Affects, and Impulses, and Object (or Interpersonal) Relationships.

In three separate studies, individuals who were addicted to narcotics showed major deficits in object relations and in the regulation and control of drives, impulses, and affects (Treece, 1984). Although addicts showed greater impairment of affect regulation in an intoxicated state, they still showed a severe lability or impulsivity in affect management in the abstinent state (Milkman & Frosch, 1973).

Another approach to assessing affect regulation capacities in narcotic addicts has been employed by Wilson *et al.* (1989). To avoid the potential biases of observer-rated and self-report measures, and to assess more adequately the preverbal manifestations of affect regulation problems, these investigators developed the Scale for Failures in Self-Regulation (SFSR), which uses responses to the nine standardly administered TAT cards (Wilson, Passik & Faude, 1990). The SFSR yields three factor scale scores – structural–non-verbal, thematic–verbal, and impulsivity.

To explore the issue of self- and affect regulation, the SFSR was administered to a control group of 25 normal subjects (mean age 22.75 years) screened for DSM-III-R Axes I and II diagnoses, and to an experimental group of 25 opiate addicted individuals (mean age 23.50 years) receiving treatment in a methadone maintenance program (Wilson *et al.*, 1989). The addicts scored higher than the control subjects on all three factors of the SFSR, especially on the structural–non-verbal factor. Although the addicts also scored higher than the controls on the BDI, the mean total depression score (12.87, SD = 9.11) was not very elevated and the correlations with the factors of the SFSR were not high. And whereas the thematic and structural manifestations of failures of self-regulation were significantly correlated in the control group, there was virtually no relationship in the group of addicts. These findings supported Wilson *et al.*'s (1989) notion that 'self-regulatory failures are not highly related to what is accessible to verbal encoding' (p. 397). The investigators concluded that:

> The particular items that load on the [structural–non-verbal factor of the SFSR] suggest that addicts, more than normal subjects, have particular difficulties in mapping their experiences temporally, with the attendant difficulties of lack of planning and poor anticipation of consequences; impaired and idiosyncratic notions of cause and effect relationships; poor impulse control and affect tolerance; a marked tendency to construe relationships in terms of either overt dependency on or exploitative intrusion by a need gratifier (p. 397).

Our own approach to assessing affect regulation capacities, and that of several other investigators, has been to examine the relationship between alexithymia and substance abuse and/or dependency in different populations. We will now review the empirical studies that have used this approach.

## Empirical studies

In an initial attempt to evaluate empirically the relationship between alexithymia and substance use disorders, a group of Polish researchers investigated a sample of 100 male inpatients with alcohol dependence using the self-report Schalling–Sifneos Personality Scale (SSPS) to measure alexithymia (Rybakowski et al., 1988). Seventy-eight percent of the sample were found to be alexithymic and patients with alexithymia did not differ from non-alexithymic patients in demographic factors and in the severity of alcohol dependence. No relationship was found between the presence of alexithymic personality characteristics and a family history of alcohol dependence (Rybakowski & Ziółkowski, 1990). This last finding contrasted with a result from a Canadian study in which Finn, Martin and Pihl (1987) found that sons of alcoholic fathers with extensive male-limited generational family histories of alcoholism had a higher level of alexithymia (also measured with the SSPS) than sons of alcoholic fathers without any family history of alcoholism. The results of these Polish and Canadian studies must be considered preliminary, however, given the psychometric limitations of the SSPS that were described in Chapter 3. Also, the Polish researchers did not indicate clearly whether their subjects were tested at the time of admission to hospital or following a period of treatment.

Further studies with substance dependent patients were conducted in Poland and Canada, and also in the United States and in other European countries, following the introduction of the Toronto

Alexithymia Scale (TAS). In Canada, for example, we investigated an inpatient group of 44 male substance abusers (Taylor et al., 1990b). Seventeen subjects had histories of chronic alcohol abuse, 5 had histories of chronic drug abuse, and 22 abused drugs as well as alcohol. In addition to a pilot scale containing items from both the TAS and the TAS-20, the subjects completed the MMPI, the BDI, the Michigan Alcoholism Screening Test (MAST), and the Drug Abuse Screening Test (DAST). The various measures were administered following a period of one to seven days of abstinence from alcohol and other addictive chemicals. Based on the TAS cutoff score of ≥74, 50% of the patients in this group were found to be alexithymic. The rate of alexithymia based on the TAS-20 cut-off score of ≥61 was 51%. The MAST, the DAST, and the MMPI MacAndrew Alcoholism Scale were used to measure the severity of alcohol and/or drug abuse. The results from these measures indicated that the alexithymic patients did not differ from the non-alexithymic patients in the mean severity of psychoactive substance dependence.

A similar rate of alexithymia (50.4%) was found in a sample of 125 male alcoholic inpatients in the United States, who completed the TAS following 1 to 21 days of sobriety (Haviland et al., 1988c). In a more recent study, however, Haviland and his colleagues (1994) found a lower rate of alexithymia in a sample of 204 substance dependent patients (84 women and 120 men) who completed the TAS-20 during their first week of hospitalization. Seventy-two subjects were being treated for alcohol dependence, 79 for drug abuse, and 53 for mixed alcohol and drug abuse. Although 41.7% of the total sample were alexithymic, the rate of alexithymia in women (50%) was significantly higher than the rate in men (35.8%). No comparison groups were used in the Canadian and American studies; however, the high rates of alexithymia found in the substance use disorder patients contrast with lower rates of 9% to 12% that have been found with the TAS-20 in normal male adult and college student samples and 8% to 12% in samples of normal female adults and college students.

Using a Polish translation of the TAS, Ziółkowski, Gruss and Rybakowski (1995) assessed 60 male alcoholic outpatients and found a rate of 48% of alexithymia, which was independent of age and the duration of alcohol dependence. The mean duration of abstinence in the Polish sample was 22 months (range = 1–108 months). Men with a shorter duration of abstinence (less than one year) had significantly higher alexithymia scores than men who had abstained from alcohol for more than one year. For comparison purposes, the rate of alexithymia found in a sample of Polish male college students (as measured by the TAS) was 8% (J. K. Rybakowski, personal communication, November, 1993).

Rather than using a clinical population, Kauhanen, Julkunen and Salonen (1992b) investigated a large community population of 2297 middle-aged men in eastern Finland and found a strong association between alexithymia and alcohol consumption. Although prevalence rates could not be calculated (because of a slight modification of the Likert scoring format in the Finnish version of the TAS), both heavy acute intake of alcohol ('binge drinking') and long-term heavy use of alcohol were related linearly with alexithymia scores. The proportion of men who reported either frequent intoxication or unpleasant after-effects of heavy drinking also increased linearly with alexithymia. Interestingly, the amount of cigarette smoking was also related linearly with alexithymia scores in this large population study (Kauhanen, 1993), although Lumley et al. (1994) found no association between alexithymia and cigarette smoking in university student and community samples in the United States.

In our investigation of substance dependent men in Canada (Taylor et al., 1990b), we selected certain MMPI scales to evaluate ego strength (the Ego Strength Scale), the use of repressive defense mechanisms (the Repression-Sensitization Scale), anxiety (the Manifest Anxiety Scale), introversion/extraversion (the Social Introversion Scale), depression (the Depression Scale), and the tendency to develop 'functional' somatic symptoms (the Hypochondriasis Scale). Consistent with the theoretical conception that alexithymia reflects a reduced ability to regulate and modulate distressing emotional states, the alexithymic patients (N = 22) were significantly more anxious and depressed than the non-alexithymic patients (N = 22) and they had more physical complaints and general psychological turmoil. In addition, the alexithymic patients showed significantly less ego strength and use of repressive defense mechanisms and were significantly more socially introverted than the non-alexithymic patients.

Due to the cross-sectional design of the above studies, it was not possible to determine whether alexithymia is an antecedent of substance abuse or a consequence of the disorder or recent abstinence. In our own study (Taylor et al., 1990b), however, the findings of lower scores on the Ego Strength Scale and higher scores on the Repression-Sensitization Scale[1] and scales assessing general psychological turmoil, are consistent with the view that alexithymia is a predisposing risk factor for substance abuse and that many addicts use alcohol and drugs

---

1. High scores on this scale indicate sensitization and low scores repression.

to compensate for defects in affect defense and in the ego's capacity to regulate and modulate emotions and drives.

As noted in Chapter 2, there are important theoretical differences between the alexithymia construct and the repressive coping style, which is a refinement of the repression–sensitization construct. However, studies with non-clinical populations have shown that both the TAS and the Repression-Sensitization Scale correlate negatively with the Ego Strength Scale and that high scorers on either scale (i.e. alexithymic or sensitizing individuals) typically report significantly greater levels of anxiety, depression, and somatic symptoms than low scorers (i.e. non-alexithymic or repressing individuals) (Bell & Byrne, 1978; Taylor & Bagby, 1988). Such findings suggest strongly that the higher levels of dysphoria and physical symptoms found in the alexithymic patients in our Canadian sample are unlikely to be a cause of their alexithymia but rather are a consequence of the ego's inability to modulate distressing affects.

The alternate view that many patients with substance use disorders develop a state of alexithymia as a result of severe anxiety and depression has been argued most strongly by Haviland and colleagues. In an initial study with a sample of recently sober alcoholics, Haviland et al. (1991) developed a causal model and found that scores on the TAS items assessing the ability to identify feelings or to communicate feelings (Factors 1 and 2) were predicted by depression. In a later study with a mixed group of alcoholics and drug addicts, who were tested within 3 to 7 days of hospitalization, Haviland et al. (1994) used the TAS-20 to measure alexithymia and again developed a causal model. State anxiety was found to predict depression and all three factors of the TAS-20; depression predicted only Factor 1 of the TAS-20. Based on these findings, the investigators concluded that in many substance dependent individuals alexithymia is a situational response to the distressing emotions that often lead them to seek treatment. In an earlier study with newly abstinent alcoholics, Haviland et al. (1988a) had speculated that alexithymia may be a defense against affective distress. As we have shown in earlier chapters, however, an association between alexithymia and negative affectivity has been found in non-clinical populations as well as in a variety of clinical populations; an association has been found also between alexithymia and the use of immature and maladaptive ego defenses (see Chapter 4). In our view, the presence of alexithymia in individuals with substance use disorders should be regarded not as a defense, but rather as signifying a deficiency in defense and a failure cognitively to self-regulate distressing affects. The apparent worsening of alexithymia when levels of anxiety and depression are high reflects the developmental and contemporary psychoanalytic perspective that personality organization is quite fluid, and subject to regressive and progressive shifts in the predominant mode of organization within the hierarchical models of affect regulation proposed by Lane and Schwartz (1987) and by Wilson *et al.* (1989).

There have been some preliminary longitudinal studies to explore the direction of causal relationships among alexithymia, substance abuse, and other associated psychopathology. In a pilot study of newly abstinent alcoholics in the United States, who were tested both before and after a 3 week period of treatment, Haviland *et al.*, (1988*b*) found no significant change in the mean TAS score despite a significant drop in the mean BDI score as the level of psychological distress subsided. Similarly, in a Canadian sample of substance dependent patients who were tested at the time they presented at a treatment center and again following a 4-6 week period of treatment and continuous abstinence, Pinard *et al.* (1996) found no significant change in mean TAS-20 total score and mean factor scores although there was a significant reduction in the mean total score on the BDI. More recently, Keller *et al.* (1995) found that the mean TAS score of a group of cocaine abusers remained stable across a 12-week period of treatment with psychotherapy alone or in combination with pharmacotherapy, but BDI scores decreased significantly over the course of treatment. Although these prospective studies are of short duration, the findings support the view that alexithymia is not merely a state phenomenon secondary to depression or withdrawal.

Further support for alexithymia being a stable trait in individuals prone to substance abuse is provided by studies of individuals who have been abstinent from psychoactive substances for long periods. We have already described the high rate of 48% of alexithymia found in a Polish sample of alcoholic men who had a mean duration of abstinence of 22 months (Ziółkowski *et al.*, 1995). Delle Chiaie *et al.* (1994) similarly found a high rate of 66.6% of alexithymia in a group of 87 young heroin addicts in Italy, none of whom was in an acute phase of withdrawal; the mean period of abstinence was 22.12 (SD = 8.25) months. Although affective distress may contribute a state-dependent component to alexithymia, the findings of high rates of alexithymia among addicts in a stable phase of rehabilitation programs and with longlasting abstinence strongly suggest an underlying trait structure as well.

Although difficult to execute, more longitudinal studies are needed, preferably with testing of subjects in their late teens or early twenties before alcohol or drug abuse or dependence develops, to determine whether alexithymia predicts their risk of subsequent development of a substance use disorder.

## Toward a comprehensive model

As we noted at the beginning of this chapter, our emphasis on alexithymia and failures in affect regulation is only one step in a field that is attempting to develop a comprehensive model that will successfully encompass the multifactorial, interactional nature of the etiology of substance use disorders (Donovan, 1986). The attainment of this goal is complicated by mounting evidence that alcoholism is a heterogeneous disorder, and by the probability that subtypes of alcoholism reflect different intensities and/or patterns of interaction among genetic, personality, and environmental risk factors (Buydens-Branchey et al., 1989; Cloninger, 1987). Although the relationship among these factors is likely to be complex, our proposal that alcoholism and other substance use disorders be reformulated as disorders of affect regulation provides an overarching concept that permits an integration of genetic, personality, and environmental factors.

It is important to remember, for example, that affect dysregulation can be a consequence of neurobiological and/or psychostructural deficits. Thus, while some individuals seem more vulnerable to alcohol dependence because of a genetically determined decreased intensity of reaction to modest doses of ethanol (Schuckit, 1994), they may also show neuropsychological deficits in language processing and emotion regulation before any exposure to alcohol (Donovan, 1986; Tarter, 1988; Tarter et al., 1984). Other individuals may be at risk because of an inherited proneness to affective disorders, or to an affective temperament which provides a substrate for the development of personality characteristics and behaviours that further heighten the risk (Akiskal, 1994; Sher & Trull, 1994). And, while deficiencies in an individual's childhood environment may result in the psychostructural deficits and difficulties in object relatedness that are often associated with substance abuse, inherited constitutional deficits influence the development of the personality both directly and secondarily through their effects on the primary caregivers within the family (Tarter, 1988; Thomas & Chess, 1977). The inclusion of hereditary and environmental factors, as well as alexithymia and other personality factors, in future studies using a prospective research design will lead to further elaboration of a comprehensive model, as Donovan (1986) has also noted.

# [9] Eating disorders

During the past 15 years, eating disorders have been the focus of increasing attention from both the general public and from medical and psychiatric researchers. While once diagnosed rather rarely, anorexia nervosa and the closely related syndrome known as bulimia nervosa are now commonly diagnosed and have become an important health problem in Western countries. Both disorders typically follow a chronic, frequently relapsing course and often lead to medical complications that produce significant morbidity and sometimes result in death. Indeed, long-term outcome studies indicate that up to 50% of anorexic patients relapse even after successful treatment in hospital (Hsu, 1980), and that between 5% and 22% of patients with eating disorders die from medical complications or commit suicide (Bruch, 1971; Deter & Herzog, 1994; Herzog, Keller & Lavori, 1988).

The extent of this public health problem is evidenced by incidence rates of around 1% to 2% for both anorexia nervosa and bulimia nervosa among adolescent and young adult females, which is the population most at risk for developing eating disorders (Crisp, Palmer & Kalucy, 1976; Drewnowski, Yee & Krahn, 1988; Fairburn & Beglin, 1990; Zerbe, 1992). Milder forms of these disorders occur in about 5% of the female population, although bulimic symptomatology may be reported by as many as 10% to 15% of high school and college-age females (Drewnowski et al., 1994; Herzog, 1991). There is evidence that the incidence rate of anorexia nervosa increased among females 15–24 years old during the past several decades; there has been no increase among older women, however, and the disorder remains rare in males (Lucas et al., 1991; Olivardia et al., 1995). Bulimia nervosa also occurs rather rarely in males, affecting approximately 0.2% of adolescent boys and young adult men; these individuals account for 10% to

15% of all bulimic subjects identified in community-based studies (Carlat & Camargo, 1991).

Although the past two decades have seen an enormous amount of research on eating disorders, still very little is known about the causes of anorexia nervosa and bulimia nervosa. As Goldbloom *et al.* (1989) have noted, most clinicians and researchers believe in a multifactorial etiology involving biological, psychological, familial and socio-cultural variables and vulnerabilities. In our view, these multiple etiological factors may be successfully integrated within a theory that conceptualizes the eating disorders as disorders of self-regulation, with impairment in affect regulation as the most salient component. We will attempt to show in this chapter how such a theoretical model can serve as a valuable heuristic tool to guide research efforts as well as treatment.

## Background

The idea that anorexia nervosa and bulimia nervosa are essentially disorders of self-regulation and affect regulation has emerged gradually as clinicians and researchers have recognized the need to revise earlier conceptual models because of serious limitations in their ability to explain the clinical features of the eating disorders and to devise effective therapies. Since Sir William Gull (1874) rediscovered and named as anorexia nervosa the condition that Richard Morton (1694) had previously described as 'a nervous consumption', many physicians have sought to understand the role of emotional factors in the pathogenesis of the disorder.

In an early psychoanalytic attempt to understand anorexia nervosa, Waller, Kauffman and Deutsch (1940) advanced a conceptual model that was derived from Freudian instinct theory and the classical psychoanalytic view of psychoneurotic symptom formation. Although these clinicians regarded anorexia nervosa as a paradigm of psychosomatic disorders, they employed a psychogenic, linear model of causality that closely resembled Freud's conception of hysteria. Like hysterical conversion symptoms, the abnormal eating behaviour and other symptoms of anorexia nervosa were given primary symbolic meaning and considered amenable to interpretation; conflict over unconscious oral impregnation fantasies was believed to be expressed through avoidance of food or alternatively through periodic gratification of the fantasy by binge eating, which generated feelings of guilt and anxiety.

Although other classical psychoanalysts later emphasized the importance of ego defects and the symbolic representation of preoedipal as well as unresolved oedipal conflicts through the illness (Mushatt, 1982/83; Sperling, 1978; Wilson, Hogan & Mintz, 1985), their psychotherapeutic approach to patients with eating disorders was mainly to offer motivational interpretations of the symptoms and abnormal eating behaviour, an approach that has still not been abandoned fully (see, for example, Schwartz, 1985).

A major critic of this theoretical conception and psychotherapeutic approach was Bruch (1973, 1982/83). Noting that treatment results from traditional insight-oriented psychotherapy were rather poor, Bruch concluded that the classical psychoanalytic formulations of anorexia nervosa were based mainly on observations of atypical cases suffering from conversion hysteria. Her conclusions were subsequently supported by Garfinkel et al. (1983), who used psychometric tests to document differences between anorexic patients and patients with conversion disorders. The latter showed fewer pervasive psychological deficits, their vomiting and weight loss were more likely to have primary symbolic significance, and they appeared better able to use fantasy and to respond to insight-oriented psychotherapy.

Bruch (1982/83, 1985) regarded the psychopathology of primary anorexia nervosa as different from psychoneurosis and more akin to narcissistic, borderline, or schizoid personality disorders. It was her opinion that the core problem lies in a deficient sense of self and involves a wide range of deficits in conceptual development, body image and awareness, and individuation. Bruch (1962) observed that anorexic patients manifest difficulty in accurately perceiving or cognitively interpreting stimuli arising in their bodies, in particular sensations of hunger and satiety, as well as fatigue and weakness as the physiological consequences of malnutrition. In addition, Bruch (1962, 1982/83) observed that patients with anorexia nervosa experience their emotions in a bewildering way and often are unable to describe them. In one case vignette, Bruch (1973) reported a male patient who 'seemed unable to identify the feelings associated with the physiological correlates of anxiety'. When asked if he had been anxious at his first day on a job, Bruch's patient 'denied this vigorously, but then added: "Why is my face so red and why are my hands so wet?"' (p. 254). As we have outlined earlier, such disconnection between the physiological and subjective feeling components of emotion is commonly observed in alexithymic individuals.

The lack of awareness of inner experiences and the failure to rely on feelings, thoughts, and bodily sensations to guide behaviour contributes to the overwhelming sense of *ineffectiveness* that Bruch (1973) identified as another outstanding feature of patients with eating disorders. Bruch (1962) observed that when the lack of body and emotional awareness is severe, patients may not experience their bodies as their own and consequently they suffer an overall lack of awareness of living their own lives. Anticipating the contemporary concept of disorders of self-regulation, she argued that the psychodynamic issues on which therapists usually focus represent the patient's efforts at compensating for these underlying deficits in the ego and the self. In Bruch's (1962) view, 'giving insight to these patients through motivational interpretations was not only useless but reinforced a basic defect in their personality structure, namely the inability to know what they themselves felt, since it has always been mother who "knew" how they felt' (p. 194). She advocated a psychotherapeutic approach aimed at increasing these patients' awareness that there are feelings and impulses that originate in themselves and that they can learn to recognize (Bruch, 1962, 1973).

Bruch (1973) also advanced a developmental model to explain the self and ego deficits she observed in eating disorder patients. In her opinion, *interoceptive confusion* is a consequence of consistently poor attunement between the innate needs of the child and the responses of the caregivers in the environment. The mother's misinterpretation of the non-verbal presymbolic communications of her infant, and the parents' 'direct mislabeling of a child's feeling state, such as that he *must* be hungry (or cold, or tired), regardless of the child's own experience . . . [leads] a child to mistrust the legitimacy of his own feelings and experiences' (p. 62).

Selvini Palazzoli (1971, 1974) independently arrived at a similar formulation that the main issues underlying anorexia nervosa stem from a *helplessness of the ego* rather than from conflicts over oral instinctual drives. Like Bruch, she emphasizes the lack of identity and sense of personal effectiveness, as well as an inability to recognize and distinguish different kinds of feeling states, impulses, and wishes. Selvini Palazzoli attributes these characteristics to the experience during childhood of consistently overintrusive parents who were unattuned to their child's actual subjective experiences and imposed their own personal and arbitrary interpretations of their child's bodily needs. Indeed, if impregnation fantasies are identified, Selvini Palazzoli attributes them not to unconscious sexual wishes toward the father, but to the patient's more primitive fear of being invaded by the mother. In her view, the anorexic patient perceives her own body as not belonging to her as she has completely equated it with the bad maternal object. The logical consequence is 'an attitude of mistrust toward the body, its stimuli and its needs' (Selvini Palazzoli, 1971,

p. 209). Selvini Palazzoli agrees with Bruch that psychotherapists must avoid making aggressive confrontations and giving motivational interpretations to eating disorder patients, as these merely repeat the insensitive attitude they experienced in past interpersonal relationships.

Bruch's ideas and also those of Selvini Palazzoli are consistent with findings from modern developmental psychology that have had an important influence on contemporary psychoanalytic theory, and helped shift the focus of interest from conflicts over libidinal and aggressive drives to ego functions and to the realization that personality development and the organization of innate neurophysiological structures arise out of the dynamic interactions between the infant and his or her primary caregivers (Taylor, 1987a, 1992b). As we outlined in earlier chapters, problems in affect development, which are associated invariably with the lack of a stable positive sense of self, can be linked to an absence from infancy of on-going positive affective exchanges with a caregiver who recognizes that the infant's emotions are signals communicating needs and satisfactions (Beebe & Lachmann, 1988; Osofsky & Eberhart-Wright, 1988; Stern, 1985).

In addition to individuals with acquired deficits in affect regulation, however, there are individuals with inherited deficits in neurobiological functions that may predispose to affective disorders or to variants of affective disorders. Acquired and/or inherited deficits may be involved in the genesis of the problems in emotion regulation that underly the eating disorders.

### Self-regulatory disturbances in eating disorders

In applying Grotstein's (1986, 1987) conceptualization of disorders of self-regulation to the eating disorders, we consider an impairment in the capacity cognitively to process and regulate emotions as the *primary* regulatory disturbance. This impairment, as we have just indicated, may reflect a constitutional–inherited deficit or be acquired through defective bonding in an inadequate nurturing environment (Grotstein, 1986). To compensate for the underlying disorder of affect regulation, eating disorder patients secondarily develop pathological eating behaviours which may lead to disordered weight regulation and other physiological disturbances. A variety of impulsive behaviours not related to food but often accompanying eating disorders (including substance abuse, promiscuity, and stealing) are also viewed as defensive reparative manoeuvres to regulate dysphoric affects.

Engaged in a relentless pursuit of thinness, patients with anorexia nervosa may lose weight only by restricting food intake (the 'restricter' subtype), or they may also periodically gorge and then lose weight by vomiting and/or purging (the 'bulimic' subtype) (Garfinkel & Garner, 1982). Patients with bulimia nervosa also engage in recurrent binge eating, but they maintain a normal body weight by vomiting, abusing purgatives, or engaging in vigorous exercise. However, like patients with anorexia nervosa, they manifest a morbid dread of fatness and many have a history of a previous episode of anorexia nervosa (Russell, 1985). A family and personal history of obesity is also common in patients with bulimia nervosa (Fairburn & Cooper, 1984a). And some obese individuals manifest bulimic behaviour (Marcus & Wing, 1987; Specker et al., 1994).

Thus, there is a spectrum of pathological eating behaviours and disturbances in weight regulation. However, the range of abnormal eating behaviours and variety of other symptoms associated with eating disorders all serve to screen the underlying disturbance in affect regulation. As Grotstein (1986) suggests, the symptoms offer 'a makeshift "floor" under, or container around, a fragmenting self to protect it from disintegrating catastrophe' (p. 104).

Several experts in the field of eating disorders have proposed similar formulations in which abnormal eating behaviours and associated symptomatology are seen as attempts to re-establish a form of self-regulation of unpleasant emotional states and other aspects of the self. According to Goodsitt (1983), for example, patients with eating disorders have severe deficits in self-organization and self-regulation and are subject to profound states of overstimulation and tension. In his view:

> They attempt to drown out these anguished feelings by frantic self-stimulatory activities. This is the common denominator to such behaviours as starvation, bingeing, vomiting, and hyperactivity. The symptoms are misguided attempts to organize affects and internal states meaningfully (p. 59).

Swift and Letven (1984) offer a similar formulation of bulimia nervosa based on Balint's (1968) concept of the 'basic fault' and Kohut's concept of disorders of the self (Kohut & Wolf, 1978). In Swift and Letven's view, severe bulimics demonstrate a 'basic fault' in their ego, specifically an impairment in functions that regulate tension. Unable to insulate themselves against overstimulation, and without the ability to soothe themselves, bulimic patients are considered prone to intolerable internal tension and a sense of deadness or emptiness pervading their inner worlds. The typical bulimic sequence of restrictive dieting, bingeing, vomiting, relaxation, and repudiation (or variations of this sequence) is conceptualized by Swift and Letven as a defensive reparative attempt to alleviate internal tension and to bridge the underlying ego defects, thereby temporarily consolidating the sense of self.

In an earlier contribution concerning psychological processes in anorexia nervosa and bulimia, Casper (1983) also makes the point that 'food and physiological processes become perversely employed to regulate emotions' (p. 390). Addressing the preoccupation of these patients with body size, Casper observes that anorexic patients, at moments of emotional tension and distress, immediately shift to a cognitive mode in which the overvalued idea 'I must not be fat' and other self-directing and self-appraising thoughts dominate and serve to regulate the affective states 'with a thin body bearing testimony to superb self-control and equanimity' (p. 390). Casper suggests that, in bulimic patients, this cognitive ideational mechanism partially fails and, in the end, becomes subservient to a bingeing–vomiting sequence. Although this sequence is initially employed to control weight and as such is under the patient's volitional command, it evolves over time into a compulsive defensive mechanism for regulating and alleviating intolerable affect and tension states. Thus, as Casper (1983) insightfully comments, anorexic patients consolidate their self experience by abstaining from food. And while bulimic patients experience comforting and a brief tension-alleviating effect during the act of overeating, the ensuing shame leads to vomiting as 'the last step in an attempt to regain a sense of self by overcoming the dependence on food through expelling and rejecting it' (pp. 391–392).

Lacking adequate self-regulating psychic structure, individuals prone to eating disorders are unduly influenced by external factors such as cultural ideals in determining their body image and thereby consolidating their self experience. Typically, they impose on themselves an ideal body weight which is somewhat lower than their optimum or 'healthy' weight and is based on the contemporary depiction in Western cultures that femininity, popularity, and success are associated with an ectomorphic physique (Nasser, 1988; Striegel-Moore, Silberstein & Rodin, 1986). The fact that the culturally determined ideal body type for men is the muscular mesomorphic physique is considered at least a partial explanation for the low prevalence of bulimia nervosa and anorexia nervosa among males (Carlat & Camargo, 1991). There are reports, however, that athletic men (and women) who engage in habitual running resemble anorexic women in terms of personality characteristics (Yates, Leehey & Shisslak, 1983), and use running as a way of regulating emotional states (Blumenthal, Rose & Chang, 1985).

Some empirical support for the conceptualization of bulimia nervosa as a disorder of self- and affect regulation was provided in a recent study by Schupak-Neuberg and Nemeroff (1993), who demonstrated that bulimic subjects report greater amounts of identity confusion, enmeshment, and overall instability in self-concept than normal controls and binge eaters (defined in the study as individuals who report one or more binges per week but who fail to meet other criteria for bulimia nervosa). For the bulimic subjects, binge eating served as an escape from self-awareness and purging was used to regulate negative affects.

Several other studies have also demonstrated that a major precipitant to bingeing is negative emotional states and that bingeing, vomiting, and purging serve the function of attempting to modulate dysphoric and fluctuating mood states (Abraham & Beaumont, 1982; Kaye et al., 1986; Johnson & Connors, 1987; Johnson & Larson, 1982; Leon et al., 1985). Abraham and Beaumont (1982) found that 34% of patients obtained relief from anxiety during episodes of bingeing and 66% reported freedom from anxious feelings after each episode of bingeing had concluded. Kaye et al. (1986) similarly found that 50% of patients reported decreased anxiety during bingeing and 67% after bingeing. However, while a reduction in anxiety or tension often occurs during or immediately after bingeing and vomiting, these behaviours are not effective mood elevators as many patients experience a general worsening of affective state in terms of greater guilt, shame, depression, and anger (Johnson & Larson, 1982). This worsening occurs during the repudiation phase of the bulimic sequence, described by Swift and Letven (1984), in which patients promise to themselves that they will not engage in any future episodes of bingeing and purging.

### Impulsivity

As noted earlier, many patients with eating disorders, especially those with bulimia nervosa, also manifest impulsive behaviours not related to food including repeated self-harm, alcohol or drug abuse, multiple overdoses, sexual disinhibition, and shoplifting. When 39 bulimic patients and 25 anorexic patients were interviewed about impulsive behaviours other than bingeing, 51% of the bulimic patients and 28% of the anorexic patients reported at least one other impulsive behaviour – usually self-harm or alcohol or drug abuse (Fahy & Eisler, 1993). In a study of 112 normal-weight bulimic women all stemming from the same urban British catchment area, Lacey (1993) found that 40% reported self-damaging and addictive behaviour, 80% of whom gave a history of three or more impulsive behaviours together. Clinical interviews revealed that the patterns of impulsive behaviour fluctuated and were usually interchangeable, and that each behaviour was associated with a similar sense of being out of control. The patients' descriptions suggested that the behaviours usually had the function of reducing or blocking unpleasant or distressing affects.

Although Lacey (1993; Lacey & Evans, 1986) has argued that there is a distinct subgroup of bulimic patients with an underlying multi-impulsive personality disorder, he acknowledges that this may be a variant of borderline personality disorder, which often is associated with impulsive self-harm, substance abuse, affective disorders, and eating disorders (Sansone et al., 1989; Skodol et al., 1993). (As we indicated in Chapter 7, the borderline personality disorders have also been conceptualized by Grotstein (1987) and others as disorders of self-regulation arising on a substrate of affective dysregulation.) Furthermore, a recent study employing multiple measures found that depression, impulsivity, obsessionality, and dyscontrol were all elevated in patients with bulimia nervosa (Newton, Freeman & Munro, 1993). This is not a contradictory finding, but is in keeping with the hypothesis that 'the problem in bulimia nervosa is one of brittle hypercontrol, so that obsessional hyper- and hypo-control are present in the same individual' (Newton et al., 1993, p. 393). Indeed, consistent with our concept of disorders of self- and affect regulation, Sohlberg (1991) suggests that the underlying abnormality is an inability to regulate impulses flexibly; Fahy and Eisler (1993) suggest that the so-called impulsive behaviours arise from an affective disturbance rather than from an underlying disorder of impulse control.

### Comorbidity with substance use disorders

As we noted in Chapter 8, there is a high comorbidity between eating disorders and substance use disorders. Many investigators have reported a high prevalence of alcohol and/or drug abuse among patients with bulimia nervosa, and some have noted that patients with anorexia nervosa are also prone to alcohol abuse (Cantwell et al., 1977; Casper et al., 1980; Crisp, 1968; Henzel, 1984; Jones, Cheshire & Moorhouse, 1985; Hatsukami et al., 1984; Lacey, 1993). In a recent survey of various published studies, Holderness et al. (1994) reported that the prevalence of substance abuse has been found to range from 2.9% to 55% in bulimic populations, and from 6% to 13% in patients with anorexia nervosa.

Studies of individuals with substance use disorders have also re-vealed a high co-occurrence of eating disorders. In a survey of 259 cocaine abusers, for example, Jonas et al. (1987) found that 32% met DSM-III criteria for either anorexia nervosa, bulimia nervosa, or both. And in a recent study in Japan of 50 young women with a diagnosis of either alcohol abuse or alcohol dependence, Higuchi et al. (1993) found that 29 of the women (58%) had eating disorders. Almost all of them had bulimia nervosa, but many had started with anorexia nervosa. The eating disorders usually preceded, and were not replaced by, the development of alcoholism. When compared with young alcoholic women who did not have eating disorders, those with eating disorders experienced significantly more major depression and almost two-thirds (62%) had borderline personality disorders (Suzuki et al., 1993). Some studies have also reported a significantly higher rate of alcohol-ism in the first- and second-degree relatives of bulimic subjects than in the relatives of control subjects, suggesting a genetic predisposition for these disorders (Bulik, 1987).

The high comorbidity of eating disorders and substance use disor-ders is not surprising given our thesis of a similar underlying deficit in affect regulation. Substance abuse and/or abnormal eating behaviours may be employed by patients in an attempt to surmount the profound distress caused by deficits in their self-regulating capacities. Although patients with bulimia nervosa abuse alcohol and drugs more frequently than patients with anorexia nervosa, some eating disorders experts have noted that much of the behaviour associated with anorexia nervosa is similar to that observed in the addictive disorders, and they have even made a case for viewing anorexia nervosa as an 'addiction to starvation' (Luby, Marrazzi & Sperti, 1987; Szmukler & Tantam, 1984). Such a proposal suggests the need for treatment modalities similar to those used for other dependence disorders.

## Relationship with affective disorders

Depressive and anxiety symptoms are common in patients with eating disorders. There is continuing debate, however, over whether the association of such symptoms with anorexia or bulimia is coincidental or causative (Levy, Dixon & Stern, 1989; Swift, Andrews & Barklage, 1986). While some investigators regard anorexia nervosa and bulimia nervosa as distinct entities (Altshute & Weiner, 1985; Levy et al., 1989; Strober & Katz, 1987), others have suggested that the eating disorders may be variants of affective disorders (Cantwell et al., 1977; Hudson,

Laffer & Pope, 1982). The latter opinion is supported by the frequent finding of a concomitant family history of affective disorder (Cantwell *et al.*, 1977; Hudson *et al.*, 1982; Strober *et al.*, 1982), by a reduction in binge eating that sometimes occurs in response to antidepressant medications (Brotman, Herzog & Woods, 1984; Pope *et al.*, 1983; Walsh *et al.*, 1982), and by a high lifetime prevalence of affective and anxiety disorders.

In a long-term follow-up study of 55 Canadian patients with anorexia nervosa, 60% had a lifetime diagnosis of major depression and/or anxiety disorder as opposed to 12% of an age- and sex-matched normal control group (Toner, Garfinkel & Garner, 1986). Recognizing that this study did not separate the anorexic patients into those who were recovered from those who were not, Hsu, Crisp and Callender (1992) conducted a pilot follow-up study in the United Kingdom and confirmed that chronic eating disorders are often associated with depressive and anxiety disorders; and that anorexia nervosa patients are more likely than members of the general population to develop a major depressive illness whether or not they have recovered from their eating disorder.

Critics of the idea that eating disorders are variants of affective disorders correctly argue that positive family history studies should be evaluated cautiously because of an absence of normal control groups and because interviewers were not blind to diagnoses of the eating disorder subjects (Levy *et al.*, 1989). In addition, a favourable response to antidepressant medication alone is not an adequate basis for inclusion in one diagnostic category or another (Swift *et al.*, 1986). However, whether or not major depression and the eating disorders are distinct entities, the strong association of eating disorders with anxiety and depressive symptoms is consistent with our view that the syndromes of anorexia nervosa and bulimia nervosa comprise symptom and behaviour complexes that have developed secondarily in an attempt to manage dysphoric affects.

Although the neurochemistry of the eating disorders is still poorly understood, the neurotransmitters and neuromodulators that regulate eating behaviour also provide important neural substrates for the regulation of anxiety and mood (Fava *et al.*, 1989; Jimerson *et al.*, 1990). Given the complex feedback loops between the networks of different neural systems, dysregulation in any one system will also influence the functioning of all other systems (Dubovsky & Thomas, 1995b; Weiner, 1989). The nature and intensity of the symptoms of anxiety and depression that accompany the eating disorders may vary depending on the neurotransmitter systems most affected; in turn, this variation may contribute to the heterogeneity of the eating disorders (Garfinkel, Moldofsky & Garner, 1980).

Patients with eating disorders may also experience alterations of mood secondary to malnutrition (Laessle, Schweiger & Pirke, 1988; Swift *et al.*, 1986) or as a consequence of bingeing and vomiting (Johnson-Sabine, Wood & Wakeling, 1984). These dysphoric mood states have been conceptualized as side-effects of the pathological behaviours employed by the patients to treat as best they can the underlying deficits in self- and affect regulation (Grotstein, 1987). Such mood states are thought to serve as a sustaining variable that perpetuates and exacerbates the basic disorder of regulation, and also may worsen the eating disorder, thereby establishing a vicious circle (Swift *et al.*, 1986).

## Object relations and ego functions

In earlier chapters we indicated some of the important ways in which developmental psychology and attachment theory have increased our understanding of the role of early family relationships in affect development and in the acquisition of self-regulatory capacities. We also outlined some of the consequences of deficient early relationships and faulty attachment patterns, in particular the failure to fully desomatize and differentiate affects and to achieve the Kleinian 'depressive position' (Segal, 1964; Stein, 1990) of stable self- and object representations.

Although many investigators have traced anorexia nervosa and bulimia nervosa to pathogenic early mother–child relationships, these disorders are clearly heterogeneous and present with varying degrees of severity suggesting different degrees and levels of developmental pathology. Indeed, some investigators identify subtypes on the basis of different personality features and different degrees of ego strength and levels of object-relating. For example, Sours (1980), Mushatt (1982/83), and Masterson (1977) each distinguish between anorexic patients who are more like psychoneurotic patients and anorexic patients who are more like patients with borderline personality disorders. They attribute these differences to different degrees of failure in resolving the developmental task of separation–individuation. The neurotic anorexics are arrested in the final subphase of separation–individuation on the way to libidinal object constancy. They have difficulty entering the second individuation phase during adolescence because of anxieties over sexuality, but their defensive regression does not lead to a loss of self-object differentiation. The borderline anorexics, who form a larger group, are arrested in the symbiotic phase or in an early separation–individuation subphase, and are therefore prone to separation anxiety, abandonment depression, and fusion with the primary infantile object (Taylor, 1987a).

Recent empirical research that analyzed a number of thoroughly assessed ego functions confirmed that there is a continuum of ego functioning among eating disordered patients and that this is unrelated to the eating disorder diagnoses and the restrictor/bulimic distinction (Norring et al., 1989). The investigators identified four clusters that reflected level differences within this continuum – higher neurotic, lower neurotic, borderline, and borderline-psychotic. Not surprisingly, interpersonal relations were found to be a greater problem for patients in the borderline clusters than for the higher neurotic patients.

The ability of 'borderline' eating disorder patients to form symbols and to think abstractly is limited, as is their ability to soothe themselves by way of inner psychological resources (Silver, Glassman & Cardish, 1988). Prone to both claustrophobic and agoraphobic anxieties, these patients oscillate between closeness and distance in their object relationships (Steiner, 1979) and are unable to establish the interactional regulation that is characteristic of mature adult relationships (Taylor, 1987a). Deprived of soothing from intimate interpersonal relations or from inner resources, they may resort to binge eating or substance abuse as a primitive and concrete way of filling the emptiness they experience within themselves. The affective and interpersonal instability of eating disorder patients with borderline personality disturbances are predictive of a poorer treatment outcome (Wonderlich et al., 1994).

Observations of the families of eating disorder patients yield some clues to the pathogenesis of these disorders as they commonly indicate patterns of enmeshment (in which family members intrude on each other's thoughts and feelings), overprotectiveness (an intrusive concern about the child's psychological and bodily functioning), lack of conflict resolution, and involvement of the child in conflict between the parents (Minuchin, Rosman & Baker, 1978; Selvini Palazzoli, 1974). These patterns of object relating all interfere with self-object differentiation and the achievement of autonomous functioning.

When the mother has misread the affect signals and failed to attend to the needs of the child, and instead fulfilled her own needs through the child, the patient-to-be feels totally responsible for fulfilling her mother's needs and is unable to experience her body as her own (Zerbe, 1993). In her attempts to achieve a degree of autonomy, the anorexic patient starves her body 'as a way of killing off the maternal object from whom she wishes to emancipate herself' (Zerbe, 1993, p. 167). As

Selvini Palazzoli (1974) posits, the patient experiences her body concretely as a persecutory maternal object which must be controlled at all costs. Although Sugarman and Kurash (1982) have proposed that the bulimic patient also uses her body to play out her unresolved conflict over individuation and separation from the maternal object, they incorrectly conceptualize the body as a transitional object representing the mother. Given that these authors postulate an arrest in the bulimic patient during a presymbolic stage of development, neither self nor object can be represented symbolically in the body; rather, the body is concretely equated with the mother and used as a 'sensation object', as one of us outlined in an earlier contribution (Taylor, 1987a). This explains partly the preoccupation of eating disorder patients with somatic experiences as well as their failure to benefit from interpretations that give symbolic meaning to their bodily symptoms and abnormal eating behaviours (Goodsitt, 1983; Zerbe, 1993). Rumination, which is sometimes associated with affective disturbances and eating disorders, particularly bulimia (Blinder, 1986; Fairburn & Cooper, 1984b; Parry-Jones, 1994), is one example of an asymbolic sensorimotor behaviour that presumably helps modulate affective states through the recapitulation of sensations reminiscent of aspects of the early feeding experience with the mother. It signifies collapse into the autistic–contiguous mode of generating experience described by Ogden (1989) and mentioned in Chapter 2.

### Clinical illustrations

The two following vignettes illustrate some of the regulatory disturbances described in the preceding sections and indicate why we have come to view eating disorders as disorders of affect regulation. Both patients had affective disturbances and borderline personality organizations, both scored in the alexithymic range on the TAS, and many of their behaviours were consistent with Lane and Schwartz's (1987) hierarchical model in which people with arrests in affect development (and associated defective self- and object representations) show a strong reliance on sensorimotor behaviours to regulate emotions.

#### Case I

Sally was in her late twenties when she sought therapy for bulimia nervosa and symptoms of depression. For many years she had been prone to states of intense anxiety, depression, and rage, which she attempted to regulate through the sensations evoked by bingeing and purging, chain-smoking cigarettes, or abusing alcohol and street drugs. Sally often complained of difficulty keeping warm, and to soothe and warm herself she frequently spent several hours soaking in a hot bath or burying herself in bed among a mound of pillows. The patient's sleep was generally disrupted, her sleep–wake cycle was altered, and she was prone to headaches, nausea, dizziness, and a variety of other 'functional' bodily symptoms.

To comfort herself at home, Sally often rocked her body, as this kinesthetic stimulation made her feel less fragmented and more in control of her thoughts. She also listened to extremely loud 'heavy metal' music in order 'to feel [her] organs vibrate'. During the early months of psychotherapy Sally frequently displayed repetitive movements as she stroked the soft fabric on the arms of the comfortable chair in which she sat; in addition, she had a tendency to cross her legs and swing one leg back and forth in a repetitive, stereotyped manner. These sensorimotor behaviours were most evident when Sally was distressed and they appeared partially to calm her. She sometimes relieved confusing states of inner tension by compulsively cleaning her apartment. Sally did not seek soothing from the therapeutic relationship, nor from her boyfriend or any other interpersonal relationships.

Evidence of an impaired symbolic function and faulty internal representations was provided by the patient's dreams, most of which were violent and non-interpretable, and similar to those reported by Levitan (1981) in a study of patients with eating disorders. Notably absent were the wish-fulfilling type of dreams described by Freud that would have helped preserve Sally's sleep and help organize and modulate her primitive emotions.

## Case 2

Jane, a 34-year-old married woman with three children, sought treatment for dysphoric symptoms, compulsive vomiting, and impulsive shopping sprees. At age 14, she had developed the restricter subtype of anorexia nervosa, but during late adolescence she began to binge and vomit and also purge with laxatives as ways of maintaining a low body weight. Jane had a normal body weight and was not bingeing at the time she requested therapy; yet she was vomiting several times daily after ingesting only small quantities of food. She described the vomiting as a habit she had acquired to control anxiety and agitation, as well as angry and unhappy feelings, but the vomiting had now become a behaviour that she could no longer control.

Evidence of this patient's longstanding problem in affect regulation was provided by a history of thumbsucking until age 7, hair-twirling since age 10, and frequent headbanging and beating of the floor with her hands in the privacy of her room during childhood to relieve states of anxiety or intense anger. Any verbal expression of anger was prohibited by her deeply religious and controlling parents, who also placed a taboo on masturbation and sexual desire. Consequently, Jane had experienced confusion and a terrible tension from the upsurge of sexual feelings at puberty, which she attempted to ward off by self-starvation. In her adult life, Jane complained of a lack of sexual gratification and of other pleasurable feelings. Sexual intercourse felt like rape and was associated strongly in the patient's mind with vivid memories of feeling her body violated during childhood by pediatricians performing vaginal and rectal examinations in search of pinworm infections, and by her mother administering enemas or washing out her mouth with soap.

During her childhood, Jane was prohibited from using toilets at school because of her mother's obsession with contagious skin infections. She therefore had to suppress the natural bodily sensations that signalled the need to empty a full bladder or bowel. Jane also reported frequent nightmares in which either her body was being mutilated or she and other people were being tortured with hot metal rods that were inserted into their bodily orifices. She recalled her parents forcing religion on her during childhood, and of being told repeatedly that she was going to hell.

Like the previous patient, Jane manifested a thermoregulatory disturbance and a need for kinesthetic stimulation to regulate inner tension; she relied on a favourite blanket to comfort and warm herself, engaged in long periods of rocking her body, and during psychotherapy sessions she often swung one leg or repetitively stroked the fabric of her chair. Episodes of self-harm were not uncommon, the first occurring at age 14 shortly before the onset of anorexia nervosa. Not appreciating her need for pleasurable bodily sensations to help comfort herself, Jane had taken a butcher's knife with the aim of cutting off her right hand to ensure that she would not masturbate. The idea of committing suicide was never far from her thoughts.

Jane had been born prematurely by Caesarean section and spent the first five days of her life in a hospital nursery incubator without any contact with her mother. She was a hyperactive child, suffered intense separation anxiety, and had a learning deficit. Prone to spontaneous panic attacks and also to prolonged states of autonomic hyperarousal, Jane reported a family history which suggested that she had an inherited neurobiological deficit, as well as acquired deficits, as her father also experienced depression and recurrent panic attacks. Indeed, during the course of several years of psychoanalytic psychotherapy, Jane manifested brief hypomanic episodes as well as episodes of major depression, which were accompanied by recurrences of frequent daily vomiting and body rocking, and were difficult to regulate even with antidepressant and mood stabilizing medications.

## Assessment of regulatory disturbances in eating disorders

As noted earlier, the reformulation of eating disorders as disorders of self- and affect regulation was anticipated by Bruch (1982/83, 1985) in her emphasis that the abnormal eating behaviours associated with anorexia nervosa and bulimia nervosa are secondary to underlying disturbances in the development of the personality. Several of the personality features described by Bruch were incorporated into the development of the Eating Disorder Inventory (EDI) (Garner et al., 1983b), which is now widely used in research as well as in clinical settings. This self-report measure comprises three subscales that assess attitudes and behaviours concerning eating, weight, and body shape (Drive for Thinness, Bulimia, Body Dissatisfaction), and five subscales that assess personality traits commonly associated with anorexia nervosa and bulimia nervosa (Ineffectiveness, Perfectionism, Interpersonal Distrust, Interoceptive Awareness, Maturity Fears). The EDI subscales have been shown to be reliable and psychometrically robust when employed with eating disorder patients (Welch, Hall & Norring, 1990).

The Interoceptive Awareness subscale and the Interpersonal Distrust subscale of the EDI provide information relevant to affect regulation, namely, the amount of 'confusion and apprehension in recognizing and accurately responding to emotional states' and 'the person's reluctance to express thoughts and feelings to others' (Garner, 1991). These traits obviously overlap with two facets of the alexithymia construct – difficulty identifying and distinguishing between feelings and the bodily sensations that accompany emotions, and difficulty communicating feelings to other people. Not surprisingly, in a recent study of female college students, Factor 1 of the TAS correlated most strongly with Interoceptive Awareness, and Factor 2 correlated most strongly with Interpersonal Distrust (Laquatra & Clopton, 1994).

To some extent Interpersonal Distrust taps the eating disorder patient's disturbance in the interpersonal domain of emotion regulation (Dodge & Garber, 1991), as this subscale of the EDI assesses an individual's general feeling of alienation and reluctance to form close relationships, as well as the person's reluctance to communicate thoughts and feelings to others (Garner, 1991). The Interoceptive Awareness subscale taps the eating disorder patient's disturbance in the cognitive–experiential domain of emotion regulation.

Studies comparing weight-preoccupied college and ballet students with anorexia nervosa patients on the EDI have found that anorexic patient groups are distinguished by higher scores on scales assessing Interpersonal Distrust, lack of Interoceptive Awareness, and Ineffectiveness (Garner, Olmsted & Garfinkel, 1983a; Garner et al., 1984). These findings help differentiate diagnosable eating disorders from milder forms or subclinical variants characterized by extreme dieting (Garner, 1991), and also provide empirical support for the idea that patients with eating disorders have basic disturbances in self- and affect regulation.

## Empirical studies

During the past decade several empirical studies have explored a possible association between alexithymia and eating disorders. As with other disorders, however, initial studies were conducted before the introduction of any reliable and valid alexithymia measure. Bourke *et al.* (1985), for example, used the $SAT_9$ to assess the ability to use symbols and to create fantasies in 20 patients with anorexia nervosa who had been admitted to a major British teaching hospital. Of the anorexic patients, 30% showed an impaired symbolic function at the time of hospitalization, and there was a tendency for further deterioration of this ego function following restoration of body weight. Although the patients showed elevated scores on both the Interoceptive Awareness subscale and the Interpersonal Distrust subscale of the EDI, the $SAT_9$ scores did not significantly correlate with either of these subscale scores or with any of the other EDI subscale scores. In another preliminary study, Pierloot, Houben and Acke (1988) administered the Rorschach and the MMPI to a group of 35 anorexia nervosa patients who had been admitted to a university hospital in Belgium. A control group of 35 inpatients with neurotic symptoms, who were matched for age and intelligence, also completed the psychological tests. Although the anorexia nervosa group scored significantly higher than the control group on the MMPI alexithymia scale (MMPI-A), only 8 of the 35 anorexic patients reached the cutoff score of 14.

Pierloot and his colleagues also selected several Rorschach indices to assess alexithymia including Human Movement, Colour, the Total Number of Responses, Originality and Variability of Content in responses, and strict Form responses. These indices have been employed by Vogt *et al.* (1977) to reflect fantasy elaboration and the expression of affect. Surprisingly, the anorexia nervosa patients did not significantly differ from the neurotic controls, except for a higher percentage of Original responses. Although one would predict neurotic patients to manifest better affect expression and fantasy elaboration on projective tests than patients with eating disorders, there is evidence from other research (Selvini Palazzoli, 1971; Wallach & Lowenkopf, 1984) that eating disorder patients show considerable individual differences in Rorschach protocols rather than a pattern typical of the disorder. None the less, future research with the Rorschach test to assess alexithymia in patients with eating disorders might evaluate the utility of the set of alexithymia indices used by Acklin and Alexander (1988) in studies with other clinical populations.

Another early investigation of alexithymia and anorexia nervosa was conducted by Engel and Meier (1988), who assessed aspects of verbal affective expression using the Gottschalk–Gleser method of analysing the content of monadic speech samples (Gottschalk & Gleser, 1969). Twenty German inpatients with a diagnosis of anorexia nervosa were compared with ten surgical inpatients on the Gottschalk–Gleser Scales measuring the verbal expression of anxiety and aggressiveness. Overall, the anorexic patients showed a general trend toward a higher affective level than the surgical patients with significantly higher scores for expressions of shame anxiety and introverted aggressiveness. Although Engel and Meier interpreted these results as failing to support an association between alexithymia and anorexia nervosa, they failed to discuss the limitations of the Gottschalk–Gleser Scales, in particular, that the scales were developed to measure immediate, labile emotional states, rather than stable traits (Gottschalk, 1974). Results from other studies have seriously questioned the validity of the Gottschalk–Gleser method of verbal content analysis for assessing alexithymia. Taylor and Doody (1985), for example, found that a combined score from several Gottschalk–Gleser Scales correlated opposite to the expected direction with other measures of alexithymia including the BIQ and a TAT index of the capacity to elaborate fantasy; there was no correlation with Human Movement scores on the Rorschach, which also indicate fantasizing ability.

Following the introduction of the TAS, empirical studies were conducted with this measure to explore alexithymia among patients with bulimia nervosa as well as among patients with anorexia nervosa. In a preliminary investigation at the Beth Israel Hospital in Boston, Jimerson et al. (1991, 1994) compared the mean TAS score of 20 medication-free female outpatients who met DSM-III-R criteria for bulimia nervosa with the mean TAS score of 20 age-matched healthy female control subjects. The bulimic patients scored significantly higher on the TAS than the control subjects with 40% of the patients meeting the TAS cutoff score for alexithymia compared with none of the control subjects. In addition, the bulimic patients scored significantly higher than the control subjects on the Revised Schalling Sifneos Personality Scale and the BIQ. Although the patients also scored significantly higher than the control subjects on both the Beck Depression Inventory (BDI) and the Hamilton Rating Scale for Depression, all of the patients were free of symptoms of major depressive illness at the time of the study. Also, none of the patients met DSM-III-R criteria for anorexia nervosa or substance dependence at the time of the study or during the six months prior to evaluation.

More recently, Cochrane et al. (1993) used the TAS to assess alexithymia in 114 female patients who were consecutively evaluated for treatment in an eating disorders program in South Carolina. The patients met DSM-III-R criteria for either anorexia nervosa (N = 19), bulimia nervosa (N = 52), both anorexia nervosa and bulimia nervosa (N = 18), or eating disorder not otherwise specified (N = 25). The mean TAS scores did not differ significantly among the various subtypes of eating disorder patients. However, the scores of the total sample of patients were significantly higher than those of published norms for female college students (Taylor et al., 1985), who were not significantly different from the age of the eating disorder patients except for the group with an eating disorder not otherwise specified. Based on the TAS cutoff score of ⩾74, alexithymia was identified in 63% of the anorexia nervosa group, in 56% of the bulimia nervosa group, in 61% of the group with anorexia nervosa and bulimia nervosa, and in 64% of the group with eating disorders not otherwise specified. TAS scores were not significantly correlated with age, percentage of average body weight, or frequency of bingeing or vomiting. However, TAS scores were significantly correlated with self-ratings of depression and anxiety as well as with crying, irritability, and difficulty falling asleep.

In another recent study, Schmidt, Jiwany and Treasure (1993) employed the TAS to investigate alexithymia in a group of 173 female eating disorder patients referred to the Maudsley Hospital Eating Disorder Clinic. The group comprised 93 subjects with bulimia nervosa, 55 subjects with the restricter subtype of anorexia nervosa, and 25 subjects with the bulimic subtype of anorexia nervosa. All patients met DSM-III-R criteria for their respective diagnosis. The TAS was also administered to a comparison group comprising 48 female students and 47 male students. Patients with the restricter subtype of anorexia nervosa had significantly higher TAS scores than patients with bulimia nervosa and all three eating disorder groups differed from the female and male comparison groups. Using the pre-established TAS cutoff scores, alexithymia was identified in 50% of the bulimic patients, in 56% of the restricting anorexic patients, and in 48% of the patients with the bulimic subtype of anorexia nervosa. In contrast, alexithymia was present in 27% of the female students and 19% of the male students. Although the rate of alexithymia in the female students was somewhat higher than has been found in samples of female students in Canada and the United States, the rate among male students (as measured by the TAS) was comparable to other reports (Loiselle & Dawson, 1988; Parker, Taylor & Bagby, 1989b). The TAS did not significantly correlate with the Body Mass Index in any of the three eating disorder groups, suggesting that the greater degree of alexithymia in the anorexic patients was not an effect of starvation on cognitive functioning. Because of the cross-sectional design of the study, however, the results could not determine whether alexithymia is a predisposing personality trait for an eating disorder or whether it is secondary to the influence of chronic illness on personality functioning.

The question of whether alexithymia is an enduring personality characteristic or a state-dependent effect of eating disorders was explored further by Schmidt *et al.* (1993) in a second part of their study. The TAS was administered to a subgroup (N = 42) of the sample of patients with bulimia nervosa before and after a 10-week interval of drug treatment (2 weeks single-blind placebo wash-out followed by 8 weeks double-blind placebo-controlled fluvoxamine). This subgroup of patients was also assessed for level of depression before and after treatment with the Hamilton Rating Scale for Depression; eating pathology was assessed with the self-rating Bulimic Investigatory Test, Edinburgh (Henderson & Freeman, 1987) and with interviewer-ratings of the frequency of bingeing and vomiting. Although there was a significant improvement in eating pathology after 10 weeks of treatment, there was no significant change in mean TAS scores and mean scores on the Hamilton Rating Scale for Depression. The investigators reported that as many as 73% of patients who had been categorized as alexithymic at baseline were still alexithymic after treatment, and 87.5% who at baseline were non-alexithymic remained in this category. Despite previous reports of an association between alexithymia and depression, the TAS did not correlate with the Hamilton Depression scale at baseline or at the end of the 10-week treatment period. While the findings suggest that alexithymia is a stable trait among patients with bulimia nervosa, Schmidt *et al.* (1993) correctly noted that the continuing high TAS scores might be explained by persistent symptoms, as the majority of patients had not fully recovered at the end of the 10 weeks.

Another recent longitudinal study was conducted by de Groot, Rodin and Olmsted (1995) who administered the TAS and the BDI to a group of 31 female patients, who met DSM-III-R criteria for bulimia nervosa, and to a comparison group of 20 female nurses who were similar in weight and slightly older than the bulimia nervosa group. The patients were new admissions to the Toronto Day Hospital Program for Eating Disorders where they received intensive group psychotherapy with a focus on nutrition, body image, and symptom management as well as on family and other relationships. The patients were retested at the time of discharge from the treatment program, the average length of treatment being 9.6 (SD = 1.9) weeks. The bulimia nervosa patient group was significantly more alexithymic and significantly more depressed than the comparison group with alexithymia being present in 61.3% of the patients compared with only 5% of the nurses. Even when the effect of depression was accounted for, there remained a trend for the bulimia nervosa patients to be more alexithymic than the nurses.

In contrast to Schmidt et al.'s (1993) findings, in the study by de Groot and her colleagues the mean TAS score at the time of discharge was significantly lower than the pre-treatment score. The patient group, however, still had a significantly higher mean TAS score than the comparison group and 32.3% of the bulimia nervosa patients were still above the TAS cutoff score for alexithymia. Interestingly, de Groot and her colleagues found no significant change in the mean TAS score for a subgroup of patients (N = 7) who were depressed both at the time of admission and at discharge; patients who were no longer depressed at discharge, and those who were not depressed either at admission or discharge, showed a significant improvement in TAS scores. Further analysis of the data revealed that only the patients who were abstinent from bingeing and vomiting at the time of discharge showed a significant reduction in TAS scores; there was a trend for those with persistent symptoms to be more alexithymic on discharge from the treatment program. The investigators were unable to conclude whether the partial reversibility of alexithymia in the bulimia nervosa women was due to a reduction in associated depression, a reduction of eating disorder symptoms, or involvement in the group therapy program.

An 8- to 10-year follow-up study of women who had recovered from restricting anorexia nervosa has provided suggestive evidence also that alexithymic characteristics may be an integral part of the personality of individuals who are at risk for eating disorders. Casper (1990) found that recovered anorexic women, despite their good outcome, scored significantly lower than age-matched normal women on the psychological mindedness subscale of the California Psychological Inventory, which has been shown to correlate negatively with the TAS (Bagby et al., 1986b), as indicated in Chapter 3. The recovered women also displayed greater restraint in emotional expression and initiative than the healthy control subjects.

Our own research team, in collaboration with Dr Michael Bourke (Bourke et al., 1992), investigated alexithymia in a sample of 48 women who had been referred to private clinics in England and who had met the DSM-III-R diagnostic criteria for anorexia nervosa at the time of initial consultation. The group was heterogeneous in that patients were tested at various stages of illness, although none could be considered recovered. The mean duration of illness was 8.5 years (range 6 months to 34 years). Of the total anorexic sample, 30 patients were of the restricter subtype, while the remaining 18 patients reported bulimic behaviour at some stage of their illness. The restricter and bulimic subgroups did not differ significantly in age, educational level, or age of onset of the illness. The bulimic subgroup, however, was significantly heavier. A control group matched for age and education comprised 30 normal female volunteers, who were recruited from among hospital employees and had no current or past history of eating disorder. In addition to completing the TAS (and a set of items subsequently used in developing the TAS-20), the subjects completed the EDI and the Crown-Crisp Experiential Index (CCEI) (Crown & Crisp, 1979). The total score of the CCEI was used as a measure of general psychoneurotic pathology (Birtchnell, Evans & .Kennard, 1988); the depression subscale provided an index of depressive symptomatology. Though the initial results of this study were based on the TAS and reported before the development of the TAS-20 (Bourke et al., 1992), we subsequently reanalyzed the data and now report results based on the improved alexithymia scale.

The anorexic patients scored significantly higher than the normal women on both the TAS-20 and the CCEI. Based on the TAS-20 cutoff score of $\geq 61$, 33 (68.8%) of the anorexic group were classified as alexithymic compared with 1 (3.3%) of the control group. (The less conservative cutoff score of the TAS yielded rates of 77.1% of alexithymia in the anorexic group and 6.7% in the control group.) In the anorexic group, alexithymia was unrelated to duration of illness, amount of weight loss, and level of depression. However, the TAS-20 total scores correlated significantly and positively with the CCEI total scores, and the bulimic anorexic patients scored significantly higher on the TAS-20 than the restricting anorexic patients.

To examine the relationships between alexithymia and other psychological traits, attitudes, and behaviours that are common in anorexia nervosa, we correlated TAS-20 scores with scores on the eight EDI subscales. To correct for item overlap, all correlations were computed after removal of four items from the TAS-20 that were derived from the Interoceptive Awareness subscale of the EDI in developing both the TAS and TAS-20 (see Chapter 3). In the anorexic group, the 'corrected' TAS-20 showed significant positive correlations with Ineffectiveness ($r = 0.33$, $p < 0.05$), Interpersonal Distrust ($r = 0.47$, $p < 0.01$), Interoceptive Awareness ($r = 0.42$, $p < 0.01$), and Maturity Fears ($r = 0.36$, $p < 0.05$); correlations were non-significant with Perfectionism, Drive for Thinness, Bulimia, and Body Dissatisfaction. The only significant correlation in the control group of normal women was with Interpersonal Distrust ($r = 0.52$, $p < 0.01$). These results suggest that the alexithymia construct is unrelated to attitudes and behaviours concerning eating, weight, and body shape, and also unrelated to the belief that only the highest standards of personal performance are acceptable. However, the results confirm that alexithymia is related to, and overlaps with, several other psychological traits associated with anorexia nervosa. The positive correlation between the TAS-20 and (lack of) Interoceptive Awareness (even after correcting for item overlap) confirms that difficulty in recognizing and accurately responding to emotional states and certain visceral sensations is a central deficit in eating disorder patients. The positive correlation between Interpersonal Distrust and the TAS-20 provides concurrent validation that eating disorder patients tend not to express feelings to others. The positive correlation between Ineffectiveness and the TAS-20 indicates that alexithymia is related to the anorexic patient's difficulty in regulating self-esteem and other aspects of self-experience including feelings of emptiness and aloneness. The finding of a positive correlation between Maturity Fears and the TAS-20 suggests that alexithymia in anorexic patients is related to an avoidance of psychological maturity.

To compare the ability of the TAS-20 and the EDI to predict those subjects in our study with a diagnosis of anorexia nervosa, we conducted separate discriminant function analyses on the combined data from the anorexic and normal control groups using the three TAS-20 factor scales as predictors in the first analysis and the eight EDI subscales in the second analysis. The TAS-20 correctly classified 85.9% of the subjects compared with 93.6% correctly classified by the EDI. While in the second analysis, Drive for Thinness made the greatest contribution to the discrimination of the anorexic and normal groups, this was followed by subscales assessing those traits most strongly related to the alexithymia construct, *viz.*, Interoceptive Awareness, Ineffectiveness, and Interpersonal Distrust.

**Summary and conclusions**

In conceptualizing eating disorders as disorders of affect regulation, we have proposed a model that is consistent with the prevailing view that eating disorders have a multifactorial etiology. As outlined in earlier chapters, neurobiological, developmental, and sociocultural factors all play a role in affect development and in the acquisition of effective affect regulating capacities. Deficiencies in affect regulation, and accompanying disturbances in self-organization, may stem from constitutional–inherited deficits and/or developmental deficiencies.

Familial and sociocultural factors may influence the choice of abnormal eating behaviours, *viz.*, self-starvation and/or bingeing and vomiting, which are viewed in this chapter as responses to, and attempts to regulate, distressing and relatively undifferentiated emotional states.

Though alexithymia is not related directly to bingeing or body image disturbances, or to a relentless pursuit of thinness, there is empirical evidence that this construct is related to several psychological traits that were identified initially by Bruch (1962, 1973) as cardinal features of eating disorders, in particular interoceptive confusion, difficulty communicating feelings, and an overwhelming sense of ineffectiveness. In addition, studies that used reliable and valid measures have shown consistently high rates of alexithymia among both anorexia nervosa patients and bulimia nervosa patients.

These findings strongly support Bruch's (1962) view that patients with eating disorders are unlikely to benefit from traditional psychodynamic psychotherapy, and require modified treatment approaches. Rather than interpreting unconscious symbolic meanings for various symptoms or abnormal eating behaviours, patients with eating disorders need assistance in developing certain ego- and self functions including clarification of bodily sensations and feeling states, which are perceived often in a vague and fleeting way, as well as help in regulating internal tension states (Bruch, 1985; Goodsitt, 1985). For bulimic patients, it is helpful also to elucidate the internal and external stimuli that heighten the urge to binge (Swift & Letven, 1984).

While there is evidence that behaviour therapy and/or pharmacotherapy with antidepressant drugs can produce significant symptomatic improvement in patients with bulimia nervosa (Mitchell, Raymond & Specker, 1993; Walsh, 1991), the benefits are often short-lived (Fairburn et al., 1995; Freeman & Munro, 1988). Intensive cognitive-behaviour therapy provides a better longer-term outcome, because it focuses on modifying cognitive distortions and faulty attitudes concerning dieting and body weight and shape, as well as on abnormal eating behaviour (Fairburn et al., 1993; Mitchell et al., 1993). Overall, however, the relapse rate is high for both anorexic patients and patients with bulimia nervosa.

It is our impression that the high relapse rate among eating disorder patients is related to alexithymia and deficits in affect regulation. In a long-term study of 76 women who had been treated for anorexia nervosa, Schork, Eckert and Halmi (1994) found at a 10-year follow-up that those women who had recovered and had no other eating disorder showed little or no psychopathology on the MMPI, whereas those who had remained anorexic or developed bulimia nervosa showed high levels of psychopathology. Consistent with our conceptualization of eating disorders as disorders of affect regulation, the psychopathology of those women with persistent eating disorders typically involved somatization and bodily preoccupation, depression and anxious dysphoria, impulsivity and low frustration tolerance, immaturity and lack of insight, interpersonal distrust, and poor social adjustment. Findings from another long-term follow-up study showed that even women who have recovered from restricting anorexia nervosa are more emotionally constrained and less psychologically minded than normal women, characteristics that are consistent with the alexithymia construct (Casper, 1990). We will elaborate on psychotherapeutic techniques for modifying alexithymia in Chapter 11.

# [10] Affects and alexithymia in medical illness and disease

In the Introduction to this book, we briefly outlined different periods in the history of medicine when prominent physicians and philosophers firmly held the belief that people's health can be influenced by their emotions. During the 19th century, many physicians attempted to evaluate this belief scientifically by investigating the direct effects of various emotions on different bodily functions. Beaumont (1833), for example, demonstrated that fear and anger reduce secretion from the gastric mucosa. The emergence of psychoanalysis at the beginning of the twentieth century led to a very different approach, as it inspired several psychoanalysts to begin to study the personality traits and psychological conflicts that were assumed to be responsible for the emotional states contributing to the development of disease. It was largely the enthusiasm and work of these psychoanalysts that led to the emergence of psychosomatic medicine as an organized movement and to the founding of the American Psychosomatic Society in the early 1940s.

During the past 50 years, however, psychosomatic theorists have proposed several different models for understanding the development of somatic disease that involve different conceptualizations for the role of affects. In this chapter, we first briefly review the different theoretical models, and then present a contemporary model in which deficient emotional processing is viewed as one of several possible factors that can dysregulate other biological systems in the body and thereby create conditions favourable for the emergence of medical illness or disease. We show the application of this model to several common medical illnesses and diseases.[1]

1. We remind the reader of the important distinction between these terms. Disease is defined by alterations in the structure of body organs or tissues; illness is defined by changes in bodily functions. Many people seeking health care are ill without having a disease (Weiner, 1987).

## Review of psychosomatic models of disease

As outlined in earlier contributions (Taylor, 1987*a*, 1992*a,b*), Alexander (1950), Deutsch (1959), and other pioneers in the field of psychosomatic medicine adopted Freud's drive–conflict–defense model of psychopathology, which was proving successful in understanding and treating psychoneurotic disorders, and applied this model to patients with somatic diseases. They gave little attention to functional physiological illnesses such as migraine, fibromyalgia, and irritable bowel syndrome, and instead focused their investigations mainly on a group of seven diseases (peptic ulcer, bronchial asthma, essential hypertension, thyrotoxicosis, ulcerative colitis, rheumatoid arthritis, and neurodermatitis), which were then of uncertain etiology and subsequently came to be referred to as the 'classical' psychosomatic diseases. Although there was disagreement among the early psychoanalytic psychosomaticists as to whether the symptoms of these diseases have primary symbolic meaning, comparable to the symptoms of conversion hysteria, the different theoretical disease models they developed were all based on the notion that intrapsychic (especially preoedipal) conflicts, and the emotions associated with them, play a central role in the pathogenesis of disease. Biological and stressful life events were also given important roles in these early psychosomatic models, but the models were based on a linear conception of causality (the so-called 'mysterious leap from the mind to the body') and psychoanalytic interest was mainly in the psychogenesis of disease.

These theoretical conceptions, together with the classical psychoanalytic view that emotions are derivatives of instincts that need to be discharged or 'tamed' (Sandler, 1972), led to a therapeutic approach to medically ill patients that attempted to release 'strangulated' affects and resolve conflicts over drive-related wishes. The outcome of this approach, however, was generally disappointing. While some patients responded favourably with a remission of their disease, others showed either no change or a worsening of physical symptoms and were found to benefit more from supportive psychotherapy and/or behavioural interventions (Karush *et al.*, 1977; Kellner, 1975; Lipowski, 1977; Reiser, 1978; Sifneos, 1975). These poor treatment results suggested serious limitations to the conflict-based psychosomatic models of disease. Research using psychological assessments, or physiological data, or both, subsequently provided some empirical support for an association between specific intrapsychic conflicts and specific psychosomatic diseases (Alexander, French & Pollock, 1968; Weiner *et al.*, 1957); however, recent advances in statistical techniques and methodology have seriously weakened this support (Friedman &

Booth-Kewley, 1987; Holroyd & Coyne, 1987). In addition, as will be elaborated later in this chapter, ongoing medical research has led to the discovery that many of the diseases that were investigated are heterogeneous, both physiologically and psychologically (Magni *et al.*, 1986; Weiner, 1977, 1992). None the less, a meta-analytic review of published studies on the personality correlates of four diseases (bronchial asthma, peptic ulcer, rheumatoid arthritis, coronary heart disease) and one somatic illness (headache) found moderate support for the construct of a 'disease-prone personality' that involves the affects of depression, anger/hostility, and anxiety (Friedman & Booth-Kewley, 1987). However, as there is yet no evidence that these affects are generated by intrapsychic conflicts, alternative explanations for their origin must be considered. For example, as suggested in earlier contributions (Taylor, 1992a,b), high levels of anger and hostility, which are now regarded as the critical components of the Type A coronary-prone behaviour pattern (Dembroski *et al.*, 1985), might be explained by an impaired ego capacity for containing and modulating narcissistic rage and for tolerating frustration rather than by conflicts over unconscious drive-related wishes. Recent research has in fact provided empirical support for an association between narcissistic personality characteristics and the Type A behaviour pattern (Fukunishi *et al.*, 1995a; Fukunishi, Moroji & Okabe, 1995b). This is consistent with Grotstein's (1986) proposal that Type A behaviour be reconceptualized as a manifestation of a disorder of self- and affect regulation.

In earlier chapters, we indicated that the concept of disorders of regulation is implicit in Freud's (1898) model of the actual neuroses. The relevance of this model for understanding the role of affects in certain medical illnesses and diseases was recognized by only a minority of early psychoanalysts, including Glover (1939) and MacAlpine (1952), who emphasized that the so-called classical psychosomatic diseases have no primary psychic content and are therefore different from the conflict-based psychoneuroses. Indeed, MacAlpine argued that 'psychosomatic' symptoms are not a result of unconscious conflicts, but stem from primitive and only partly expressed emotions that are related to the preconceptual and preverbal phase of development.

MacAlpine's conceptualization of psychosomatic symptom formation was consistent with Ruesch's (1948, 1957) observations that many patients with classical psychosomatic diseases (and also patients with posttraumatic syndromes) manifest a rather primitive level of psychological organization and show a lack of imagination in their responses to projective psychological tests such as the Rorschach and the TAT. Ruesch observed also that psychosomatic patients show an absence of verbal, gestural, and other symbolic expressions of affects, and a tendency to discharge emotional tension through action. He contrasted these characteristics with the cognitive/affective style of psychoneurotic patients, who generally show a high level of emotional expressiveness and relatively easy access to a rich inner life of drive-related fantasies.

Though Ruesch and MacAlpine raised the possibility that problems in emotional processing might play a more important role than neurotic conflicts in the pathogenesis of the classical psychosomatic diseases, psychosomatic medicine largely ignored investigating this possibility. As already noted, most psychosomaticists merely adopted the prevailing psychoanalytic view that emotions are drive derivatives, and failed to consider that some patients might manifest arrests in affect development and associated deficits in affect regulation. One exception was Schur (1955), who proposed that somatic disorders are partly a consequence of a regression of affects to an undifferentiated 'psychosomatic' phase of development that occurs when the ego is unable to defend adequately against stress. However, Schur's formulations were highly abstract and were never subjected to empirical evaluation.

An alternative psychosomatic model that emphasized a role for affects in the onset of disease was introduced during the 1960s by Engel and Schmale (1967; Schmale, 1972). Through studying patients with a wide variety of diseases (not just the classical psychosomatic diseases), and by shifting their focus of inquiry from intrapsychic conflicts to the life setting in which people become ill, Engel (1955, 1968) and Schmale (1958, 1972) discovered that the onset or exacerbation of disease is associated frequently with the affects of helplessness and hopelessness that are evoked by a recent separation or loss of an important relationship.

Engel and Schmale postulated that there is a heightened susceptibility to disease in individuals who are unable to grieve or otherwise cope with separations and other object losses. Such individuals develop the specific depressive affects of helplessness and hopelessness, attitudes of 'giving up' and 'given up', and a conservation–withdrawal physiological response. Engel and Schmale called this intervening psychobiological state the 'giving up/given up complex'. They postulated that once the complex develops it initiates autonomic, endocrinologic, and immunologic changes that might lead to the emergence of disease if the necessary constitutional and/or environmental factors are also present.

In exploring why some disease-prone individuals adapt poorly to separations and other object losses, Engel (1955, 1958) identified defects in ego function which appeared to stem from developmental arrests and were compensated for by excessive dependency on a symbiotic relationship. The disruption of such a relationship exposed the defects in the personality, including an inability to modulate the depressive affects evoked by the loss. Additional evidence that close relationships can function as external regulators of emotions and other biological processes was provided by Engel and Reichsman's (1956) parallel studies of Monica, an infant who was fed through a gastric fistula for the first two years of her life because of an oesophageal atresia. Lacking a strong emotional bond with her mother, who was depressed and unable to relate warmly to the child, Monica developed an anaclitic depression and severe marasmus during her second half-year and was subsequently hospitalized. Engel and Reichsman observed that Monica did not display the usual crying response to strangers but instead lapsed into a seemingly depressed and unresponsive state during which gastric secretions ceased and became unresponsive to histamine stimulation. When reunited with a favourite nurse or doctor, however, to whom she had become quite attached, Monica showed a joyful response and gastric secretion rose.

Although clinical and empirical studies have yielded considerable support for the validity of Engel and Schmale's (1967) psychobiological model, the model did little to advance the psychotherapeutic treatment of medically ill patients. Despite the identification of ego defects and compensatory regulatory functions provided by close human relationships, Engel and Schmale's conceptualizations of object loss and affects were limited by a rigid adherence to classical psychoanalytic drive theory. It was not until the 1970s that psychosomatic medicine began to revise its conceptualization of affects and to systematically investigate the possibility that somatic diseases might be associated with deficits in emotional processing.

In a preliminary observational study of randomly selected patients with classical psychosomatic diseases, Sifneos (1967) reported that some of the patients showed a marked difficulty in finding appropriate words to describe how they were feeling. Though they commonly mentioned anxiety or complained of depression, in contrast to most psychoneurotic patients, some of the physically ill patients were unable to describe associated thoughts, fantasies, conflicts, or higher level affects. Inspired by these observations, and by Marty and de M'Uzan's (1963) earlier description of pensée opératoire in many physically ill patients, Nemiah and Sifneos (1970) decided to re-examine verbatim transcripts of psychiatric interviews with 20 patients who had a current or past history of two of the classical psychosomatic diseases. The interviews had been carried out 15 years earlier, and were conducted in a manner designed to stimulate free association and fantasy production. Nemiah and Sifneos (1970, p. 28) found that 16 of the patients showed a 'marked difficulty in verbally expressing or describing their feelings', 'an absence or striking diminution of fantasy', and a thought content that was mundane, utilitarian, and tied to reality. As we indicated in Chapter 2, these observations led to the initial formulation of the alexithymia construct.

After developing the BIQ to assess alexithymia, Sifneos (1973) investigated a randomly selected group of 25 medically ill patients (with diagnoses of ulcerative colitis, bronchial asthma, peptic ulcer, or rheumatoid arthritis) and a randomly selected comparison group of 25 patients with neurotic symptoms and a variety of psychiatric diagnoses (including depression, alcoholism, borderline personality disorder, and hysterical personality disorder). The medically ill patients scored significantly higher on the BIQ than the control group. The study was limited, however, by a failure to match the psychiatric and medically ill groups on sociodemographic variables. In addition, inter-rater reliability of the BIQ was not determined as the questionnaire was completed by several different psychiatrists who were acquainted with different patients.

The emphasis given by Sifneos (1973) and Apfel and Sifneos (1979) to differences in the cognitive/affective style between psychosomatic patients and patients with neurotic symptoms unfortunately led some investigators and critics of the alexithymia construct to make the erroneous assumption that there exists a specific etiologic relationship between alexithymia and the classical psychosomatic diseases (e.g. Ahrens & Deffner, 1986; Vollhardt, Ackerman & Shindledecker, 1986). These investigators overlooked the earlier reports by Sifneos (1967) and Nemiah and Sifneos (1970) that not all patients with psychosomatic diseases manifest alexithymic characteristics; they also overlooked reports by other clinicians of alexithymic features among patients with those psychiatric disorders that we have conceptualized in this book as disorders of affect regulation. Furthermore, findings from several studies began to suggest that alexithymia could be associated with a variety of somatic illnesses and diseases, not just with those traditionally regarded as 'psychosomatic' (Heiberg, 1980; Keltikangas-Järvinen, 1985, 1987). Currently, like the giving up/given up complex and other risk factors, alexithymia is conceptualized as increasing a person's general susceptibility to disease, which is specified by other variables (Weiner & Fawzy, 1989).

With regard to its clinical implications, the presence of alexithymia was thought to explain the lack of psychological mindedness and poor response of many 'psychosomatic' patients to analytical psychotherapies. Sifneos (1974, 1975) and Nemiah et al. (1976) therefore recommended the use of supportive psychotherapies for the majority of alexithymic patients with physical illnesses, but controlled outcome studies have never been conducted.

It can be seen from this overview that the conceptualizations of emotion within different psychosomatic models of disease have varied from an emphasis on intrapsychic conflicts thought to generate pathogenic affects, to an emphasis on specific depressive affects and the life situations that evoke them, or to an emphasis on deficits in the cognitive processing of distressing affects. Let us now consider more recent research on relationships between disease and different personality types, as this field of inquiry adds further to our understanding of how emotions might influence health.

## Personality, emotions, and disease

Over the past two decades, psychosomatic researchers have become increasingly interested in identifying personality factors that might alter resilience and general susceptibility to disease (Adler & Matthews, 1994; Friedman & Booth-Kewley, 1987; Marshall et al., 1994; Smith & Williams, 1992). Much of this interest stems from investigations of the Type A behaviour pattern, which was described initially by Friedman and Rosenman (1959) as a characteristic of many patients suffering from coronary heart disease (CHD). The behaviours that comprise the Type A pattern include a sense of time urgency, competitiveness, aggressiveness, impatience, excessive achievement striving, and vigorous voice and psychomotor mannerisms. Individuals who do not exhibit these behaviours are called Type B; they are rather relaxed, deferent, and satisfied, their behaviour generally unhurried (Rosenman & Chesney, 1982).

Evidence suggesting that the Type A behaviour pattern is a risk factor for CHD was provided first from the Western Collaborative Group Study, an 8.5-year prospective study of over 3000 men (Rosenman et al., 1975). Men who were classified as Type A at the beginning of the study showed twice the risk of developing CHD, independent of other known risk factors, than men classified as Type B. Other large epidemiological studies, and also some smaller studies, yielded additional support for an association between the Type A behaviour pattern and the risk of CHD (Booth-Kewley & Friedman, 1987). However, some studies failed to demonstrate a relationship, especially when angina was excluded as a CHD outcome (e.g. Shekelle et al., 1985), and enthusiasm for the Type A concept began to wane (Thoreson & Powell, 1992). Much of the inconsistency in findings can be attributed to problems in measuring Type A behaviour and to a failure to validate the multidimensional Type A construct (Smith & Williams, 1992).

A subsequent reanalysis of data from the Western Collaborative Group Study (Matthews et al., 1977), and findings from several other studies, suggested that anger and hostility were the critical components of the Type A pattern (Dembroski et al., 1985; Shekelle et al., 1983; Williams et al., 1980). There are now considerable prospective data linking anger and hostility to CHD incidence, events, and mortality, as well as to other cardiac risk factors such as smoking (Littman, 1993; Scheier & Bridges, 1995). It is important to note, however, that hostility itself is also a multidimensional construct; whereas antagonistic hostility, which is related to the Agreeableness/Disagreeableness dimension of personality described in Chapter 4, has been found to predict incidence of CHD, neurotic hostility, which is related to the broader dimension of Neuroticism or negative affectivity, does not (Dembroski & Costa, 1987; Dembroski et al., 1989; Smith, 1992).

With their focus almost exclusively on CHD, however, researchers largely ignored the question of whether hostility and the Type A behaviour pattern might also be risk factors for other diseases. Given that atherosclerosis is a disease process that occurs throughout the body, Stevens et al. (1984) not surprisingly demonstrated that the Type A pattern is associated also with carotid artery atherosclerosis. And although not all Type A individuals are hypertensive, some researchers found an association between the Type A behaviour pattern and essential hypertension (Shekelle, Schoenberger & Stamler, 1976; Smyth et al., 1978). More recent studies that measured hostility rather than the global Type A pattern found an association with peripheral arterial disease (Deary et al., 1994; Julkunen et al., 1994) and with hypertension (Jamner et al., 1993).

It was a group of Belgian investigators, however, who eventually provided data suggesting that the Type A behaviour pattern is a general disease-prone condition rather than merely a risk factor specific to cardiovascular diseases. In a study with a large general population of both men and women, Rimé et al. (1989) found that Type A individuals, as compared with Type B persons, 'reported more frequently having suffered not only from coronary disease, but also from peptic ulcers, asthma, rheumatoid arthritis and thyroid problems' (p. 233). Such findings are consistent with the results of Friedman and Booth-Kewley's (1987) meta-analytic review, which support the construct of a generic 'disease-prone personality' rather than 'coronary-prone' and other specific disease-prone personalities.

One limitation of the Belgian study is that Type A behaviour was assessed with the self-report Jenkins Activity Survey (JAS), which is considered inferior to the structured interview method of assessment, as it does not adequately evaluate the hostility component of this behavioural pattern (Thoreson & Powell, 1992). There is some evidence that hostility is associated not only with CHD but also with a proneness to other diseases (Scheier & Bridges, 1995; Smith, 1992). Using MMPI data from one of the earlier epidemiological studies on Type A behaviour, Shekelle et al. (1983) scored the Cook-Medley Hostility Scale (Ho) and demonstrated that hostility scores were significantly associated with increased risk of CHD death, cancer death, and all-cause mortality over a 20-year follow-up. After controlling for deaths from CHD and adjusting for major CHD risk factors, there was still a positive association between hostility and 20-year mortality rates from all other causes, excluding cardiovascular-renal diseases and malignant neoplasms. Given that the significance of the positive association between Ho scores and cancer deaths diminished when the data were adjusted for smoking and other major CHD risk factors, the link between hostility and cancer is considered somewhat tenuous (Scheier & Bridges, 1995). A similar 25-year follow-up study of 255 male physicians also found that higher Ho scores were associated with mortality from all causes (Barefoot, Dahlstrom & Williams, 1983), but this study did not determine whether the effect of hostility on all-cause mortality was independent of its association with death from CHD.

Over the years researchers working with cancer patients have come to define a Type C behaviour pattern characterized by suppression of emotion, particularly anger, as well as conformity/compliance, unassertiveness, and patience (Bahnson, 1982; Bahnson & Bahnson, 1969; Baltrusch, Stangel & Waltz, 1988; Morris & Greer, 1980; Temoshok, 1987). Although the Type C behaviour pattern has been less well researched, partly because of measurement problems, there are some data that support viewing it as a predisposition for cancer; we will review this evidence later. In related but more controversial research, Grossarth-Maticek and Eysenck (1990; Eysenck, 1991b) have reported findings from three large prospective studies, which suggest that different 'behaviour' types are related more strongly to CHD and cancer, and that health also is associated with a specific behaviour type. These researchers used a personality inventory that was devised on the basis of theoretical considerations and clinical experience to predict cancer and cardiovascular disease in people who react in certain ways to certain types of stress (Eysenck, 1991c; Grossarth-Maticek, Eysenck & Vetter, 1988).

The inventory divides the population into four types, which reflect different affective styles as well as different modes of object relating.[1] Type 1 individuals tend to suppress emotion, are highly dependent on a person, goal, or situation that is inaccessible to them, and react to losses with helplessness and hopelessness. Type 2 persons are dependent on a person or goal which is experienced as rejecting and distressing, and they react in angry, hostile, and aggressive ways. Individuals who show a tendency to shift back and forth between the typical behaviours of Type 1 and the typical behaviours of Type 2 are classified as Type 3; they alternate between feelings of hopelessness/helplessness and anger/arousal. Type 4 persons are characterized by autonomy and a capacity to regulate their emotions. In other words, as Grossarth-Maticek et al. (1988, p. 480) explain, 'persons of Types 1 and 2 show a dependence on important objects that engage their emotions, but cannot remain autonomous when these emotional objects withdraw or remain unattainable.' In contrast, Type 4 persons 'are able to deal with this situation by virtue of their autonomy-preserving ability.' The results from the prospective studies conducted by Grossarth-Maticek and his colleagues (1988; Eysenck, 1991b) suggest that Type 1 persons are cancer-prone, that Type 2 persons are CHD-prone, and that Type 4 persons enjoy the best health. Type 3 persons were found to be protected to some extent from cancer and CHD, perhaps because of their alternating affective style, but were prone to chronic anxiety.

Although the work of Eysenck and Grossarth-Maticek has been harshly criticized for inconsistencies, methodological defects, and inappropriate statistical analyses (Pelosi & Appleby, 1992; see also a collection of commentaries in *Psychological Inquiry* 2, 233–93, 1991), these criticisms, in our opinion, appear to have been responded to reasonably by Eysenck (1991c, 1992) and Grossarth-Maticek (1991), who acknowledge certain limitations to their research, including the need for improving their personality inventory psychometrically, and a need for replication of their findings. As Eysenck (1991c) points out, 'the Type A-Type B classification [initially] also lacked proper psychometric foundations' (p. 302). Furthermore, Eysenck (1991b) and Grossarth-Maticek et al. (1988) point to obvious overlaps between Type 2 in their typology and the anger/hostility component of the Type A behaviour pattern, and between Type 1 and the Type C behaviour pattern. They suggest that their Type 4 corresponds to the Type B behaviour pattern. Recent studies by independent investigators have found that Type 4 is related negatively to alexithymia (Sandin

1. In later years of the research, Grossarth-Maticek and his colleagues defined two additional 'behaviour types' (Eysenck, 1991b; Schmitz, 1992), but most of their analyses involve only the first four types.

*et al.*, 1993; Schmitz, 1992); it also shows a pattern of correlations with measures of neuroticism, extraversion, and closed-mindedness that is opposite to the pattern we have found for alexithymia (see Chapter 4) (Schmitz, 1992). This at least is consistent with our view that non-alexithymic persons, perhaps because of their greater autonomy and emotional processing abilities, are less susceptible to medical illness and disease than alexithymic persons. Grossarth-Maticek and Eysenck (1995) recently reached a similar conclusion that autonomy and the capacity to regulate affects and other aspects of the self dispose a person to good physical health.

Though not commented on by Eysenck (1991*b*) and Grossarth-Maticek *et al.* (1988), it is important to recognize certain similarities between their conceptualization of the interaction between personality and emotionally stressful events in the development of disease and the model developed by Engel and Schmale (1967; Schmale, 1972). Both groups of researchers link a greater susceptibility to disease with a lack of autonomy, but they also regard the activation of certain negative emotions by a highly important person or situation as a necessary component of the predisposition to disease. Whereas Engel and Schmale specified the affects of helplessness and hopelessness in response to losses, Grossarth-Maticek and his colleagues include Type 2 persons who experience a reaction of anger as well as Type 1 persons who experience helplessness and hopelessness.

A similar interaction between personality and emotionally distressing life events is contained in Bahnson's (1982) conceptualization of the pathogenesis of cancer; in addition to the constellation of behaviours now referred to as Type C, Bahnson assigns an important role to depressive affects evoked by object loss. Temoshok (1987) proposes that Type C persons, as a consequence of suppressing their needs and feelings, harbour chronic feelings of hopelessness, but these are hidden behind a mask of normalcy until the defensive style is overwhelmed by an accumulation of stressful life events. She suggests that this might explain why some studies find Type C behaviour related to cancer outcome measures, and other studies find helplessness and hopelessness associated with cancer outcome.

We remind the reader that the results of Friedman and Booth-Kewley's (1987) meta-analytic study supported a generic disease-prone personality involving a mixture of negative affects; however, the studies included in the meta-analysis used a wide variety of both state and trait measures to assess these affects.

The conceptualization that an increase in a person's susceptibility to disease requires an interaction between a personality predisposition and an emotionally stressful life event is recognized also in a recent review article on personality variables and health by Scheier and Bridges (1995), who refer to 'personality predispositions and acute psychological states as shared determinants for disease' (p. 255). It is our view that the alexithymia trait is one such personality predisposition, and that alexithymic individuals are more prone to developing medical illnesses and diseases than non-alexithymic individuals because of their deficient emotional processing, in particular their difficulty in modulating states of acute emotional arousal (Lane & Schwartz, 1987).

What we must now consider are the neural mechanisms whereby deficient emotional processing might lead to dysregulation of biological systems in the body and thereby create conditions favourable for the emergence of disease. There is, of course, an alternative pathway through which poorly regulated negative emotions might influence health; some individuals attempt to cope with unregulated distressing emotions by increasing consumptive behaviours such as smoking, use of alcohol, and overeating, which are all risk factors for disease.

## A dysregulation model of illness and disease

Over the past decade, several psychosomatic theorists and researchers have made considerable progress in devising a new integrative model which conceptualizes many medical illnesses and diseases as disorders of psychobiological regulation (Schwartz, 1989; Taylor, 1987a, 1992b; Weiner, 1989). This dysregulation model is derived from general systems theory and a synthesis of findings from developmental biology and the biomedical sciences; in addition, the model incorporates recent theoretical developments in psychoanalysis and findings from infant-observational studies, in particular those pertaining to affects, object relations, and the development of the self. The reader will find a detailed description of the model and its clinical application in earlier publications (Taylor, 1987a, 1992a,b, 1993b).

The essence of the dysregulation model is its conception of human beings as self-regulating cybernetic systems, each person being comprised of a hierarchy of reciprocally regulating subsystems that interface via the brain with the larger social system. There is ample evidence that the various subsystems that comprise the organism regulate each other's activities as well as their own. Recent research has shown, for instance, that not only can the neuroendocrine system regulate immunologic functions, but also the immune system can regulate neuroendocrine functions (Blalock, 1989). The regulatory mechanisms seem to include peptide hormones that are produced by both systems and interact with receptors that are common to the two systems (Pert *et al.*, 1985; Smith & Blalock, 1986).

But what about emotions and the psyche? These too are conceptualized as components within the hierarchical arrangement of reciprocally regulating subsystems. Furthermore, as we indicated in Chapter 5, the psyche is itself conceptualized by Ciompi (1991) as a complex hierarchical structure of affective/cognitive systems of reference that are generated by repetitive concrete action. These systems have corresponding operational neuronal systems, store past experience in their structure, and regulate feelings, thoughts, and behaviour. That is, affects and their neurobiological equivalents have mobilizing, organizing, and integrating functions, and are always accompanied by cognitions. Furthermore, through descending connections from the hypothalamic and limbic systems, affects always involve the whole body, and are evidenced by physiological changes such as alterations in heart rate, blood pressure, and muscle tone (Ciompi, 1991).

A transition from health to illness or disease is likely to occur within the self-regulating system when there are perturbations in one or more components of the feedback loops, which lead to changes over time in the rhythmic functioning of one or more of the subsystems (Schwartz, 1983, 1989; Weiner, 1989). Perturbations can arise at any level in the system, from the cellular or subcellular level (as with viral infections, sensitivity to allergens, and variations in the expression of genes) to the psychological and social level (as with intrapsychic conflicts, attachment disruptions, and loss of self-esteem). Through complex feedback loops, these initial perturbations may trigger perturbations at other levels; if the ensuing dysregulation is sustained it may initiate a transition from health to illness or disease.

Although Hogan (1995) or other critics of the dysregulation model might accuse us of Cartesian interactionism, we emphasize again that emotions are conceptualized in this model (and throughout this book) not as psychological phenomena that cause bodily changes, but as part of the biological response of the organism as a whole to environmental events. Emotions generate measurable physiological effects and observable facial expressions and other motor behaviours. However, as we elaborated in Chapter 1, emotions are accessible also by introspection and, during childhood development, come to be represented by cognitive schemata that permit the reporting of subjective experience of moods and feelings, as well as the creation of fantasy, all of which provide regulatory feedback (Ciompi, 1991; Dodge & Garber, 1991; Lane & Schwartz, 1987). Although cognitive and representational deficits and/or constitutional-inherited factors may influence a person's style of emotion regulation and produce a tendency to emotional dysregulation, it is the autonomic nervous system arousal and neuroendocrine activation components of emotional responding (i.e. biological events) that can contribute potentially to the development of medical illness or disease through their effects on other biological subsystems and/or bodily structures.

Let us now consider the influence of emotions on some specific medical diseases.

### Coronary heart disease

Physicians have long known that states of acute emotional arousal can have an immediate deleterious effect in individuals with existing cardiovascular disease and sometimes produce sudden cardiac death. Engel (1971) and his colleagues (Adler, MacRitchie & Engel, 1971; Greene, Goldstein & Moss, 1972) found that individuals were likely to suffer an ischemic stroke or sudden cardiac death when experiencing emotional distress evoked by disruption of an important relationship. Other researchers (Perlman et al., 1971) found that emotional upsets due to violent arguments or threatened separation from family members, or both, could precipitate the onset of congestive heart failure. It has been the work on hostility and the Type A behaviour pattern, however, that has led to an awareness that styles of emotional processing might influence the predisposition to CHD.

What are the mechanisms whereby hostility and/or other components of Type A behaviour might influence the cardiovascular system? Several studies have demonstrated that Type A or high hostile individuals exhibit greater cardiovascular and neurohormonal reactivity in response to stressors than low hostile or Type B individuals, as reflected by elevated catecholamine levels in plasma and urine and greater heart rate and blood pressure changes (Suarez & Williams, 1989; Weidner et al., 1989; Williams et al., 1991). There is evidence also that persons scoring high on Type A behaviour and hostility have elevated levels of plasma total and LDL cholesterol (Weidner et al., 1987). According to Williams (1994), research suggests that the increased catecholamine release in high hostile persons stimulates a mobilization of fat that is then converted into cholesterol. Other studies have shown that hostility is associated strongly with smoking, alcohol consumption, and excess eating (Scherwitz et al., 1992). It is known that smoking and other health-related behaviours such as alcohol and dietary lipids impact on the functioning of macrophages, which are key cells in the development of atherosclerosis (Adams,

1994). In fact, after reviewing a large number of published studies, Littman (1993) concluded:

> . . . there is a great deal of evidence to implicate hostility as a patho-genic factor in the development of atherosclerosis, precipitation of silent ischaemia, induction of coronary vasospasm by mental stress, reduction of parasympathetic-to-sympathetic autonomic balance, risk of sudden cardiac death by ventricular fibrillation, and the continuation of smoking (p. 160).

The discovery that aggressive behaviour is associated with low levels of brain serotonin has led recently to the suggestion that the hostility trait may be associated with deficient central nervous system serotonergic function (Littman, 1993; Williams, 1994). There is evidence that such a deficiency could cause the autonomic nervous system imbalance (i.e. increased sympathetic nervous system and decreased parasympathetic nervous system function) found in hostile persons (Williams, 1994). This proposal has led to the suggestion that pharmacological agents such as selective serotonin reuptake inhibitors (e.g. fluoxetine and sertraline) might be used to raise central serotonin activity and thereby reduce Type A behaviour and hostility. Littman et al. (1993) found that a specific serotonin receptor agonist buspirone, reduced Type A behaviour, hostility, and perceived stress in cardiac patients.

Surprisingly, there has been little empirical research exploring the relationship between alexithymia and the Type A behaviour pattern and CHD. In a preliminary study, Defourney, Hubin and Luminet (1976/77) used the TAT to assess alexithymic characteristics in male civil service employees who were categorized into Type A and Type B groups on the basis of results from Rosenman's structured interview method of assessment. The Type A men expressed significantly fewer words in response to selected TAT cards than Type B men, with the content of their responses revealing a lack of emotional investment in their personal activities and interpersonal relationships and a certain poverty of fantasy activity. Such findings were suggestive of a positive relationship between alexithymia and the Type A behaviour pattern. In a later study, however, Keltikangas-Järvinen (1990) used the BIQ to measure alexithymia in a group of consecutive non-acute surgical patients who were assessed for Type A behaviour with the JAS. No relationship was found between alexithymia and the Type A behaviour pattern. However, inter-rater reliability for the BIQ was not reported and, as noted earlier, the JAS does not assess adequately the hostility component of the Type A behaviour pattern. Moreover, in a study of Finnish adolescents, Keltikangas-Järvinen and Jokinen (1989) found little relationship between Type A behaviour and somatic risk factors for CHD, whereas an inability to recognize and express negative emotions and a coping style characterized by a denial of problems and refusal to ask for help correlated positively and significantly with somatic risk.

As part of their large epidemiological study of middle-aged Finnish men, Kauhanen *et al.* (1994) found that alexithymia, measured with the TAS, was associated with a prior diagnosis of CHD, but not with greater prevalence of ischemia on an exercise tolerance test, nor with evidence of greater atherosclerosis of the carotid artery. In fact, alexithymic men with a prior diagnosis of CHD tended to have less atherosclerosis. These results, together with findings that alexithymia was associated with higher perceived exertion and more symptom reporting during the exercise tolerance test, suggested that alexithymia affects illness behaviour rather than pathophysiological changes in CHD. On the other hand, findings from a prospective study with a small group of Polish men and women (N = 25) suggest that alexithymia does influence CHD, if not through a direct effect on pathophysiology, then through altering behaviours detrimental to health; alexithymic persons in the study were reported to have fivefold more myocardial infarctions over an 8 year period than non-alexithymic persons (Brzeziński & Rybakowski, 1993). This finding must be regarded cautiously, however, as alexithymia was measured with the Schalling–Sifneos Personality Scale (SSPS). The study requires replication with larger samples and with reliable and valid measures of the alexithymia construct.

Though hostility is now considered the critical component of the Type A behaviour pattern, our own preliminary research suggests that alexithymia is unrelated both to antagonism and neurotic hostility as measured by the NEO PI and NEO PI-R (see Table 4.1 and Figs. 4.2 and 4.3 in Chapter 4). However, some individuals may be both alexithymic and high on the trait of cynical or antagonistic hostility. For example, one of our patients, a 40-year-old man with a history of marital conflict and frequent job losses because of his disagreeable style of relating to his colleagues, manifested both alexithymic characteristics and features of the Type A behaviour pattern in clinical interviews. He obtained a score of 70 on the TAS-20 and scored in the very low range on the Agreeableness dimension of the NEO PI-R; as with other alexithymic patients, he also obtained a moderately elevated score on Neuroticism, and low scores on Openness to Experience and on the warmth and positive emotions facets of Extraversion. This patient's competitiveness, cynicism, and mistrust, together with his alexithymic difficulty in understanding his own emotions and empathizing with the feelings of others, explained his tendency to create interpersonal conflicts that were leading to social isolation. Thus, as empirical studies have found (Fukunishi & Rahe, 1995; Smith & Frohm, 1985), both alexithymia and antagonistic hostility may contribute to a lack of supportive relationships, a factor that independently predicts mortality from CHD in Type A men (Orth-Gomér & Undén, 1990). Future prospective studies might compare the effects of alexithymia and hostility alone and in combination on CHD outcomes.

Another way in which alexithymia might influence the behaviour of cardiac patients is through confusion over feelings and somatic sensations; this has the potential for creating delays in responding to symptoms of an acute myocardial infarction. In a study examining factors affecting the time between symptom onset and hospital arrival for patients suffering an acute myocardial infarction, Kenyon et al. (1991) found that patients with low emotional or somatic awareness (measured by the TAS and a measure of general bodily awareness) sought treatment significantly later than patients who were more capable of identifying inner experiences of emotions and/or bodily sensations. No significant differences in delay times were found between Type A and Type B patients.

### Essential hypertension

It is well established that acute stress can cause a transient rise in blood pressure, and that exposure to prolonged stress can increase the risk of developing sustained hypertension, as in the well-known example of air traffic controllers. These stress-induced changes in blood pressure are thought to be mediated by increased sympathetic activity in the autonomic nervous system (Pilgrim, 1994).

There is evidence also that blood pressure can be influenced by the communication of feelings. Studies have demonstrated an inverse relationship between blood pressure and the awareness and expression of anger (Goldstein et al., 1988), as well as reductions in blood pressure while talking about and describing feelings of helplessness and hopelessness (Lynch, Lynch & Friedman, 1992) and after talking about extremely emotional topics (Pennebaker & Susman, 1988). Though difficulty communicating feelings is only one component of the alexithymia construct, the findings of blood pressure changes with both inhibition and expression of affects suggests a relationship also between alexithymia and essential hypertension.

Based on his findings from psychoanalytic case studies, Alexander (1948) concluded that hypertensive individuals struggle with a specific conflict between passive, dependent, receptive tendencies and over-compensatory competitive, aggressive, hostile impulses. Although his emphasis was on interpreting and resolving the intrapsychic conflict, Alexander recognized the role of unregulated affect in his proposal that 'a *chronic* inhibited rage may lead to a *chronic* elevation of the blood pressure' (p. 293). Although later psychosomatic researchers identified an association between the Type A behaviour pattern and essential hypertension, as with CHD, subsequent research has demonstrated that blood pressure is linked more strongly with the anger/hostility component of Type A behaviour. Studies have shown that high hostility is associated with greater blood pressure reactivity in response to stressful experiences (Christensen & Smith, 1993), and also with more consistently elevated blood pressure in patients with mild hypertension (Jamner et al., 1993). There is evidence, however, that blood pressure is influenced also by the way individuals cope with their anger, i.e. by their mode of regulating this affect. In an investigation of a community sample, for example, Harburg et al. (1991) found that older black men who employed a reflective mode of coping with anger (i.e. constraining their anger and trying to solve the problem) had significantly lower blood pressure than those who scored low on this mode. In contrast, older black men with a strong tendency to impulsively express or act out their anger (e.g. slam doors, say nasty things, lose their temper) had significantly higher blood pressure than those who scored low on this mode.

Recognizing that individuals who become hypertensive show a heightened physiological reactivity in response to stress, Melamed (1987) formulated an intervening personality variable which he called *emotional reactivity*. This personality construct was designed to denote 'a tendency to more easily enter and maintain a state of emotional arousal' (p. 218). The characteristics of emotional reactivity are a tendency to experience intrusive images, feelings, and thoughts following an emotional event, a lack of ability to control becoming emotionally aroused, a tendency to experience unpleasant emotional responses in anticipation of forthcoming emotional events, and emotional responses that are excessive in magnitude and/or duration following stressful stimuli. The construct obviously overlaps with our concept of deficits in the cognitive processing and regulation of affects.

After developing a reliable measure of emotional reactivity (the ER scale), Melamed (1987) tested a large population of factory workers in Israel who were divided into controls and those with elevated blood pressure. Individuals with elevated systolic blood pressure (both men and women) over the age of 40 years scored significantly higher on the ER scale than the controls. Individuals below the age of 40 years scored in the same direction, but the results were not statistically significant. Interestingly, control subjects who had a family history of hypertension scored higher on the ER scale than control subjects without such a history. Melamed concluded that emotional hyperreactors are probably physiologic hyperreactors as well, and that the process whereby emotional reactivity contributes to the development of essential hypertension is gradual. However, not all individuals over the age of 40 years with high ER scale scores (including some with a family history of hypertension) had elevated blood pressure.

Although several studies have attempted to explore the relationship between alexithymia and essential hypertension, most of the empirical findings are of questionable validity because of the poor psychometric properties of the instruments that were used to measure the alexithymia construct. Osti, Trombini and Magnani (1980), for example, found that patients with essential hypertension were significantly more alexithymic than patients with other cardiovascular disorders; however, alexithymia was measured with the SSPS, which was shown later to lack adequate reliability and validity. A strong association between hypertension and alexithymia was reported also by Gage and Egan (1984), but alexithymia was assessed with the MMPI alexithymia scale, which also lacks reliability and validity. A finding with stronger validity was reported by Paulson (1985), who investigated a sample of 53 hypertensive patients with the BIQ and found a prevalence rate of 41% of alexithymia. However, no comparison goup was used in this study.

Although Safar et al. (1978) did not use the concept of alexithymia, they assessed similar characteristics in groups of male patients with borderline and sustained hypertension and in a group of normal men. Compared with the normal men, patients with sustained hypertension manifested significantly less fantasy activity, as well as a more rational thinking style and a stereotyped approach to reality. Similar tendencies were noted in the patients with borderline hypertension, but these were not statistically significant.

In a more recent study, Todarello et al. (1995) investigated a sample of 114 essential hypertensive patients using a validated Italian translation of the TAS-20. The patients were recruited from a hospital clinic for the management and prevention of hypertension. Alexithymia was assessed also in a group of 113 general psychiatric outpatients and a group of 130 normal adults. The hypertensive patients scored significantly higher than the psychiatric patients on the total TAS-20, and the psychiatric patients scored significantly higher than the normal adults. Based on the TAS-20 cutoff score, a rate of 55.3% for alexithymia was found in the hypertensive group compared with significantly lower rates of 32.7% in the psychiatric group and 16.3% in the normal group. Interestingly, the hypertensive patients scored significantly higher than the normal adults on all three factors of the TAS-20, not just on the factor assessing difficulty communicating feelings.

Though the results of the Italian study indicate a strong association between alexithymia and essential hypertension, this was in a selected sample of patients receiving medical care and may not be representative of the hypertensive population at large. It is possible that individuals who have been diagnosed as hypertensive and are concerned about their health may differ psychologically from those whose condition remains undetected in the general population (Pilgrim, 1994; Steptoe, 1986). Also, because of the cross-sectional design of this study, it was not possible to draw conclusions concerning the causality of the relationship between alexithymia and essential hypertension. The relationship should be more thoroughly evaluated using community samples of individuals who do not know that they are hypertensive, and taking care to identify subtypes of hypertension, as these may be associated with different personality traits. For example, consistent with the heterogeneity of essential hypertension, several investigators have found that hypertensive patients with high plasma renin activity score differently on a range of psychological tests than those with low or normal plasma renin activity (Esler *et al.*, 1977; Perini, Rauchfleisch & Bühler, 1985; Thailer *et al.*, 1985).

## Diabetes mellitus

Emotions have long been suspected as having an influence on blood sugar control and the course of diabetes mellitus (Helz & Templeton, 1990; Surwit & Schneider, 1993). This influence may be mediated directly through a release of stress hormones (catecholamines, cortisol, glucagon, and growth hormone) that counter-regulate the action of insulin, or indirectly by invoking poor compliance with diet, exercise regimes, insulin doses, or self-monitoring of glucose and acetone levels (Barglow *et al.*, 1984; Fonagy & Moran, 1994). Baker and Barcai (1970), for example, demonstrated a direct neurohumoral pathway by showing that the ketoacidosis evoked by emotional stress in superlabile juvenile diabetics can be blocked by administration of beta-adrenergic blocking agents. And Rodin *et al.* (1991) demonstrated a behavioural pathway in finding that some adolescent Type I diabetics with eating disorders intentionally omit insulin to produce hyperglycemia and weight loss. There is also suggestive evidence that Type I diabetics have a heightened sensitivity to cortisol and catecholamines, and therefore a more marked hyperglycemic response to stressful situations that increase the levels of these hormones (Gilbert et al., 1989). However, insulin-dependent diabetics show considerable variation in their response to stressful stimuli; while some show a hyperglycemic response to acute psychologic stress, others become hypoglycemic, or show no change at all in blood sugar levels (Surwit & Schneider, 1993). This variation suggests a role for personality factors in mediating between emotional stress and glucose regulation in diabetic individuals. Although there is no support for a specific diabetic personality, there is some evidence that glucose regulation in diabetic individuals is associated with personality factors that reflect different styles of emotional processing. In a study of insulin-dependent diabetic children, for example, Stabler et al. (1987) found that children with Type A personalities had a hyperglycemic response to playing a stressful video game that did not occur in children with Type B personalities. A more comprehensive study was conducted by Peyrot and McMurray (1985), who administered several measures of psychosocial adjustment to 20 Type I insulin-dependent diabetic adults, all of whom were married and living with their spouse. The subjects were categorized into 'good' and 'poor' control groups on the basis of their blood glycosylated hemoglobin concentration, which is a measure of long-term glucose control. The poor control patients demonstrated higher scores on measures of anger and impatience, which are elements of the Type A behaviour pattern that has been found to increase the psychophysiologic response to stress. Although there was no significant difference between the two groups on a measure of anxiety, the poor control group was significantly more prone to anxiety extremes (high or low), while the good control group experienced more moderate levels of anxiety.

In a more recent study, Abramson et al. (1991) used the TAT to assess alexithymic characteristics in a group of 30 Type I diabetic adults and in a control group of 49 healthy adults. The diabetic subjects produced significantly fewer affect words than the control subjects in response to six TAT cards, suggesting that they were more alexithymic. In addition, a strong negative correlation between the number of affect words and glycosylated hemoglobin in the diabetic group indicated that alexithymic characteristics are associated with poorer metabolic control.

Fonagy and Moran (1994) have recently offered some interesting psychoanalytic observations on young people with 'brittle' diabetes, which is 'a form of insulin-dependent diabetes characterised by extreme and chronic failure to maintain blood glucose control' (p. 63).

Their clinical observations suggest that such patients fail to create mental representations of the self and primary caretakers as thinking, feeling, and experiencing persons; such deficits parallel Marty and de M'Uzan's (1963) concept of *pensée opératoire*. According to Fonagy and Moran, 'The incomplete structuralisation of the self enables patients to disavow ownership of their body' (p. 68) and to enact through self-destructive diabetic mismanagement conflicts over separation from, or closeness to, an internal representation of an important figure that is experienced as dangerously invading the self or abandoning it. Fonagy and Moran's observations are consistent with our view that deficits in affect regulation are associated invariably with deficits in the internal representation of the relationship between the self and primary caregivers.

## Rheumatoid arthritis

At one time classified among the seven classical psychosomatic diseases, rheumatoid arthritis is now known to be an autoimmune disease in which inflammatory reactions are set up in the body, especially in the joints. The disease is thought to be initiated by an abnormal immune response to a common virus or bacterium, which then becomes self-perpetuating (Baker, 1987). As with other diseases traditionally regarded as psychosomatic, subtypes of rheumatoid arthritis have now been identified that differ in clinical and immunological features as well as course characteristics. Several studies have suggested that there is a psychological heterogeneity among rheumatoid patients as well. Rimon (1969; Rimon & Laakso, 1985), for example, identified a subtype that was less connected with genetic factors and more influenced by emotionally stressful life events, and a second subtype that was more associated with a hereditary predisposition and less influenced by stressful events. Subtypes of the disease were identified also by Crown, Crown and Fleming (1975), who found that patients whose serum was positive for rheumatoid factor scored low on a measure of neurotic psychopathology, in contrast to seronegative patients who scored significantly higher.

Similar subgroups were identified by Vollhardt et al. (1982), who found that patients with rheumatoid serum factor and erosive joint changes evident by X-ray were the most homogeneous in regard to psychometric measures of symptom distress and mood disturbance, but they showed significantly less psychopathology than rheumatoid patients who lacked the combination of the serum rheumatoid factor and erosive joint changes. The psychological profile of the seropositive patients could not be considered a feature of adaptation to chronic joint disease, as a group of patients with other types of arthritis and matched for illness duration and functional impairment showed significantly more psychopathology. Moreover, a follow-up study that used several indices from the TAT to assess alexithymic characteristics found the seropositive patients were no more or less alexithymic than the other groups (Vollhardt, Ackerman & Shindledecker, 1986).

Two other studies have explored a possible association between alexithymia and rheumatoid arthritis, but patients were not categorized into physiologically distinguishable subgroups. In a study conducted in India, Fernandez et al. (1989) used both the BIQ and the TAS to assess alexithymia in a group of patients with rheumatoid arthritis and in a sociodemographically-matched comparison group of healthy adults. The rheumatoid arthritis patients scored significantly higher than the healthy subjects on both the BIQ and the TAS, and there was a significant positive correlation between the two measures. Based on the established TAS cutoff score, 27.5% of the rheumatoid arthritis patients were alexithymic compared with only 7.5% in the healthy group. Although alexithymia was unrelated to the duration of illness, rheumatoid arthritis patients with greater functional impairment showed significantly higher alexithymia scores.

In a more recent study, Jordan and Lumley (1993) administered the TAS to a group of rheumatoid arthritis patients who were receiving treatment at the outpatient rheumatology clinic of a large metropolitan hospital in the United States. The patients also completed measures of negative affectivity, perceived pain severity, perceived pain control, pain coping strategies, and psychosocial functioning and activity level. Although there was no comparison group in this study, the mean TAS score for the arthritis patients was not significantly different from the mean TAS score that has been reported for a North American community sample. Consistent with findings from other research on alexithymia and emotional coping or coping with stress (Fukunishi & Rahe, 1995; Paez et al., 1995), however, TAS scores were associated strongly with negative affect, the highest level of distress being found in patients with elevated alexithymia scores who failed to use active coping strategies such as ignoring or reinterpreting pain, using coping self-statements, or increasing activity.

Given the pathophysiology of rheumatoid arthritis, and the highly complex biological mechanisms that underly immunoregulation in healthy individuals, it is perhaps not surprising that empirical research has failed to show a strong association between alexithymia and this disease, apart from a possible influence of this personality trait on the coping style of some patients with the disease. Although rheumatoid arthritis must involve some imbalance in immunoregulation, exactly why a person's immune system loses the capacity to differentiate between self and foreign macromolecules is not known (Shoenfeld & Schwartz, 1984). As with other autoimmune diseases, such as ulcerative colitis and juvenile onset (Type I) diabetes mellitus, a high percentage of patients with rheumatoid arthritis report experiencing an emotionally stressful life event prior to the onset of symptoms (Baker 1982; Rimon, 1969); however, the evidence for a personality predisposition involving high negative affectivity in rheumatoid arthritis patients is rather weak (Friedman & Booth-Kewley, 1987). And while there is increasing evidence that emotions can influence the immune system through their impact on the sympathetic nervous system and endocrine functions (Baker, 1987; Camara & Danao, 1989; Kiecolt-Glaser & Glaser, 1995), it is much less certain that such changes are sufficiently sustained and of a kind that could lead to an autoimmune disease. Individuals who show the greatest cardiovascular reactivity to stressors seem also to show the largest immune alterations (Herbert *et al.*, 1994); however, the pathways discussed earlier through which emotions can influence cardiovascular reactivity and metabolic functions are far less complex than those mediating between emotions and immune functions; the latter involve a host of neuropeptides and neurotransmitters that are still in the process of being understood (Blalock, 1989; Daruna & Morgan, 1990; Felten *et al.*, 1993).

## Inflammatory bowel diseases

Also linked with autoimmune processes are the inflammatory bowel diseases, ulcerative colitis and Crohn's disease, although genetic and environmental factors are implicated in their etiology as well. The observation that affects could influence the course of these diseases was made initially by Engel (1955, 1958), who observed that the onset or exacerbation of ulcerative colitis was associated frequently with feelings of helplessness and hopelessness in response to disruption of an important attachment relationship (i.e. the giving up/given up complex). Although Engel (1955) recognized that the intense dependency of many ulcerative colitis patients on a 'key relationship' compensated for 'serious defects in ego function', his allegiance to classical psychoanalytic drive theory diverted him from elaborating further on the psychic structure of these patients and from recognizing that the ego defects sometimes involve problems in self- and affect regulation. In a later study, Karush *et al.* (1977) were able to categorize patients with moderate to severe chronic ulcerative colitis into three groups – individuated, symbiotic, and transitional – according to the degree to which unresolved symbiotic needs dominated their object relationships. After examining the clinical descriptions provided by Karush and his coworkers, Nemiah (1982) inferred that the symbiotic patients (who were clingingly dependent) manifested alexithymic characteristics, in contrast to the individuated patients, whose personality organization resembled that of psychoneurotic individuals. This should not be surprising, in that excessive dependency implies deficits in the inner representations of self and object along with associated deficits in the representation and regulation of affects.

Although the type of object relating was not assessed, an early empirical study of alexithymia yielded results that were consistent with Nemiah's impression that the cognitive–affective style of some patients with inflammatory bowel disease is markedly different from that of psychoneurotic patients. Using responses to nine cards of the TAT to assess alexithymic characteristics, Taylor *et al.* (1981) found a group of patients with inflammatory bowel disease (ten with ulcerative colitis and ten with Crohn's disease) were significantly less verbally productive and used significantly fewer affect words than a sociodemographically matched group of psychoneurotic patients. Significant differences between the two groups were still found in a subsequent analysis that used a simple frequency count of different affect words (Taylor & Doody, 1985).

More recently, Porcelli *et al.* (1995) used the TAS-20 to measure alexithymia in a group of patients with inflammatory bowel disease (89 with ulcerative colitis and 23 with Crohn's disease) and in a control group of healthy adults matched for gender, age, and education. The bowel disease group was significantly more alexithymic than the control group, and no significant difference was found between the ulcerative colitis and Crohn's disease patients. Alexithymia was unrelated to the duration of illness and the level of disease activity. In a follow-up assessment with the same group of bowel disease patients, which was referred to in Chapter 4, Porcelli *et al.* (1996) found no significant change in the mean TAS-20 score over a six-month period, suggesting that alexithymia is a stable trait in these patients.

Although 35.7% of the bowel disease patients in this study scored within the alexithymic range of the TAS-20, compared with only 4.5% of the control group, the results indicate that about two-thirds of patients with inflammatory bowel disease may not manifest difficulties in the cognitive regulation of affects. Further studies are needed to determine whether the alexithymic bowel disease patients are more symbiotic than their non-alexithymic counterparts and more likely to develop a giving up/given up complex in response to loss of their key relationships. It is likely that subforms of inflammatory bowel disease will be detected that are distinguishable in terms of styles of object relating and emotional processing, and in regard to the role of stressful events in the onset and exacerbation of the disease.

## Cancer

Although the field of psychoneuroimmunology is capturing a great deal of attention, a major problem in studying the role of emotions in the development and course of cancer is that there are numerous forms of this disease. According to Weiner (1992), 'a minimum of 100 forms of malignant disease are recognized [and] their initiating factors are far from uniform' (p. 571). Furthermore, as Kiecolt-Glaser and Glaser (1995) point out, the stage of cancer can profoundly affect how a patient feels, as can the side-effects from chemotherapy and radiation treatment.

The idea that certain personality traits might predispose to cancer stemmed partly from Kissen and Eysenck's (1962) finding of emotional suppression in a study of men with lung cancer, and partly from Greer and Morris's (1975) finding that women aged under 50 who were tested the day before breast biopsy and were subsequently diagnosed as having breast cancer showed significantly higher levels of suppressed anger than women who turned out to have benign tumours. Similar findings of emotional suppression were reported in other studies of women with breast cancer, and also in women with cancers of the cervix, body of the uterus, and ovary (Mastrovito et al., 1979). Kneier and Temoshok (1984) subsequently demonstrated that patients with malignant melanomas were significantly more repressed than patients with cardiovascular diseases; and in a later study of malignant melanoma patients, Temoshok et al. (1985) operationalized the construct of a Type C behaviour pattern and found it correlated significantly with the thickness of the initial skin lesions.

Notwithstanding the methodological problems in the prospective studies by Grossarth-Maticek and his colleagues (1988; Eysenck, 1991b), their finding that Type 1 behaviour was a major predictor of cancer incidence is consistent with results reported by other investigators (Graves & Thomas, 1981). As Eysenck (1991c) emphasizes, however, 'suppression of emotion is only one of two suggested risk factors, the other being poor coping when faced with stress, leading to feelings of hopelessness and helplessness' (p. 297). In a study of women admitted to hospital for cone biopsy following discovery of suspicious cervical cytology, Schmale and Iker (1966) found that women who reported feelings of helplessness and hopelessness were significantly more likely to have cancer of the cervix than women without those affects, despite little difference in the incidence of recent stressful experiences.

Although the majority of women with breast cancer in the Greer and Morris (1975) study showed marked suppression of affect, there was a subgroup who lost control and suffered from difficulty modulating affects. Graves and Thomas (1981), in a prospective study of Johns Hopkins medical students, also found that men who later developed cancer were not a homogeneous group. While a proneness to cancer was associated with a pattern of relatedness in which emotions are controlled and rather restricted (as measured by a Rorschach Interaction Scale), a strong association was found also with an 'ambivalent' style of relating which is characterized by emotional lability. This prospective study also found an association between the development of cancer and perceived closeness to parents as measured by a Family Attitude Questionnaire that was completed while the men were in medical school (Thomas, Duszynski & Shaffer, 1979).

There have been few attempts to explore the relationship between alexithymia and cancer. In a preliminary study, Todarello et al. (1989) administered the SSPS and a measure of neurotic psychopathology to 200 women prior to their undergoing mammography either for suspected carcinoma of the breast or for a routine checkup. The examination revealed positive evidence of breast cancer in 13 of the women. A comparison of the mean psychological test scores for these women with the mean scores of the healthy women and women with benign pathology revealed significantly more alexithymia in the former group but no difference in neurotic psychopathology. Given the small number of women with breast cancer, and the psychometric properties of the scale used to measure alexithymia, these findings are of limited value. Furthermore, a high proportion of women, some of whom tested positive for cancer, refused to participate in the study.

In a more recent study, Anagnostopoulos et al. (1993) used the TAS to assess alexithymia in 100 women attending two breast-screening clinics for a routine checkup or for suspected breast pathology. The TAS was administered before clinical and mammographic examinations or biopsies were made. No relationship was found between alexithymia and the presence or absence of breast cancer.

In an effort to explore further the relationship between alexithymia and the development of cancer, Todarello et al. (1994) conducted a study with 26 women affected by cervical dysplasia who were not aware of their medical status and a control group of 36 healthy women. Women with cervical dysplasia showed higher alexithymia scores than women with an unsuspicious PAP smear. Recognizing that the finding must be interpreted cautiously because of the small sample size and the psychometric limitations of the Revised SSPS which was used to measure alexithymia, Todarello *et al.* (1997) recently repeated the study with larger groups of women and using a validated Italian translation of the TAS-20. Again, women affected by cervical dysplasia (N = 43) had significantly higher alexithymia scores than healthy women (N = 67).

Although there is now evidence of bidirectional communication pathways between the brain and the immune system, as well as considerable evidence that emotional and other stress can produce alterations in immune function (Herbert & Cohen, 1993; Kiecolt-Glaser & Glaser, 1995; Maier, Watkins & Fleshner, 1994), it is still difficult to say definitively whether such alterations can trigger the onset of cancer. As Weiner (1992) points out, the initiation of tumours by the transformation of cells involves a dysregulation of highly complex mechanisms (oncogenes, growth factors, second messenger systems, etc.) that are quite specific to a particular tumour. Furthermore, the cellular mechanisms involved in the progression and metastasis of tumours differ from those that initiate the transformation of cells. Improved measures and more prospective studies are needed, as well as specification of the exact type, nature, and stage of cancer.

### Functional physiological disorders

In Chapter 6, we noted that many patients who present to physicians with somatic symptoms and no identifiable medical disease suffer from functional physiological disorders such as fibromyalgia syndrome, irritable bowel syndrome, and chronic fatigue syndrome (CFS). Although the term *functional* is often contrasted with the term *organic* and given the added meaning of psychogenic, it really denotes a disturbance of physiological function that is present in medical illnesses that do not have the structural tissue and organ changes that occur in medical diseases (Kirmayer & Robbins, 1991b). An advantage of the dysregulation model outlined earlier in this chapter is that it eliminates the usual distinction between organic diseases and functional disorders, and also the distinction between physical disorders and psychiatric disorders (Taylor, 1992a; Weiner, 1989). With the emphasis on the functioning of biological systems (including the affect system) rather than the structure of cells and organs, the model allows us to reconceptualize many illnesses and diseases as 'disorders of regulation' which may or may not be associated with actual structural changes.

Unfortunately, the tendency for medical physicians to regard somatic symptoms as psychogenic when there is no detectable 'organic' disease is paralleled by a tendency in many psychiatrists to view all puzzling somatic syndromes as manifestations of primary psychiatric disorders and/or abnormal illness behaviour. These tendencies are evidenced in earlier views that fibromyalgia is a form of 'psychogenic rheumatism' (Shulman & Bunim, 1962), and that patients with irritable bowel syndrome are essentially neurotics who use their symptoms as a socially more acceptable way to express distress (Latimer, 1981). More recently, several authors have argued that CFS corresponds to the nineteenth century diagnosis of neurasthenia and that the symptoms in most patients can be attributed to a psychiatric disorder, most commonly major depression, dysthymia, or somatization disorder (Abbey & Garfinkel, 1991; Greenberg, 1990; Manu, Lane & Matthews, 1992; Stewart, 1990). Such opinions led one medical historian to adopt the simplistic and reductionistic position that fibromyalgia, irritable bowel syndrome, and CFS are psychogenic disorders, the 'choice' of symptoms being determined by the patient's unconscious mind (Shorter, 1992).

Although several review articles report a high comorbidity between functional physiological disorders and psychiatric disorders (Abbey & Garfinkel, 1991; Hudson & Pope, 1989; Kellner, 1991; Walker, Roy-Byrne & Katon, 1990), a number of studies have found the prevalence of psychiatric disorders to be no higher than that found in community groups and groups of patients with other medical diseases (Goldenberg, 1989; Hickie et al., 1990; Kirmayer, Robbins & Kapusta, 1988; Shanks & Ho-Yen, 1995), or elevated only among those sufferers who seek medical help (Drossman et al., 1988; Smith et al., 1990). It is thus incorrect to argue that the symptoms of functional physiological disorders can be solely accounted for by psychiatric disorders. This does not exclude the possibility that emotional distress may intensify patients' symptoms or reduce their ability to cope with somatic symptoms.

Rather than attributing the symptoms of fibromyalgia and irritable bowel syndrome to associated psychopathology, Hudson and Pope (1989, 1990) proposed that the functional physiological disorders (including migraine) and several psychiatric disorders may arise from a common pathophysiologic abnormality and represent a family of related conditions, which they provisionally named *affective spectrum disorder* (ASD). The choice of the word 'affective' does not imply that major depression plays a special causal role, but reflects the fact that all forms of ASD have shown favourable responses to antidepressant medications, this having been demonstrated first in major depression. The psychiatric disorders in the spectrum include major depression, bulimia, panic disorder, and obsessive–compulsive disorder. The concept of ASD is based not only on the response to pharmacologic treatment, but also on the frequent comorbidity among the various disorders, and reports of high rates of major depression among the relatives of patients with fibromyalgia.

Although the validity of the ASD concept is yet to be established, the concept is consistent with clinical observations of marked similarities between fibromyalgia and CFS, as well as an inconsistent, but not uncommon, finding of concurrent irritable bowel syndrome, major depression, or panic disorder among patients with these disorders. The ASD concept is congruent also with the dysregulation model of illness and disease in that the different forms of ASD involve dysregulations in different biological subsystems. There is evidence, for example, that CFS and fibromyalgia 'have similar disordered sleep physiology, which shows features of an arousal disturbance within NREM sleep . . .' (Moldofsky, 1993, pp. 149-150). Recent research findings suggest a reciprocal relationship between the immune (sub)system and the sleep–wake (sub)system so that perturbations in one will affect the other and over time result in sleep abnormalities, fatigue, diffuse muscle pains, and emotional distress. Any of these symptoms may further disturb sleep physiology and lead to continuing alterations in immune function (Moldofsky, 1989, 1993).

There is evidence also that different forms of irritable bowel syndrome involve disturbances in colonic motility (and sometimes in other parts of the gastrointestinal tract), alterations in the perception of sensations from the gut, or both (Weiner, 1992). Some patients suffer also from migraine headaches, bladder dysfunction, or dysmenorrhoea. Reciprocal connections between the brain and the enteric nervous system (which is a rich neuronal network in the gut), and the presence of similar neurotransmitters and neuropeptides in both sites, permit numerous brain–gut interactions whereby perturbations in the central nervous system (including those associated with various emotional states) may affect gastrointestinal functions, and afferent input from the gut may cause perturbations within the brain, such as increased firing of the locus coeruleus that could result in anxiety (Lydiard, 1992; Walker *et al.*, 1990). Such reciprocal interactions, as Lydiard (1992) points out, 'potentially create a vicious positive feedback cycle' (p. 615).

It will be evident to the reader that we do not regard emotions as being a primary cause of functional physiological disorders; however, the dysregulation model provides a way of conceptualizing how poorly modulated emotional distress can dysregulate other biological subsystems and thereby be one factor that can potentially influence the onset or course of these illnesses. As with medical diseases, we predict that empirical studies will not find a strong association between alexithymia and functional physiological disorders. None the less, some patients may be more prone to states of affective dysregulation and exacerbations of illness because of an alexithymic deficit. We conclude the chapter with a brief description of such a patient.

### Clinical illustration

James, a man in his late 20s, presented to his family physician with symptoms of generalized anxiety, an unpleasant and constant feeling of pressure in his head, diffuse muscle pains, lack of energy and drive, and severe gastrointestinal discomfort. He had experienced these symptoms intermittently for about 18 months and had a prior history of recurrent panic attacks which had responded to treatment with antipanic medication. Although James did not complain of a depressed mood, he showed evidence of a moderate clinical depression on the Beck Depression Inventory. Consultation with a gastroenterologist confirmed a diagnosis of irritable bowel syndrome; other physicians identified multiple tender points on physical examination and attributed the patient's muscle pains to fibromyalgia. A psychiatric consultant made a diagnosis of major depression with an associated somatization disorder, and a past history of panic disorder.

Although James obtained some symptom relief from antidepressant medication and a variety of stress management techniques, over the next several years he had several recurrences of his fibromyalgia and/or irritable bowel syndrome, and frequently complained of severe headaches that sometimes lasted several days. On psychological testing, the patient scored in the alexithymic range of the TAS-20, very high on the Neuroticism dimension of the NEO PI-R, very low on the positive emotion subscale of Extraversion, and in the low average range on the fantasy and feelings subscales of Openness to Experience. Projective testing with the Rorschach and TAT revealed that James lacked psychological mindedness and had difficulty dealing with affect-laden issues. There was evidence that he was inclined not to reflect or introspect, and that his cognitive style was oriented toward external events. The patient's responses to TAT cards revealed a sense of inner impoverishment and difficulty in forming close relationships; mother figures were described as undemonstrative, and father figures were experienced as remote, emotionally ungiving, and difficult to communicate with.

In addition to pharmacotherapy and behavioural therapies, James was treated with psychotherapy that was modified in some of the ways that will be described in the next chapter. During the early months of psychotherapy it became evident that James struggled with a great deal of anger and rage, but usually he was unaware of such feelings until he lost control. On one occasion, he impulsively punched his fist through a wall. Exploration of this event revealed that he had been bothered a few hours earlier by pressure from a salesperson but had failed to identify his feelings; nor had he linked his impulsive outburst with this situation. Although James described many stresses and misunderstandings in his job and family relationships, rather than experience distressing feelings and communicate them to others, he mostly complained of a recurrence or intensification of fibrositic or irritable bowel symptoms.

Over the course of several years of treatment, James became increasingly aware of, and able to describe, his subjective feelings. He formed a strong emotional attachment to the psychotherapist and began, especially during separations from therapy, to experience overwhelming feelings of sadness, and hopelessness, and even a fear that he might commit suicide. Such feelings largely replaced the patient's somatic symptoms and enabled the therapist to begin to address James's emotional neediness and difficulty in establishing a satisfying and intimate relationship with a woman.

# [11] Treatment considerations

Medical and psychiatric patients with alexithymia or other deficits in emotional processing typically present major treatment problems for physicians and mental health professionals. In addition to deficits in affect expression and affect regulation, such patients manifest disturbances in inner self- and object representations and other aspects of self-regulation, which often lead to countertransferential or other interpersonal difficulties within therapeutic relationships. Their proneness to somatization may result in medical overinvestigation that can add an iatrogenic component to their illnesses; and their 'affect storms' or difficulty in relinquishing unhealthy affect regulatory behaviours, such as alcohol abuse or binge eating, may lead to feelings of frustration, anger, and helplessness in their treating physicians, nurses, or psychotherapists.

Based on extensive clinical observations, several therapists have concluded that alexithymic patients respond poorly to psychoanalysis or other insight-oriented forms of psychotherapy. Before the term 'alexithymia' was coined to describe these patients, Ruesch (1948) reported a poor response to insight psychotherapy which he attributed to an inability to connect verbal, gestural, or other symbols with affects and feelings. Horney (1952) similarly viewed a paucity of inner experience and the associated externally orientated mode of thinking and living a major impediment to psychoanalytic therapy. Krystal (1982/83), who has extensive experience in treating patients with substance use disorders, PTSD, and other disorders of affect regulation, regards alexithymia as 'possibly the most important single factor diminishing the success of psychoanalysis and psychodynamic psychotherapy' (p. 364); and McDougall (1972) warns of the potential for prolonged periods of 'stagnation' if such patients are taken into psychoanalysis. Moreover, as Sifneos (1972/73, 1975) has pointed out, alexithymic patients with somatic diseases may be made worse as a result of anxiety-provoking psychotherapeutic interventions. Consequently, Sifneos (1975), Freyberger (1977), and Nemiah et al. (1976) recommend the use of supportive rather than interpretive psychotherapies for alexithymic patients, an approach that may be as successfully pursued by primary care physicians as by psychiatrists. Others advise the use of pharmacologic, cognitive–behavioural, or multiple modes of therapeutic intervention including modified forms of psychodynamic psychotherapy (Flannery, 1978; Schraa & Dicks, 1981; Taylor et al., 1991).

## A lack of psychological mindedness

The poor response of alexithymic patients to traditional insight-oriented psychotherapies is generally attributed to their lack of psychological mindedness (Singer, 1977). Research evaluating the validity of the alexithymia construct has provided empirical support for this clinical impression (Taylor, 1995; Taylor & Taylor, 1997). As noted in Chapter 3, both the TAS and the TAS-20 were found to correlate significantly and negatively with measures of psychological mindedness. The strongest correlations were between the TAS-20 and its three factors and the recently developed Psychological Mindedness Scale (PMS) which, in a preliminary study, successfully predicted outcome from psychodynamically oriented individual psychotherapy (Conte et al., 1990). Both alexithymia measures also negatively correlate with the short form of the Need-for-Cognition Scale (NCS), which assesses a person's tendency to engage in and enjoy effortful and analytical cognitive endeavours (Cacioppo & Petty, 1982), a characteristic essential for insight-oriented psychotherapies. In addition, as was outlined in Chapter 4, research with the TAS and TAS-20 has shown that alexithymia is related inversely to the openness to experience dimension in the five-factor model of personality, which encompasses a broad range of traits associated with suitability for psychodynamic psychotherapy. These include intellectual curiosity, behavioural flexibility, receptivity to inner feelings, and a creative imagination (McCrae & Costa, 1985). Openness to experience, as Miller (1991) has pointed out, influences the patient's reactions to the therapist's interventions, in particular the ability to understand and accept psychodynamic interpretations. The psychological mindedness construct is generally associated with ego strength (Lake, 1985); indeed, Conte et al. (1995) recently reported a high positive correlation between the

PMS and an ego strength scale derived from items on Bellak's (1984) modified version of Ego Function Assessment. In our own research, we found that the TAS correlates negatively with the MMPI Ego Strength Scale (Es), a test that was designed to predict successful response to psychotherapy (Barron, 1953), and that alexithymic patients score significantly lower on the Es than non-alexithymic patients (Bagby et al., 1988b; Taylor et al., 1990b; Taylor et al., 1992b).

Although empirical studies have yet to be conducted to determine whether alexithymia is a useful predictor of outcome from psychodynamic psychotherapy, clinical experience and the findings from correlational studies strongly suggest the need to employ modified forms of psychotherapy and/or alternative treatment approaches for alexithymic patients. This recommendation also applies to non-alexithymic patients with disorders of affect regulation, such as many patients with borderline personality features who, though capable of genuine affective experience and expression, show poor affect tolerance and an inability to use affects as signals (Brown, 1993; Robbins, 1989).

### Modified psychotherapy

Several clinicians have devised parameters or modifications of psychodynamic psychotherapy for alexithymic patients who seek treatment for disorders of affect regulation. In general, these modifications focus on the form, rather than on the content of the patient's communications, and they attempt to enhance the patients' awareness of deficits in the way they process and experience emotions. As outlined by Krystal (1979, 1982/83, 1988), for example, the therapist might first explain to alexithymic patients that they differ from other people in that they often experience their emotions as physiological reactions and bodily sensations rather than as feelings. Patients are then helped to develop affect tolerance by being taught that states of emotional arousal are self-limited in duration and intensity. The therapist helps these patients to recognize, differentiate, label, and manage their own feelings. This is a slow and tedious process, but it is assumed that patients will begin to know their own feelings only as they learn to desomatize and differentiate emotions and to externalize them in verbal patterns. Directing patients' attention to behavioural expressions of emotion, such as sighs, gestures, and movements, can provide an important source of information that may help connect them with feelings (Greenberg & Safran, 1989). Patients are taught that emotions are not discrete entities to be suppressed or discharged through immediate action, but, rather, valued aspects of experience that signal important information which, when reflected upon, can help them respond more effectively to stressful events and to the vicissitudes of their interpersonal relationships. That is, the acquisition of an ability to use affects as signals permits a greater cognitive appraisal of the evoking events. There is evidence that teaching alexithymic patients to attend to their dreams also increases their access to feelings and other aspects of inner life, and leads to better progress in psychotherapy (Cartwright, 1993; Cartwright, Tipton & Wicklund, 1980).

Attention is given also to the tendency for these patients to amplify and misinterpret the bodily sensations accompanying states of emotional arousal. For this purpose, it has been found helpful sometimes to combine psychotherapeutic interventions with behavioural techniques, such as relaxation training, autogenic training, or biofeedback, which focus directly on bodily sensations and which increase both the patient's awareness of the relationship of these sensations with environmental events and their capacity to self-regulate various physiological functions (Stephanos, Bieble & Plaum, 1976; Taylor, 1987a). In addition, as observed originally by Ruesch (1948), and later by several other clinicians (Krystal, 1982/83; McDougall, 1985; Taylor, 1987a; Wolff, 1977), these patients can learn much about emotional processing from therapists who express how they feel more openly than is the rule in traditional psychodynamic psychotherapy and who attempt to enhance and share fantasy, humour, and other imaginal activity during psychotherapeutic sessions.

While these psychotherapeutic techniques are mainly educational, clarification and interpretation of the cognitive and affective deficits are also required inasmuch as these patients are directed to attend to their inner experiences and to the way they relate to other people. As was noted in Chapter 2, alexithymic individuals tend to employ symbiotic relationships adaptively to compensate for their deficits and to help regulate dysphoric states. Consequently, they appear to be prone to exacerbations of their illnesses when these relationships are threatened or disrupted (Taylor, 1987a). This problem also manifests itself in the type of transference many of these patients form. As Krystal (1982) has described, they quickly assume the dependent patient role and expect their illnesses to be cured according to the medical model of transaction. At the same time, their communicative style often evokes countertransference dullness, boredom, and frustration (Krystal, 1982/83; Sifneos et al., 1977; Taylor, 1977, 1984b). While this type of transference is difficult to interpret and work through, some therapists report that progress can be achieved with some patients by a creative use of countertransference responses and analysis of primitive internalized object relations (Krystal, 1982/83; McDougall, 1985; Taylor, 1987a, 1994; Wolff, 1977). In particular, attention must be given to correcting these patients' distorted self- and object representations and inhibitions in self-care that contribute to the difficulties therapists generally encounter when they attempt to implement the various treatment modalities (Krystal, 1982/83, 1990). We will elaborate on the use of a more psychoanalytically oriented psychotherapy to alter the inner world of selected patients later in this chapter.

Clearly, the above treatment approach contrasts markedly with traditional psychodynamic psychotherapy, which attempts to influence both psychological and somatic symptoms by interpreting conflicts over drive-related wishes. The therapeutic approach for alexithymic patients attempts to elevate emotions from a level of perceptually bound experience (a world of sensation and action) to a conceptual representational level (a world of feelings and thoughts) where they can be used as signals of information, thought about, and sometimes communicated to others (Frosch, 1995; Lane & Schwartz, 1987). The organization and representation of emotions as conceptual abstractions that go beyond immediate experience not only allows emotions to come more under the control of thoughts, as Frosch (1995) has described, but also to be used symbolically in dreams, fantasy, and creative play which provide additional affect-regulating functions. The enhanced capacity to self-regulate emotions prevents prolonged states of emotional arousal that might be conducive to somatic disease, and also reduces the tendency to somatize and the tendency to 'discharge' emotional tension through binge eating, substance abuse, or other compulsive affect-regulating behaviours (Gross & Muñoz, 1995). Movement away from a motoric and sensation-bound existence to a world of mental representations (that can *stand for* experience rather than be the experience) allows for increased differentiation of self- and object representations and an ability to move freely between imagination and the world of 'objective' reality (Frosch, 1995).

In conducting a modified type of psychotherapy the therapist functions initially as an 'auxiliary ego' to the patient, helping the patient to bear his or her affects and also leading the patient toward recognizing the *possibility* of experiencing new states of mind and eventually to actually experience states of mind that were unfamiliar to him or her (Margulies, 1993). To this end, in our own clinical work we have sometimes found it useful to be guided by test results from the NEO Personality Inventory (NEO PI; Costa & McCrae, 1985) and by the models of emotion regulation of Tomkins (1962) and Izard and Kobak (1991) that were mentioned in Chapter 1. According to these models, the minimization of negative emotions (neuroticism) involves *feedback mechanisms* whereby interests and imaginal activity (i.e. aspects of openness to experience) help maintain and enhance positive emotions; these, in turn, motivate further interests and imaginal activity, which help strengthen emotional bonds with others that enhance interpersonal emotion regulation.

These concepts of emotion regulation and the modified type of psychotherapy were employed successfully in the treatment of Mr J, a patient whose clinical history and NEO PI profile were outlined in Chapter 4 (Case 1). Over the course of two years of once-weekly psychotherapy, Mr J became less alexithymic and developed a greater capacity to tolerate and modulate the negative affective states to which he had been extremely prone. He developed a wider range of interests, a capacity to create pleasurable fantasies, and an ability to derive solace from transitional objects and transitional phenomena, such as listening to music. Mr J even began occasionally to recall dreams. The expansion of his interests not only generated feelings of enjoyment, but also broadened his network of social relationships which added further to his experience of positive emotions. With the overcoming of his anhedonia, Mr J gradually also began to experience the feeling of being in love with his girlfriend; they became married and subsequently developed the desire to have a child. The establishment of pleasurable interests and a capacity to use imaginal processes, and the development of warm relationships, enhanced the cognitive and interpersonal domains of emotion regulation in this patient and thereby reduced considerably his vulnerability to high levels of emotional distress.

### Group therapy

Group therapy is considered a useful alternative or adjunct to individual psychotherapy for many alexithymic patients (Apfel-Savitz, Silverman & Bennett, 1977; Swiller, 1988). Whereas individual sessions are ideal for educating patients about their affect regulating problems, the group setting provides a broader range of interpersonal situations for alexithymic patients to experience and learn about emotions. It is important, however, to avoid placing more than two or three alexithymic patients in the same group; even then it is preferable for them to be at different stages of treatment (Swiller, 1988). While it is essential that the alexithymic patients experience the group as a safe and supportive setting, candid feedback from other group members should be encouraged, to the extent that it does not threaten the patients' self-esteem, as this can help them learn about the impact of their lack of empathy on other people. At the same time, the group therapist can direct an alexithymic patient's attention to communications between other group members that demonstrate more successful and sensitive ways of relating.

The effectiveness of group therapy in modifying alexithymia was evaluated by Fukunishi *et al.* (1994) in a recent study in Japan. Based on the finding from an earlier study that alexithymia is often present among family members of alcoholics (Fukunishi *et al.*, 1992*a*), the investigators used a method of family group psychotherapy with 14 alcoholic families. They selected for the study only the person in each family who was closest to the alcoholic person in daily life. This was usually the spouse, but sometimes a child, parent, or sibling. The subjects were divided into three treatment groups, which comprised four or five members and met once weekly for two hours. Before group therapy began, all subjects completed the TAS and the Family Environment Scale which contains 10 subscales assessing various aspects of family functioning such as cohesiveness, expressiveness, and conflict. The psychological tests were readministered after six months of group therapy, and the effects of treatment were assessed by comparing mean scores before and after treatment. The mean TAS score after treatment was significantly lower than that before group therapy; and, based on the TAS cutoff score, seven subjects (50%) were alexithymic before group therapy compared with only three subjects (21.4%) at the end of treatment. Group therapy also increased family cohesion and allowed anxiety and conflict to be expressed more easily within the family. Unfortunately, other than indicating that patients were expected to express their feelings in the group, Fukunishi and his associates did not describe the therapeutic techniques they employed; nor did they assess the long-term benefits for the alcoholic member of the families.

In another innovative study, which was conducted in Lithuania, Beresnevaité (1995) evaluated the effectiveness of group therapy in modifying alexithymia in a sample of 20 postmyocardial infarction patients. The patients attended the group once weekly for 90 minutes over a period of four months. A variety of therapeutic techniques were employed. To decrease stress and focus attention on inner experiences, patients were first taught Jacobson's technique of progressive relaxation. Then, to improve their ability to identify and communicate subjective feelings, patients were required to participate in role playing and non-verbal communication of emotion (e.g. mimicry and eye communication), to draw their inner world and describe the inner worlds of other group members, and to describe the feelings they experienced while reporting dreams. To enhance fantasy and other imaginal activity, the group listened to music while in a relaxed state, and patients were encouraged to write down any dreams and fantasies they had. If patients seemed preoccupied with the details of external events rather than inner experiences, the therapist used a gestalt therapy technique of directing them to replace utilitarian statements with statements that expressed wishes and desires. At the end of each group therapy session, a hypnotic method of relaxation was used to reduce any heightened physiological activity. Patients were required to practise the techniques they learned in the group in the course of their daily lives.

The cardiac patients completed the TAS prior to entering the group, at the end of four months of group therapy, and again at six-month and one-year follow-ups. Any changes in the somatic status of the patients were observed by recording complications of coronary heart disease (such as reinfarction, sudden death, development of an arrhythmia, or hospitalization for severe angina pectoris), and the frequency of anginal attacks. There was a statistically significant reduction in the mean TAS score of the group immediately following the four months of group therapy and this remained significantly lower than the pre-treatment score at the retesting six months and one year later. At the end of the one-year follow-up period, patients who had shown a stable decrease in TAS score in response to the group therapy also had a more favourable medical outcome with significantly fewer cardiac complications and significantly less disability than those patients whose TAS score was not changed by group therapy.

Although the Lithuanian study is the only study we are aware of that has used group therapy to modify alexithymic characteristics in patients with coronary heart disease, several researchers have used group behavioural counselling to modify Type A behaviour in postmyocardial infarction patients. In a large Recurrent Coronary Prevention Project carried out in the San Francisco Bay area, patients who received Type A behavioural counselling in addition to group standard cardiological counselling had a cardiac recurrence rate (infarction or cardiac death) significantly lower than patients who received group cardiological counselling only (Friedman et al., 1986). While the group behavioural techniques enhance patients' self-monitoring of Type A behaviours, there are data suggesting that the beneficial effect on cardiovascular health is through an improvement of the Type A coronary-prone patient's familial and other social relationships (Friedman et al., 1986; Orth-Gomér & Undén, 1990). It is possible that behavioural counselling attenuates the antagonistic hostility component of the Type A behavioural pattern, thereby rendering patients

more agreeable and more able to establish secure attachments and a
sense of being loved.

## Integrating pharmacotherapy with psychotherapy

Over the past decade increasing knowledge of the brain mechanisms
underlying affective states has been accompanied by the development
of an array of pharmacologic agents that can aid in modulating unstable
affective states. Although there is a tendency in psychiatry for polariza-
tion of biological and psychological perspectives, we hold the firm
opinion that the treatment of disorders of affect regulation often
requires an integration of pharmacologic and psychotherapeutic approaches. An integrated treatment approach is consistent with the
psychobiologic nature of emotions and with our view that the etiology
and pathogenesis of disorders of affect regulation involve complex
interactions between psychosocial and neurobiological factors.

A wide variety of psychoactive drugs have been found useful in the
treatment of disorders of affect regulation including benzodiazepines,
tricyclic antidepressants, MAO inhibitors, selective serotonin reuptake
inhibitors (SSRIs), mood stabilizers (such as lithium carbonate, car-
bamezapine, and valproate), and neuroleptics. Medications are selected to target specific symptoms such as anxiety, panic, depression,
instability of mood, irritability, impulsivity, or intrusive thoughts. By
their nature, pharmacological interventions often produce rapid symptom relief with a minimum of time devoted to treatment; however,
without parallel psychotherapeutic and/or cognitive–behavioural
treatment of the psychological vulnerability, there is frequently relapse
or recurrence of the disorder when pharmacotherapy is discontinued.
Moreover, different treatments seem to affect different aspects of an
illness. In panic disorder, for example, antipanic drugs (e.g. imipramine, phenalzine, sertraline, and alprazolam) block brainstem-
provoked panic attacks, relaxation training reduces anticipatory anxiety, cognitive–behavioural therapies relieve phobic avoidance as well
as panic attacks triggered by catastrophic misinterpretations of normal
bodily sensations, and psychotherapy resolves conflict and promotes
the development of psychic structure that enhances self-regulation
(Gorman et al., 1989; Shear et al., 1993; Taylor, 1989). And while drug
treatment might attenuate the intrusive or hyperarousal symptoms of
PTSD, and reduce the affective instability and impulsive–aggressive
behaviour of many patients with borderline personality disorders, its
main value is in making patients with these disorders more amenable to
psychotherapy (Friedman, 1988; Soloff, 1994).

While the efficacy of psychoactive drugs seems due to their ability to restore efficient regulation of dysregulated neurotransmitter systems in the brainstem or limbic system (Siever & Davis, 1985, 1991), because of multiple neural connections, it is impossible to effect a change in any one neuronal system without altering others. Indeed, as Dubovsky and Thomas (1995b) recently pointed out, the specificity of different neurotransmitter subsystems and selectivity of drug treatments is far from absolute. Serotonin, for example,

> is a cotransmitter with gamma-aminobutyric acid (GABA) and norepinephrine. Serotonergic and noradrenergic neurons can take up each other's transmitter, altering the functioning of the parent neuron (p. 432).

Not only is it proving naive to consider serotonin actions separate from the actions of other neurotransmitters, but observations in clinical settings indicate that serotonergic dysfunction and a favourable response to SSRIs are not specific to depression. The SSRIs can be effective in a number of other psychiatric disorders including panic disorder, PTSD, obsessive–compulsive disorder, body dysmorphic disorder, eating disorders, and alcoholism. These findings have led Dubovsky and Thomas (1995b) to conclude that it is inaccurate to describe the SSRI's as 'antidepressants'. While they consider symptom overlap and comorbidity as possible reasons for the lack of clinical selectivity of the SSRI's, Dubovsky and Thomas (1995b) suggest that these medications 'alter basic psychobiological processes in directions that correct or compensate for faults that transcend specific diagnoses' (p. 438–439). They attribute this effect to the diffuse projections of serotonin pathways in the brain that 'allow them to contribute to the regulation of many core psychobiological functions that are disrupted in psychiatric disorders, including mood, anxiety, arousal, vigilance, irritability, aggression, suicide, intrusive and obsessional thinking, cognition, appetite, the sleep–wake cycle, circadian and seasonal rhythms, nocioception, and neuroendocrine functions' (Dubovsky & Thomas, 1995b, p. 439).

Employing a conceptual model very similar to our dysregulation model of illness and disease, Dubovsky and Thomas (1995a, 1995b) propose that the interactions between these basic psychobiological functions may permit alterations in any one subsystem to cause significant shifts in the overall pattern and thereby produce different disorders.

> For example, when arousal is sufficient to overwhelm regulation of aggression and impulsivity that has been impaired by suboptimally active 5-HT systems, suicide, various forms of outwardly directed aggression, or generalized impulsivity may be the predominant

problem, or they may complicate depression, anxiety, schizophrenia, or personality disorders. If obsessionality is the primary problem, a diagnosis of obsessive compulsive disorder is made, but if it interacts with a significant disturbance of mood, ruminative depressive states may emerge; if the interaction is with the consequences of traumatic experiences, the intrusive recall of posttraumatic stress disorder may develop (Dubovsky & Thomas, 1995a, p. 39).

Similarly, an alteration in the serotonergic appetitive subsystem may result in an eating disorder, but interactions with other basic functions could produce associated behavioural impulsivity and/or depressive symptoms (Jimerson et al., 1990). A malfunction of the subsystem regulating anxiety could result in panic disorder as the major problem, but interactions with subsystems regulating mood and cognition could produce an overlap with major depression and obsessive–compulsive disorder. As Dubovsky and Thomas (1995a) indicate, 'What appears to be comorbidity may represent an overlap of dimensional malfunctions driven by dysfunction of one or more 5-HT systems . . .' (p. 39).

It will be evident to the reader that Dubovsky and Thomas's proposals fit with our shift from categorical DSM-III-R and DSM-IV diagnoses to the broader reconceptualization of certain psychiatric disorders as disorders of affect regulation. Serotonin and other neurotransmitters play a role in affective dysregulation and in the dysregulation of other psychobiological functions that produce a variety of clinical symptoms that differentiate the disorders.

Although there have been a number of studies evaluating individual drugs for the treatment of various disorders of affect regulation, there have been relatively few studies comparing drugs from more than one class. As success has been claimed for many different drugs and no compound has been established as the single drug of choice for treating any one of the disorders, it is recommended that therapists select medications that target specific symptom domains (Rosenbaum et al., 1995; Soloff, 1994; van der Kolk, 1994). This often involves trial and error and sometimes combinations of drugs from different classes are needed. Therapists must be aware of the side-effects and risks of the different medications, and need also to recognize the psychological meanings that patients often give to medications, a common one being endowing a drug with the significance of a transitional object.

The following case vignette illustrates the value of combining pharmacotherapy with psychotherapy, as well as the commonly encountered overlap of traditional diagnostic categories.

A childless accountant of 43, whom we shall call Mrs Y, was referred for treatment of chronic pain and depressive symptoms. Her symptoms had emerged following a relatively minor motor vehicle accident several years earlier but had intensified in recent months after she had a hysterectomy. Psychiatric assessment revealed that the patient had a tendency to binge eating and alcohol abuse; her depressive symptoms met the DSM-IV criteria for a diagnosis of a major depressive episode. However, the patient also had several symptoms characteristic of PTSD, which seemed related both to her hysterectomy and to an event at her workplace that she had experienced psychologically as extremely traumatic; Mrs Y complained of intrusive recollections of the hysterectomy and the traumatic event at work, recurrent distressing dreams of pregnancy and surgery and of people attempting to kill her, and intense psychological distress whenever she encountered mothers with young children or colleagues from her office who had been responsible for the distressing event. Medical assessment revealed a diagnosis of fibromyalgia, and past psychiatric records indicated that the patient had many features of a borderline personality disorder.

Because of an inadequate response to high doses of an SSRI antidepressant drug, the patient was prescribed a tricyclic antidepressant as well. Although her depressive and PTSD symptoms gradually improved, Mrs Y continued to experience chronic pain and now met the DSM-IV criteria for a diagnosis of pain disorder. Relaxation training, exercise programs, and other behavioural strategies produced only partial and transitory relief of her pain.

Although this patient expressed a considerable amount of affect verbally, she scored in the alexithymic range on the TAS-20 and showed a marked inability to use affects as signals and to modulate their intensity through cognitive processing. Instead, affects led directly to actions, including excessive talking which served an evacuative function rather than as a vehicle for meaningful communications. Because she experienced her affects as concrete and dangerous entities rather than as objects of thought, Mrs Y was unable to see that her reactions to other people, including the psychiatrist, were often based on distortions. Her emotions and the images they conjured up held more meaning for her than words or thoughts mediated by language. Consequently the patient's fear of being injured sometimes led to a mistrust and paranoid view of the psychiatrist, as well as to a perception of herself as a helpless victim; her concretely-experienced emotions lent conviction to these distortions. Once Mrs Y's depression and PTSD symptoms had improved in response to pharmacotherapy, psychotherapeutic interventions became more effective. These focused mainly on the patient's failure to think about her emotions and on her attempts to regulate distressing states through alcohol abuse or evacuation into others via a misuse of language.

## The transformation of unmentalized experience

As demonstrated by Mrs Y, and as was outlined in Chapter 2, some individuals who fail to process emotions cognitively employ a type B mode of communication in which speech is used to discharge unbearable mental states into others rather than as a vehicle for meaningful communications (Langs, 1978/79). This communicative mode makes extensive use of the primitive defense of projective identification and implies a defect in the person's inner 'container', a concept we mentioned in Chapter 1. As elaborated by Bion (1962), a defective inner container is a consequence of consistent failures in the containing function of the parents during a person's early childhood. Instead of being transformed into mental representations by the cognitive processing (or *alpha function*) of the parents with which the child could have identified, the emotions of the older child and adult remain organized on a preconceptual level as perceptions, sensations, and impulses to action (Frosch, 1995), or what Bion referred to as *beta elements*. Whereas *alpha elements* are capable of being thought about, beta elements are only suitable for discharge through projective identification or acting out.

Patients who are functioning at this level cast the psychotherapist into the role of container for their projected split self- and object representations and their attendant unmodulated affects. By internalizing the patient's projective identifications, transforming and giving them meaning, and returning them to the patient, the therapist facilitates the development of a containing capacity in the patient (Grotstein, 1981; Hamilton, 1990). The experience over time by the patient of the therapist transforming his or her projections (as opposed to being transformed by them), and an identification by the patient with the therapist's containing and analyzing functions, lead to the emergence of a greater capacity in the patient to think abstractly and to communicate symbolically (Langs' type A communicative mode). In Kleinian theory, this corresponds to a shift from the paranoid–schizoid position of mental functioning to the depressive position, which involves an advance in cognitive functioning (Brown, 1985; Segal, 1957) and a change in the way affects are regulated (Stein, 1990), and results in a greater ability to tolerate affects.

The ability to represent experience mentally and to conceive of conscious and unconscious mental states in oneself and others is referred to by Fonagy (1991) as the capacity to *mentalize*, a capacity necessary for the regulation and control of affects. In his view, 'The ability to represent the idea of an affect is crucial in the achievement of control over the overwhelming affect' (p. 642). The development of affect tolerance in the alexithymic patient thus requires not only the development of a greater capacity to fantasize and to verbalize affects, but also an improvement in the state of the inner container and in the capacity to mentalize, as Sashin (1985) also has emphasized.

Mitrani (1995), who has provided a comprehensive review of the concept of *unmentalized experience*, traces the origin of the concept to

Freud's early notion of actual neurosis; she indicates how distressing preverbal experiences, as well as traumatic experiences that happen after the development of language but fail to be mentalized, are encoded as body memories that may find expression in somatization or mindless actions. The aim of psychoanalysis or psychoanalytic psychotherapy, therefore, is not to interpret repressed unconscious ideas, wishes, and fantasies, but to shift somatosensory and iconic memories from the body into the mind, i.e. to build psychic structure (Mitrani, 1995; Taylor, 1993b). In the terminology of classical psychoanalysis (described in earlier chapters), therapeutic interventions are directed at reconstructing and transforming traumatic experiences that have been managed psychically through the mechanism of primal repression (as opposed to repression proper) or primitive denial (Dorpat, 1985; Kinston & Cohen, 1986) into mental representations (word presentations) that can give them logical meaning and modulate associated affective distress by *standing for* the experiences.

Though access to unmentalized experience may be gained often through analysis of countertransference responses to the projective identifications of alexithymic patients (Taylor, 1977, 1984b), severely alexithymic patients use predominantly the type C communicative mode described by Langs (1978/79) in which language is used to construct impenetrable barriers by destroying meaning and links between the patient's internal world and the external real world. The type C alexithymic patient, as Brown (1985) explains, 'must rupture any affective links to the analyst [or psychotherapist] in order to avert the emergence of intensely painful material by remaining interactionally concrete' (p. 396). It is this type of patient who can paralyze the therapist's analytic function and produce the prolonged periods of 'stagnation' described by McDougall (1972).

Though the alexithymia and symptomatology of these patients is often unresponsive to treatment, attempts to reconstruct early trauma can sometimes lead to a breakthrough in psychoanalytic therapy. The process of reconstruction, as outlined by Cohen (1993) and Kinston and Cohen (1986, 1988), is not the same as genetic interpretations, which explain the present in terms of the past as remembered by the patient, but addresses defects of memory resulting from traumatic experiences that have not been represented mentally but were managed by primal repression. The reconstruction is based on inferences from the patient's reports of past events or screen memories, enactments, bodily postures, and somatic symptoms, as well as from observations of the transference and countertransference and information from other important people in the patient's life. There is usually a paradoxical worsening of the patient's condition as the trauma is relived, and this can occur only after the patient has developed a sense of safety and primary relatedness with the therapist which permits the emergence of primal repression.

## Clinical illustration

An example of the use of reconstruction in the psychotherapy of an alexithymic patient with a type C mode of communication is provided by our patient Nick, whom we described in Chapter 6 (Case 2). The reader will recall that Nick had overlapping diagnoses of somatization disorder, hypochondriasis, obsessive–compulsive disorder, and body dysmorphic disorder. Though he was an accomplished musician, Nick enjoyed listening to his music only intermittently; most of the time he heard a defect in the 'flow' of the music, which convinced him that he was a totally inadequate performer and left him feeling completely devastated and prone to a resurgence of somatic symptoms and hypochondriacal concerns. Nick also spent a great deal of time examining his reflection in a mirror; while sometimes he was satisfied with his appearance, he mostly viewed himself as unattractive and therefore unable to capture the interest of women. Friends, relatives, and other musicians could not hear this supposed defect in the music; nor did they consider Nick unattractive. However, Nick could not be reassured.

As there were certain gaps in the patient's early history, the therapist had several interviews with his father. It was discovered that Nick's parents had immigrated to a new country shortly before he was conceived. His mother returned to work as a busy physician one month after her son was born, and for the next eight years Nick was reared throughout the day by his maternal grandmother. It was only in the evenings that the parents provided a few hours of caregiving.

Nick's father described the grandmother as an extremely selfish and unreliable woman; she spent most of her time watching television, smoking cigarettes, playing cards, or entertaining neighbours rather than being attuned to and attending to the baby's needs, or playing with Nick as he developed. The parents, on the other hand, found their child beautiful and adorable, even having his baby portrait displayed in the window of the photographer's shop. There were frequent arguments between the grandmother and Nick's father, who recalled an incident when the grandmother had cruelly slapped the child's face when he approached her from behind and began playing with her hair. Nick had no memory of any of these events. After nine years, the father insisted that the grandmother return to Europe.

In the course of psychotherapy (which was combined with pharmacotherapy), Nick's symptoms came to be understood as derivatives of the alternating and vastly different affective states associated with the two styles of parenting. The predominant and overwhelming unpleasant state, which had the effect of invalidating the patient's sense of self, was linked to the greater time spent with the grandmother, who was unattuned and not visually engaged with the baby's face. The pleasurable, but less reliable affective state, was linked to early experiences with the emotionally attuned parents, especially the mother. The patient's experience of shifting bidirectionally between distorted and undistorted visual and auditory perceptions seemed to stem from an encoding of these early affective experiences as representations that were exclusively perceptual, motor, and sensational.

Listening to recordings of some of the patient's music, the therapist detected a narrow range of emotional expression, an impression that Nick indicated was corroborated by several of his music teachers. According to Nick, all of his music was melancholic in tone and it was always played softly and tenderly. This suggested to the therapist a deep yearning in the patient for the warmth and love of his mother, which the infant Nick had presumably experienced for a short time in the evenings. Indeed, the rare occasions when Nick enjoyed listening to himself playing the cello suggested a state of mind resembling the imagined experience of the infant merging with the sensual mother, an experience that generates the precursors of positive affects and perhaps music itself, which may thereafter *reinstate*, rather than represent, the original experience. In contrast, the patient's experience of intrusive perceptions and thoughts that his music sounded 'bad' were suggestive of primitive, inchoate emotions stemming from the long periods of exposure to the grandmother, who had shown minimal interest in the boy and failed to provide selfobject mirroring that would contribute to the development of a self representation that was basically good and lovable. The therapist proposed that Nick's inability to control the intrusiveness of his obsessional thoughts reflected the helplessness he must have experienced as a young child in being unable to effect any change in the grandmother's behaviour and emotional tone of his early environment. Along with the helplessness, there was assumed to be a primitive rage that threatened the patient internally and was manifested in obsessive–compulsive and passive–aggressive behaviours.

Further evidence to support this reconstruction was provided by enactments such as an occasion when Nick turned his head away from an attractive female bank teller when she smiled at him as he approached her counter. Nick insisted that he had looked away because he believed that the woman's smile was a mask covering her true feelings about him. The therapist interpreted Nick's use of projective identification, his disavowal of the woman's entitlement to her own feelings and of the reality that someone could view him favourably, and the enactment in reverse of the childhood relationship with his grandmother. It was pointed out that his fantasy that no woman could like him became his view of reality, whereas the reality of the woman smiling at him became his fantasy. Nick's somatic symptoms and frequent visits to doctors and hospital emergency departments were also conceptualized as enactments of the pleasurable times he had experienced with his mother in the evenings during early childhood. As an adolescent, he frequently experienced somatic symptoms and hypochondriacal worries and regularly sought reassurance by making an appointment to see his mother in her medical office. As noted in Chapter 6, Nick's belief that he had multiple sclerosis and the obsessional doubting over his music began soon after his mother's death from heart disease. He regularly reported feeling reassured immediately after he arrived at hospital emergency departments, just as he had been reassured by visits with his mother.

The reconstruction of the patient's early experience led the therapist to suggest to Nick that his perception of 'something wrong' with his music was probably a memory of a disturbing emotional state that he had experienced persistently with his grandmother in infancy and early childhood. In contrast, the times when the music sounded good to the patient were interpreted as reflecting an emotional state equivalent to the pleasurable but brief moments he spent with his mother. Such moments were compared with glimmers of sunlight that were rapidly displaced by encroaching black clouds of despair signifying a state equivalent to the presence of the grandmother.

For the first three years of psychotherapy, Nick avoided any affective involvement with the therapist. He showed no curiosity about the therapist or even about objects in the therapist's office. Employing a type C communicative mode, the patient either complained endlessly about various obsessional or somatic preoccupations, or argued about the need for more medical investigations, thereby blocking all attempts to access his inner life. Dreams were rarely recalled and interpretations had no impact on the patient. As he did with his father and friends, Nick often attempted to engage the therapist in debates about his musical ability and physical appearance. While he sought reassurance that he was talented musically and attractive enough to get a girlfriend, he could not believe that the therapist would speak truthfully; at the same time, the failure to offer reassurance was taken as evidence that the therapist considered him unattractive and hopeless as a musician. Though it was not always possible to avoid falling into these verbal traps, the therapist endeavoured to interpret the patient's defensive use of language and arguments to avoid developing a more personal and meaningful relationship with him. The therapist also regularly confronted Nick about his self-neglect – his poor hygiene, lack of grooming, and unkempt clothing, and his frequent declining of invitations to play with other musicians and to live audiences. These behaviours were interpreted as serving to validate the negative convictions about himself by not permitting new interpersonal experiences to have any corrective impact. In addition, Nick was confronted repeatedly with his unacknowledged primitive rage, his unknown terror of falling into an empty psychic space [or 'black hole' as Grotstein (1990) has referred to it], and his unknown dread both of entering into the therapist's mind and of allowing the therapist to enter into his mind.

Consistent with Kinston and Cohen's (1986, 1988) formulations, the turning point in Nick's psychotherapy was marked by an intensification of somatization and hypochondriacal symptoms; this indicated an emergence of primal repression and a reliving of the early trauma in the transference relationship. Nick became extremely fearful that he was going to die, he began to have panic attacks, and he made frequent phone calls to the therapist between sessions to seek emotional support and reassurance about his physical health. Recognizing that the patient had now established a state of primary relatedness with him, the therapist responded directly to mediate Nick's need for an immediately available and genuinely concerned and responsive person, a need that had not been met during the traumatization in early childhood. These developments paved the way for Nick to begin to acquire a new understanding of the events in his childhood that had affected him, and to modify and build psychic structure that would enable him to experience new states of mind. The mentalization of primitive affective experience gradually permitted also an analysis of Nick's narcissistic pathology, especially an infantile form of omnipotence against which he measured himself, but which served also to elevate self esteem by the fantasy of defeating his psychotherapist and physicians through developing a fatal disease that they all had failed to detect. That is, imbedded in the patient's hypochondriacal concerns were both the unmentalized affects from his earliest relationship experiences and a phallic grandiosity that compensated for, and oscillated with, an image of the self as castrated and totally worthless.

While only a minority of alexithymic patients will endure a psycho-analytic therapy that attempts to transform unmentalized experience, it is a treatment that sometimes can be helpful in selected cases when other treatments have failed.

## Empirical studies comparing different therapeutic modalities

To date, only two empirical studies have been reported that compared the response of alexithymic patients to different types of treatment. In a preliminary study, Pierloot and Vinck (1977) compared psychiatric outpatients presenting with anxiety symptoms who were randomly assigned to short-term psychodynamic psychotherapy or behaviour therapy (systematic desensitization). The dropout rate with the former treatment was related to the presence of alexithymia which had been assessed with the BIQ.

In a more recent study, Keller *et al.* (1995) compared the response of alexithymic and non-alexithymic cocaine abusers to psychotherapy plus a placebo and to psychotherapy combined with the tricyclic antidepressant desipramine. The psychotherapy was of two types – cognitive–behavioural treatment (which taught coping skills, but re-quired patients to identify affects and cognitions) and clinical manage-ment (which included education and medication management as well as provision of a supportive therapeutic relationship). The treatments were administered for a period of 12 weeks. Alexithymic patients did not differ from non-alexithymic patients in overall retention in treatment, initiation of abstinence from cocaine, or percentage of days abstinent, and patients who received psychotherapy combined with desipramine had no better outcome than those who received psychotherapy and a placebo. Desipramine was superior to placebo in alleviating depression, but this effect was not related to the presence of alexithymia. However, the alexithymic and non-alexithymic patients did respond differently to the two types of psychotherapy. The alexithymic patients had better outcomes when treated with clinical management, whereas the non-alexithymic patients had a better response when treated with a cognitive–behavioural approach.

While the results of these studies support the general clinical impression that alexithymic patients respond better to psychotherapies that do not demand access to internal affective and cognitive states, much more research is needed to evaluate the efficacy of different treatment approaches, especially the modified forms of psychotherapy that have been described in this chapter.

# [2] Future directions

The central thesis of this book is that affect regulation and its failures have a major influence on mental and physical health. We have based this thesis on a synthesis of recent concepts and research findings from a broad range of disciplines, and have focused specifically on alexithymia as a deficit in the cognitive–experiential domain of emotion response systems. However, despite numerous studies on the development of emotion regulation and emotion dysregulation, and accumulating evidence supporting the validity of the alexithymia construct, a great deal more interdisciplinary research is required before the concept of disorders of affect regulation can be realized fully as a new paradigm for psychiatry and medicine.

In our reviews of empirical studies on alexithymia in previous chapters, we drew attention to some of the limitations and deficiencies in the research including the poor psychometric properties of several of the alexithymia measures, the paucity of prospective, longitudinal studies, and the need to further explore the developmental antecedents and neurobiological underpinnings of alexithymia. Of particular importance are the need (i) to extend the experimental approaches to construct validation; (ii) to investigate further the relationships between alexithymia and physiological responsiveness to emotional stimuli; (iii) to conduct large epidemiological studies to compare the prevalence of alexithymia in different cultures; and (iv) to evaluate the effectiveness of modified psychotherapy and other treatments in changing alexithymic characteristics and altering susceptibility to disorders of affect regulation or the course of existing illnesses (Salminen, Saarijärvi & Äärelä, 1995; Taylor et al., 1991). In this closing chapter we will offer some additional suggestions for future research that may further clarify ways in which affective dysregulation and alexithymia contribute to the development of medical and psychiatric disorders.

Given that alexithymia is conceptualized as an arrest at, or regression to, a preconceptual (sensorimotor) level of emotion organization (Lane & Schwartz, 1987), and that this is thought to result in a proneness to somatization, it is necessary to investigate systematically the way in which alexithymic individuals process affects. Such studies might evaluate alexithymic individuals' cognitive appraisal of emotion-inducing stimuli, the intensity and perception of their physiological responses to such stimuli, whether specific cognitive–affective schemata are activated, and whether these schemata are linked with an awareness of autonomic arousal.

Other studies might evaluate whether alexithymic and non-alexithymic individuals process emotional and non-emotional information differently. Although in Chapter 3 we reported results of some preliminary studies that used the emotional Stroop Test task and the ability to identify facial emotional expressions in photographs, other information processing tasks have yet to be employed. In general, such information processing methodologies are designed to identify and specify existing schemata. Investigations that systematically evaluate differences in attention, retrieval, recognition, and recall of emotional and non-emotional stimuli have the potential to delineate more clearly the mechanisms underlying failures in affect regulation. Some of these proposed studies might take advantage of recent developments in instruments designed to elicit differentiated emotional states. For example, Philippot (1993) has spliced together a number of short film segments that have proven capable of eliciting a diversity of predictable emotions.

To date, as was reviewed in Chapter 5, research on the neurobiology of alexithymia has relied mainly on indirect methods for studying the functioning brain. A direction for future research is to employ modern brain imaging techniques, including magnetic resonance spectroscopy (MRS), positron emission tomography (PET), and single photon emission computed tomography (SPECT), to compare changes in regional brain chemistry and activity between alexithymic and non-alexithymic individuals during the elicitation and processing of emotional states (Cohen, Renshaw & Yurgelun-Todd, 1995; Woods, 1992). Such studies might establish whether alexithymia is associated with reduced interhemispheric communication, and possibly identify other abnormalities in higher brain activity that affect the regulation of emotion. For example, George, Ketter and Post (1994), based on a number of different studies examining patients suffering from major depression with SPECT and PET, surmised major depression to be related to dysfunction of the prefrontal cortex in its role as a modulator of limbic activity.

Another promising recent innovation for future research on alexithymia and affect regulation is the quantitative electroencephalogram
(QEEG), a computer driven EEG that produces a two-dimensional
colour-coded print of electrical brain activity. The QEEG offers
several advantages over PET and SPECT: it can be used to assess
sustained brain activity (instead of a brief abnormal discharge); it
allows for the probing of brain activity under relatively normal
conditions; and it does not require the use of ionizing radiation. Ouellet
*et al.* (1994) recently used the QEEG in a preliminary study in which
they assessed 'coherence' (a quantitative index of the degree of functional connectivity between brain regions) during the REM sleep of a
small group of women who were categorized as alexithymic or non-
alexithymic on the basis of TAS cutoff scores. Coherence over the
lateral–frontal cortex was significantly higher in the alexithymic women, which suggested that their REM sleep was associated with
greater activation of both cerebral hemispheres. Other sleep laboratory
researchers are investigating the relationship between alexithymia and
dreaming by comparing the dream reports of alexithymic and non-
alexithymic individuals when they are awakened during REM sleep.

Although findings from several recent long-term follow-up studies
(reviewed in Chapters 4 and 8) have yielded strong support for
alexithymia being a stable trait in some individuals, the question of
whether alexithymia is an antecedent of medical and psychiatric illnesses can be solved unambiguously only by prospective, longitudinal
studies of large populations that commence *before* the onset of any
illness (Weiner, 1977). The follow-up period may be 20 years or
longer, but models for this type of epidemiological research are
provided by several studies mentioned in Chapter 10 that helped
identify hostility as a predictor of coronary heart disease. With the use
of projective test measures, such longitudinal studies also provide the
opportunity to investigate further the relationships between the inner
representational world and changes in health. For example, a preliminary but long-term prospective study of medical students (described
also in Chapter 10) found evidence of an association between mental
representations that reflect unstable patterns of attachment and poor
affect modulation and the subsequent development of cancer (Graves
& Thomas, 1981). And while attachment researchers are now studying
attachment styles over the course of the life cycle, their longitudinal
studies might include additional measures of affect regulation, as well
as an exploration of the extent to which secure and insecure attachment
styles predict the later development of disorders of affect regulation.

An important consideration in future research on affect regulation is
the appropriateness of the measurement models used to explain and

predict behaviour and feeling states. Virtually all of the research examined in this book has utilized models that involve stable linear relationships. A number of writers have pointed out, however, that linear models may be inappropriate for the study of affect regulation and state transitions in other natural systems (Margulies, 1993; Sashin, 1985; Spruiell, 1993). The relevant behaviours and causal variables involved in the regulation of affects are dynamic; these variables may change rapidly over time in intensity and frequency, often in an unpredictable and non-linear pattern. Thus, the study of affect regulation may be improved by utilizing concepts and ideas from chaos theory and non-linear dynamical modelling.

Many of the conceptual benefits from using non-linear dynamical models to study the regulation of affective states have been outlined by Sashin (1985) and Callahan and Sashin (1987), and subsequently elaborated by Margulies (1993). Consider, for example, the problem of developing a mathematical model to account for particular affect responses in stressful situations (e.g. anger outbursts, or a continuous rise in anxiety until there is a discontinuous jump to panic). According to Sashin, an appropriate model must take into account the simultaneous effects of at least four underlying variables: the level of environmental stimulation; individual differences in the capacity to verbalize affect; individual differences in the capacity to fantasize; and the condition of the inner 'container', which, as was outlined in Chapter 1, is derived from the child's relationship with an empathically attuned mother who could herself tolerate affect. Sashin noted that a mathematical affect–response model must be constructed in such a way that some causal relationships are allowed to exist at some time periods and not at others. The model must also be able to capture several important features of affect responses: gradually changing forces may produce sudden effects, while a comparable set of circumstances may generate different emotional states. All of these features can be incorporated into non-linear dynamical models that can evaluate the complex interrelationships among the variables and also test predictions when one or more of the variables is altered. Though the development of non-linear dynamical models of affect response is still in an early stage, we anticipate that the rapidly advancing field of non-linear mathematics will open up research possibilities for the future.

Finally, despite the great deal of research that has yet to be done, the concept of disorders of affect regulation is consistent with a growing realization in medicine and psychiatry that most illnesses and diseases are the result of dysregulations within the vast network of communicating systems that comprise the human organism (Weiner, 1989). Whereas in psychiatry the categorical ICD-10 and DSM-III-R and

DSM-IV diagnoses have their usefulness in identifying relatively homogeneous groups for research purposes, it has become clear that an atheoretical approach with regard to etiology or pathophysiologic process has limitations. Affect dysregulation is an overarching concept that helps explain the high comorbidity between some Axis I disorders and between some Axis I and Axis II disorders, as well as why some drug treatments are equally effective for seemingly different diagnoses (Dubovsky & Thomas, 1995b). The concept of disorders of affect regulation can be considered part of a second medical revolution; this revolution is leading toward a more comprehensive model of health, illness, and disease that is likely to make the traditional division between subspecialties (endocrinology, immunology, neurology, psychiatry, etc.) a historical artefact (Foss & Rothenberg, 1987; Pert et al., 1985).

# Appendix Twelve-item modified version of the Beth Israel Hospital Psychosomatic Questionnaire

Based on the interview you have just completed (or viewed) rank th patient on each of the descriptions listed below using the scale provided

| Not true | | Somewhat true | | | | Very tru |
|---|---|---|---|---|---|---|
| 1 | 2 | 3 | 4 | 5 | 6 | 7 |

1. The patient mostly described details concerning symptoms rather than feelings.

2. The patient had difficulty communicating feelings to the interviewer.

3. The patient was able to use appropriate words to describe emotions.

4. The patient described circumstances and details surrounding events rather than expressing feelings about how he/she may have felt about the event.

5. The patient expressed affect more in physical terms rather than in thoughts.

6. The patient's thought content was associated more with external events rather than with fantasy or feelings.

7. The patient had a rich affective vocabulary.

8. The patient could easily recall dreams.

9. When talking about close friends or loved ones, the patient showed a lack of emotional expressiveness.

10. The content of the patient's dreams closely resembles everyday thoughts or events rather than being more symbolic or abstract in nature.

11. The patient indicated that he/she did *not* daydream very much.

12. The patient indicated that he/she readily shared his/her feelings with others.

*Scoring:* Items 3, 7, 8 and 12 are negatively keyed. In addition to a total BIQ score, there are two subscale scores – (a) Affect Awareness (items 2, 3, 5, 7, 9 and 12); (b) Operatory Thinking (items 1, 4, 6, 8, 10 and 11).

*Adapted from Sifneos, 1973, with permission of the publisher S. Karger AG, Basel.*

# References

Abbey, S.E. & Garfinkel, P.E. (1991). Neurasthenia and chronic fatigue syndrome: the role of culture in the making of a diagnosis. *American Journal of Psychiatry*, **148**, 1638–46.

Abraham, S.F. & Beaumont, P.J.V. (1982). How patients describe bulimia or binge eating. *Psychological Medicine*, **12**, 625–35.

Abramson, L., McClelland, D.C., Brown, D. & Kelner, S., Jr. (1991). Alexithymic characteristics and metabolic control in diabetic and healthy adults. *Journal of Nervous and Mental Disease*, **179**, 490–4.

Acklin, M.W. (1991). Alexithymia, somatization, and the Rorschach response process. *Rorschachiana*, **17**, 180–7.

Acklin, M.W. & Alexander, G. (1988). Alexithymia and somatization: a Rorschach study of four psychosomatic groups. *Journal of Nervous and Mental Disease*, **176**, 343–50.

Acklin, M.W. & Bernat, E. (1987). Depression, alexithymia, and pain prone disorder: a Rorschach study. *Journal of Personality Assessment*, **51**, 462–79.

Adams, D.O. (1994). Molecular biology of macrophage activation: a pathway whereby psychosocial factors can potentially affect health. *Psychosomatic Medicine*, **56**, 316–27.

Adler, N. & Matthews, K. (1994). Health psychology: why do some people get sick and some stay well? *Annual Review of Psychology*, **45**, 229–59.

Adler, R., MacRitchie, K. & Engel, G.L. (1971). Psychologic processes and ischaemic stroke (occlusive cerebrovascular disease) I. Observations on 32 men with 35 strokes. *Psychosomatic Medicine*, **33**, 1–30.

Adler, R.H., Zlot, S., Hurny, C. & Minder, C. (1989). Engel's 'psychogenic pain and the pain-prone patient': a retrospective, controlled clinical study. *Psychosomatic Medicine*, **51**, 87–101.

Ahrens, S. & Deffner, G. (1986). Empirical study of alexithymia: methodology and results. *American Journal of Psychotherapy*, **40**, 430–47.

Akiskal, H.S. (1992). Delineating irritable and hyperthymic variants of the cyclothymic temperament. *Journal of Personality Disorders*, **6**, 326–42.

Akiskal, H.S. (1994). The temperamental borders of affective disorders. *Acta Psychiatrica Scandinavica*, **89** (suppl. 379), 32–7.

Akiskal, H.S., Downs, J., Jordan, P., Watson, S., Daugherty, D. & Pruitt, D.B. (1985). Affective disorders in referred children and younger siblings of manic-depressives. Mode of onset and prospective course. *Archives of General Psychiatry*, **42**, 996–1003.

Akiskal, H.S., Hirschfeld, R.M.A. & Yerevanian, B.I. (1983). The relationship of personality disorders to affective disorders. *Archives of General Psychiatry*, **40**, 801–10.

Akiskal, H.S., Khani, M.K. & Scott-Strauss, A. (1979). Cyclothymic temperamental disorders. *Psychiatric Clinics of North America*, **2**, 527–54.

Alexander, F. (1948). Emotional factors in essential hypertension: presentation of a hypothesis. In F. Alexander, & T.M. French (Eds.), *Studies in psychosomatic medicine*, pp. 289–97. New York: Ronald Press.

Alexander, F. (1950). *Psychosomatic medicine*. New York: Norton.

Alexander, F., French, T.M. & Pollock, G.H. (1968). *Psychosomatic specificity, vol. I: experimental study and results*. Chicago: University of Chicago Press.

Allport, G.W. & Odbert, H.S. (1936). Trait-names: a psycho-lexical study. *Psychological Monographs*, **47**, No. 211.

Altshute, K.Z. & Weiner, M.F. (1985). Anorexia nervosa and depression: a dissenting view. *American Journal of Psychiatry*, **142**, 328–32.

American Psychiatric Association (1987). *Diagnostic and statistical manual of mental disorders*, 3rd ed., rev. Washington, DC: American Psychiatric Association.

American Psychiatric Association (1994). *Diagnostic and statistical manual of mental disorders*, 4th ed. Washington, DC: American Psychiatric Association.

Anagnostopoulos, F., Vaslamatzis, Gr., Markidis, M., Katsouyanni, Kl., Vassilaros, St. & Stefanis, C. (1993). An investigation of hostile and alexithymic characteristics in breast cancer patients. *Psychotherapy and Psychosomatics*, **59**, 179–89.

Anderson, C.D. (1981). Expression of affect and physiological response in psychosomatic patients. *Journal of Psychosomatic Research*, **25**, 143–9.

Andreason, N.C. (1995). Posttraumatic stress disorder: psychology, biology, and the manichaean warfare between false dichotomies. *American Journal of Psychiatry*, **152**, 963–5.

Andrews, G., Pollock, C. & Stewart, G. (1989). The determination of defense style by questionnaire. *Archives of General Psychiatry*, **46**, 455–60.

Antrobus, J. (1987). Cortical hemisphere asymmetry and sleep mentation. *Psychological Review*, **94**, 359–68.

Apfel, R.J. & Sifneos, P.E. (1979). Alexithymia: concept and measurement. *Psychotherapy and Psychosomatics*, **32**, 180–90.

Apfel-Savitz, R., Silverman, D. & Bennett, M.I. (1977). Group psychotherapy of patients with somatic illnesses and alexithymia. *Psychotherapy and Psychosomatics*, **28**, 323–9.

Applebaum, S.A. (1973). Psychological-mindedness: word, concept, and essence. *International Journal of Psychoanalysis*, **54**, 35–45.

Argyle, N. & Roth, M. (1989). The phenomenological study of 90 patients with panic disorder, part II. *Psychiatric Developments*, **3**, 187–209.

Aronoff, J., Stollak, G.E. & Woike, B.A. (1994). Affect regulation and the breadth of interpersonal engagement. *Journal of Personality and Social Psychology*, **67**, 105–14.

Aronson, T.A. & Logue, C.M. (1988). Phenomenology of panic attacks: a descriptive study of panic disorder patients' self-reports. *Journal of Clinical Psychiatry*, **49**, 8–13.

Atchison, M. & McFarlane, A.C. (1994). A review of dissociation and dissociative disorders. *Australian and New Zealand Journal of Psychiatry*, **28**, 591–9.

Bach, M. & Bach, D. (1995). Predictive value of alexithymia: a prospective study in somatizing patients. *Psychotherapy and Psychosomatics*, **64**, 43–8.

Bach, M., Bach, D., Böhmer, F. & Nutzinger, D.O. (1994*a*). Alexithymia and somatization: relationship to DSM-III-R diagnoses. *Journal of Psychosomatic Research*, **38**, 529–38.

Bach, M., Bach, D., de Zwaan, M., Serim, M. & Böhmer, F. (1996). Validierung der Deutshen version der 20-item Toronto Alexithymie Skala bei normalpersonen und psychiatrischen patienten. *Psychotherapie, Psychosomatik, Medizinische Psychologie*, **46**, 23–8.

Bach, M., de Zwaan, M., Ackard, D., Nutzinger, D.O. & Mitchell, J.E. (1994*b*). Alexithymia: relationship to personality disorders. *Comprehensive Psychiatry*, **35**, 239–43.

Bacon, N.M.K., Bacon, S.F., Atkinson, J.H., Slater, M.A., Patterson, T.L., Grant, I. & Garfin, S.R. (1994). Somatization symptoms in chronic low back pain patients. *Psychosomatic Medicine*, **56**, 118–27.

Bagby, R.M., Parker, J.D.A. & Taylor, G.J. (1991*a*). Reassessing the reliability and validity of the MMPI Alexithymia Scale. *Journal of Personality Assessment*, **56**, 238–53.

Bagby, R.M., Parker, J.D.A. & Taylor, G.J. (1991b). Dimensional analysis of the MMPI Alexithymia Scale. *Journal of Clinical Psychology*, **47**, 221–6.

Bagby, R.M., Parker, J.D.A. & Taylor, G.J. (1994a). The Twenty-Item Toronto Alexithymia Scale – I. Item selection and cross-validation of the factor structure. *Journal of Psychosomatic Research*, **38**, 23–32.

Bagby, R.M., Parker, J.D.A., Taylor, G.J. & Acklin, M.W. (1993). *Alexithymia and the ability to distinguish different emotional states*. Poster presentation at the Annual Meeting of the American Psychosomatic Society, Charleston, SC, March.

Bagby, R.M., Taylor, G.J. & Atkinson, L. (1988a). Alexithymia: a comparative study of three self-report measures. *Journal of Psychosomatic Research*, **32**, 107–16.

Bagby, R.M., Taylor, G.J. & Parker, J.D.A. (1988b). Construct validity of the Toronto Alexithymia Scale. *Psychotherapy and Psychosomatics*, **50**, 29–34.

Bagby, R.M., Taylor, G.J. & Parker, J.D.A. (1994b). The Twenty-Item Toronto Alexithymia Scale – II. Convergent discriminant, and concurrent validity. *Journal of Psychosomatic Research*, **38**, 33–40.

Bagby, R.M., Taylor, G.J., Parker, J.D.A. & Loiselle, C. (1990). Cross-validation of the factor structure of the Toronto Alexithymia Scale. *Journal of Psychosomatic Research*, **34**, 47–51.

Bagby, R.M., Taylor, G.J. & Ryan, D. (1986a). The measurement of alexithymia: psychometric properties of the Schalling–Sifneos Personality Scale. *Comprehensive Psychiatry*, **27**, 287–94.

Bagby, R.M., Taylor, G.J. & Ryan, D. (1986b). Toronto Alexithymia Scale: relationship with personality and psychopathology measures. *Psychotherapy and Psychosomatics*, **45**, 207–15.

Bahnson, C.B. (1982). Psychosomatic issues in cancer. In R.L. Gallon (Ed.), *The psychosomatic approach to illness*, pp. 53–87. New York: Elsevier Biomedical.

Bahnson, M.B. & Bahnson, C.B. (1969). Ego defenses in cancer patients. *Annals of the New York Acadamy of Science*, **164**, 546–59.

Bakan, P. (1969). Hypnotizability, laterality of eye movements and functional brain asymmetry. *Perceptual and Motor Skills*, **28**, 927–32.

Bakan, P. (1978). Dreaming, REM sleep, and the right hemisphere: a theoretical integration. *Journal of Altered States of Consciousness*, **3**, 285–307.

Bakan, P. & Glackman, W.G. (1981). Brain hemisphericity and response to the Imaginal Processes Inventory. In E. Klinger (Ed.), *Imagery: concepts, results, and applications*, vol. 2, pp. 177–87. New York: Plenum.

Baker, G.H.B. (1987). Psychological factors and immunity. *Journal of Psychosomatic Research*, **31**, 1–10.

Baker, G.H.B. (1982). Life events before the onset of rheumatoid arthritis. *Psychotherapy and Psychosomatics*, **38**, 173–7.

Baker, L. & Barcai, A. (1970). Psychosomatic aspects of diabetes mellitus. In O.W. Hill (Ed.), *Modern trends in psychosomatic medicine*, vol. I, pp. 105–23. London: Butterworths.

Balint, M. (1968). *The basic fault*. London: Tavistock Publications.

Balswick, J.O. (1988). *The inexpressive male*. Lexington, MA: Lexington Books.

Baltrusch, H.J.F., Stangel, W. & Waltz, M.E. (1988). Cancer from the biobehavioural perspective: the Type C pattern. *Activitas Nervosa Superior*, **30**, 18–21.

Banich, M.T. (1995).Interhemispheric interaction: mechanisms of unified processing. In F.L. Kitterle (Ed.), *Hemispheric communication: Mechanisms and models*, pp. 271–300. Hillsdale, NJ: Erlbaum.

Barchas, J.D., Elliot, G.R., Berger, P.A., Barchas, P.R. & Solomon, F. (1985). Research on mental illness and addictive disorders: progress and prospects. *American Journal of Psychiatry*, **142** (suppl.), 9–41.

Bard, P. (1934). On emotional expression after decortication with some remarks on certain theoretical views (parts I and II). *Psychological Review*, **41**, 309–29, 424–49.

Barefoot, J.C., Dahlstrom, W.G. & Williams, R.B., Jr. (1983). Hostility, CHD incidence, and total mortality. *Psychosomatic Medicine*, **45**, 59–63.

Barglow, P., Hatcher, R., Edidin, D.V. & Sloan-Rossiter, D. (1984). Stress and metabolic control in diabetes: psychosomatic evidence and evaluation of methods. *Psychosomatic Medicine*, **46**, 126–44.

Barker, C., Pistrang, N., Shapiro, D.A. & Shaw, I. (1990). Coping and help seeking in the UK adult population. *British Journal of Clinical Psychology*, **29**, 271–85.

Barron, F. (1953). An ego-strength scale which predicts response to psychotherapy. *Journal of Consulting Psychology*, **17**, 327–33.

Barsky, A.J. (1992). Amplification, somatization, and the somatoform disorders. *Psychosomatics*, **33**, 28–34.

Barsky, A.J., Goodson, J.D., Lane, R.S. & Cleary, P.D. (1988). The amplification of somatic symptoms. *Psychosomatic Medicine*, **50**, 510–19.

Barsky, A.J. & Klerman, G.L. (1983). Overview: hypochondriasis, bodily complaints and somatic styles. *American Journal of Psychiatry*, **140**, 273–83.

Barsky, A.J. & Wyshak, G. (1990). Hypochondriasis and somatosensory amplification. *British Journal of Psychiatry*, **157**, 404–9.

Barsky, A.J., Wool, C., Barnett, M.C. & Cleary, P.D. (1994). Histories of childhood trauma in adult hypochondriacal patients. *American Journal of Psychiatry*, **151**, 397–401.

Barsky, A.J., Wyshak, G. & Klerman, G.L. (1990). The somatosensory amplification scale and its relationship to hypochondriasis. *Journal of Psychiatric Research*, **24**, 323–34.

Basch, M.F. (1976). The concept of affect: a re-examination. *Journal of the American Psychoanalytic Association*, **24**, 759–77.

Bass, C. & Murphy, M. (1990). The chronic somatizer and the government white paper (Editorial). *Journal of the Royal Society of Medicine*, **83**, 203–5.

Bass, C. & Murphy, M. (1995). Somatoform and personality disorders: syndromal comorbidity and overlapping developmental pathways. *Journal of Psychosomatic Research*, **39**, 403–27.

Baumbacher, G.D. (1989). Signal anxiety and panic attacks. *Psychotherapy*, **26**, 75–80.

Bear, D.M. (1983). Hemispheric specialization and the neurology of emotion. *Archives of Neurology*, **40**, 195–202.

Beaumont, W. (1833). *Experiments and observations on the gastric juice and the physiology of digestion*. Plattsburg, NY: F.P. Allen.

Beebe, B. & Lachmann, F.M. (1988). The contribution of mother–infant mutual influence to the origins of self- and object representations. *Psychoanalytic Psychology*, **5**, 305–37.

Bell, C.M. & Khantzian, E.J. (1991). Contemporary psychodynamic perspectives and the disease concept of addiction: complementary or competing models? *Psychiatric Annals*, **21**, 273–81.

Bell, P.A. & Byrne, D. (1978). Repression-sensitization. In H. London & J. Exner (Eds.), *Dimensions of personality*, pp. 449–85. New York: Wiley.

Bellak, L. (1984). Basic aspects of ego function assessment. In L. Bellak & L.A. Goldsmith (Eds.), *The broad scope of ego function assessment*, pp. 6–19. New York: Wiley.

Bellak, L., Hurvich, M. & Gediman, H. (1973). *Ego functions in schizophrenics, neurotics, and normals*. New York: Wiley.

Berenbaum, H. & James, T. (1994). Correlates and retrospectively reported antecedents of alexithymia. *Psychosomatic Medicine*, **56**, 353–9.

Berenbaum, H. & Prince, J.D. (1994). Alexithymia and the interpretation of emotion-relevant information. *Cognition and Emotion*, **8**, 231–44.

Beresnevaité, M. (1995). Efficacy of alexithymia's correction and its relation with the course of ischaemic heart disease. Paper presented at the Annual Congress of Lithuanian Cardiologists, Kaunas, Lithuania, May.

Beresnevaité, M., et al. (1998). Cross validation of the factor structure of a Lithuanian translation of the 20-item Toronto Alexithymia Scale. *Acta Medica Lituanica*, **5**, 146–9.

Bernstein, E.M. & Putnam, F.W. (1986). Development, reliability, and validity of a dissociation scale. *Journal of Nervous and Mental Disease*, **174**, 727–35.

Berry, D.S. & Pennebaker, J.W. (1993). Nonverbal and verbal emotional expression and health. *Psychotherapy and Psychosomatics*, **59**, 11–19.

Beutler, L.E. *et al.* (1986). Inability to express intense affect: a common link between depression and pain? *Journal of Consulting and Clinical Psychology*, **54**, 752–9.

Bibb, J. & Chambless, D.L. (1986). Alcohol use and abuse among diagnosed agoraphobics. *Behaviour, Research and Therapy*, **24**, 49–58.

Bibring, E. (1953). The mechanism of depression. In P. Greenacre (Ed.), *Affective disorders: Psychoanalytic contributions to their study*, pp. 13–48. New York: International Universities Press.

Bihrle, A.M. *et al.* (1988). Humour and the right hemisphere: a narrative perspective. In H.A. Whitaker (Ed.), *Contemporary reviews in neuropsychology*, pp. 109–26. New York: Springer.

Bion, W.R. (1962). *Learning from experience*. London: Heinemann.

Bion, W.R. (1965). *Transformations*. London: Heinemann.

Bion, W.R. (1970). *Attention and interpretation*. London: Tavistock Publications.

Bion, W.R. (1992). *Cogitations*. London: Karnac Books.

Birtchell, J. *et al.* (1988). The total score of the Crown-Crisp Experiential Index: a useful and valid measure of psychoneurotic pathology. *British Journal of Medical Psychology*, **61**, 255–66.

Blalock, J.E. (1989). A molecular basis for bidirectional communication between the immune and neuroendocrine systems. *Physiological Reviews*, **69**, 1–32.

Blanchard, E.B., Arena, J.G. & Pallmeyer, T.P. (1981). Psychometric properties of a scale to measure alexithymia. *Psychotherapy and Psychosomatics*, **28**, 36–46.

Blatt, S.J., Berman, W., Bloom-Feshbach, S., Sugarman, A., Wilber, C. & Kleber, H.D. (1984). Psychological assessment of psychopathology in opiate addicts. *Journal of Nervous and Mental Disease*, **172**, 156–65.

Blatt, S.J. & Lerner, H. (1983). Investigations in the psychoanalytic theory of object relations and object representations. In J. Masling (Ed.), *Empirical studies of psychoanalytical theories*, vol. 1, pp. 189–249. Hillsdale, NJ: Analytic Press.

Blau, A. (1952). In support of Freud's syndrome of 'actual' anxiety neurosis. *International Journal of Psychoanalysis*, **33**, 363–72.

Blinder, B.J. (1986). Rumination: a benign disorder? *International Journal of Eating Disorders*, **5**, 385–6.

Blumenthal, J.A., Rose, S. & Chang, J.L. (1985). Anorexia nervosa and exercise: implications from recent findings. *Sports Medicine*, **2**, 237–47.

Blumer, D. & Heilbronn, M. (1982). Chronic pain as a variant of depressive disease: the pain-prone disorder. *Journal of Nervous and Mental Disease*, **170**, 381–406.

Bonanno, G.A. & Singer, J.L. (1990). Repressive personality style: theoretical and methodological implications for health and pathology. In J.L. Singer (Ed.), *Repression and dissociation: implications for personality theory, psychopathology and health*, pp. 435–70. Chicago: University of Chicago Press.

Bond, M. (1986). Defense Style Questionnaire. In G.E. Vaillant (Ed.), *Empirical studies of ego mechanisms of defense*, pp. 146–52. Washington, DC: American Psychiatric Press.

Bond, M., Gardiner, S.T., Christian, J. & Sigal, J.J. (1983). An empirical examination of defense mechanisms. *Archives of General Psychiatry*, **40**, 333–8.

Booth-Butterfield, M. & Booth-Butterfield, S. (1990). Conceptualizing affect as information in communication production. *Human Communication Research*, **16**, 451–76.

Booth-Kewley, S. & Friedman, H.S. (1987). Psychological predictors of heart disease: a quantitative review. *Psychological Bulletin*, **101**, 343–62.

Borens, R., Grosse-Schulte, E., Jaensch, W. & Kortemme, K.H. (1977). Is 'alexithymia' but a social phenomenon? An empirical investigation in psychosomatic patients. *Psychotherapy and Psychosomatics*, **28**, 193–8.

Borod, J.C. (1992). Interhemispheric and intrahemispheric control of emotion: a focus on unilateral brain damage. *Journal of Consulting and Clinical Psychology*, **60**, 339–48.

Borod, J.C., Martin, C.C., Alpert, M., Brozgold, A. & Welkowitz, J. (1993). Perception of facial emotion in schizophrenic and right brain-damage patients. *Journal of Nervous and Mental Disease*, **181**, 494–502.

Bourke, M.P., Taylor, G.J. & Crisp, A.H. (1985). Symbolic functioning in anorexia nervosa. *Journal of Psychiatric Research*, **19**, 273–8.

Bourke, M.P., Taylor, G.J., Parker, J.D.A. & Bagby, R.M. (1992). Alexithymia in women with anorexia nervosa: a preliminary investigation. *British Journal of Psychiatry*, **161**, 240–3.

Bowers, D., Bauer, R.M., Coslett, H.B. & Heilman, K.M. (1985). Processing of faces by patients with unilateral hemisphere lesions. *Brain and Cognition*, **4**, 258–72.

Bowlby, J. (1969). *Attachment and loss. Vol. I: Attachment*. New York: Basic Books.

Bowlby, J. (1973). *Attachment and loss. Vol. II: Separation: anxiety and anger*. New York: Basic Books.

Bowlby, J. (1980). *Attachment and loss. Vol. III: Loss: sadness and depression.* New York: Basic Books.

Bowlby, J. (1988a). *A secure base: clinical applications of attachment theory.* London: Routledge and Kegan Paul.

Bowlby, J. (1988b). Developmental psychiatry comes of age. *American Journal of Psychiatry,* 145, 1-10.

Bradshaw, J.L. (1989). *Hemispheric specialization and psychological function.* Chichester: Wiley.

Brady, K.T. *et al.* (1993). Gender differences in substance use disorders. *American Journal of Psychiatry,* 150, 1707-11.

Bräutigam, W. & von Rad, M. (1977). Towards a theory of psychosomatic disorders. In W. Bräutigam & M. von Rad (Eds.), *Proceedings of the 11th European Conference on Psychosomatic Research,* pp. xi–xiii. Basel: Karger.

Bremner, J.D. *et al.* (1995). MRI-based measurement of hippocampal volume in patients with combat-related posttraumatic stress disorder. *American Journal of Psychiatry,* 152, 973-81.

Brenner, C. (1975). Affects and psychic conflict. *Psychoanalytic Quarterly,* 44, 5-28.

Brenner, C. (1991). A psychoanalytic perspective on depression. *Journal of the American Psychoanalytic Association,* 39, 25-43.

Breslau, N., Davis, G. & Andreski, P. (1991). Traumatic events and post-traumatic stress disorder in an urban population of young adults. *Archives of General Psychiatry,* 48, 216-22.

Breslau, N., Davis, G. & Andreski, P. (1995). Risk factors for PTSD-related traumatic events: a prospective analysis. *American Journal of Psychiatry,* 152, 529-35.

Bressi, C. *et al.* (1996). Cross validation of the factor structure of the 20-item Toronto Alexithymia Scale: An Italian multicenter study. *Journal of Psychosomatic Research,* 41, 551-9.

Bretherton, I. (1985). I. Attachment theory: retrospect and prospect. In I. Bretherton, & E. Waters (Eds.), *Growing points of attachment theory and research. Monographs of the Society for Research in Child Development,* 50, 1-2, Serial No. 299, 3-35.

Bretherton, I. *et al.* (1986). Learning to talk about emotions: a functionalist perspective. *Child Development,* 57, 529-48.

Bretherton, I., Fritz, J., Zahn-Waxler, C. & Ridgeway, D. (1986). Learning to talk about emotions: a functionalist perspective. *Child Development,* 57, 529-48.

Breuer, J. & Freud, S. (1893). On the psychical mechanism of hysterical phenomena. *Standard Edition,* 2, 3-17. London: Hogarth Press, 1958.

Breuer, J. & Freud, S. (1895). Studies on hysteria. *Standard Edition,* 2, 3-305. London: Hogarth Press, 1958.

Bridges, K.W. & Goldberg, D.P. (1985). Somatic presentation of DSM III psychiatric disorders in primary care. *Journal of Psychosomatic Research*, **29**, 563–9.

Briggs, S.R. (1989). The optimal level of measurement for personality constructs. In D.M. Buss & N. Cantor (Eds.), *Personality psychology: recent trends and emerging directions*, pp. 246–60. New York: Springer–Verlag.

Briggs, S.R. & Cheek, J.M. (1986). The role of factor analysis in the development and evaluation of personality scales. *Journal of Personality*, **54**, 106–48.

Briquet, P. (1859). *Traite de l'Hysterie*. Paris: J. Bailliere.

Brotman, A.W., Herzog, D.B. & Woods, S.W. (1984). Antidepressant treatment of bulimia: the relationship between bingeing and depressive symptomatology. *Journal of Clinical Psychiatry*, **45**, 7–9.

Brown, C.T., Yelsma, P. & Keller, P. (1980). Communication-conflict predisposition: development of a theory and an instrument. *Human Relations*, **34**, 1103–17.

Brown, D. (1993). Affective development, psychopathology, and adaptation. In S.L. Ablon, D. Brown, E.J. Khantzian & J.E. Mack (Eds.), *Human feelings: explorations in affect development and meaning*, pp. 5–66. Hillsdale, NJ: Analytic Press.

Brown, F.W., Golding, J.M. & Smith, R. (1990). Psychiatric comorbidity in primary care somatization disorder. *Psychosomatic Medicine*, **52**, 445–51.

Brown, H.N. & Vaillant, G.E. (1981). Hypochondriasis. *Archives of Internal Medicine*, **141**, 723–6.

Brown, L.J. (1985). On concreteness. *The Psychoanalytic Review*, **72**, 379–402.

Brown, P. (1991). *The hypnotic brain: hypnotherapy and social communication*. New Haven: Yale University Press.

Bruch, H. (1962). Perceptual and conceptual disturbances in anorexia nervosa. *Psychosomatic Medicine*, **24**, 187–94.

Bruch, H. (1971). Death in anorexia nervosa. *Psychosomatic Medicine*, **33**, 135–44.

Bruch, H. (1973). *Eating disorders. Obesity, anorexia nervosa, and the person within*. New York: Basic Books.

Bruch, H. (1982/83). Treatment in anorexia nervosa. *International Journal of Psychoanalytic Psychotherapy*, **9**, 303–12.

Bruch, H. (1985). Four decades of eating disorders. In D.M. Garner, & P.E. Garfinkel (Eds.), *Handbook of psychotherapy for anorexia nervosa & bulimia*, pp. 7–18. New York: Guilford Press.

Brzeziński, R. & Rybakowski, J. (1993). *Alexithymia as a possible risk factor in ischaemic heart disease*. Presented at the 12th World Congress of Psychosomatic Medicine, Bern, Switzerland.

Buchanan, D.C., Waterhouse, G.J. & West, S.C. (1980). A proposed neurophysiological basis of alexithymia. *Psychotherapy and Psychosomatics*, **34**, 248–55.

Buck, R. (1994). The neuropsychology of communication: spontaneous and symbolic aspects. *Journal of Pragmatics*, **22**, 265–78.

Bukstein, O.G., Brent, D.A. & Kaminer, Y. (1989). Comorbidity of substance abuse and other psychiatric disorders in adolescents. *American Journal of Psychiatry*, **146**, 1131–41.

Bulik, C.M. (1987). Drug and alcohol abuse by bulimic women and their families. *American Journal of Psychiatry*, **144**, 1604–6.

Burton, R. (1621). *The anatomy of melancholy*. Oxford: H. Cripps.

Busch, F.N., Cooper, A.M., Klerman, G.L., Penzer, R.J., Shapiro, T. & Shear, M.K. (1991). Neurophysiological, cognitive–behavioral, and psychoanalytic approaches to panic disorder. *Psychoanalytic Inquiry*, **11**, 316–32.

Buss, D.M. (1990). Toward a biologically informed psychology of personality. *Journal of Personality*, **58**, 1–16.

Buydens-Branchey, L., Branchey, M.H., Noumair, D. & Lieber, C.S. (1989). Age of alcoholism onset II. Relationship to susceptibility to serotonin precursor availability. *Archives of General Psychiatry*, **46**, 231–6.

Cacioppo, J.T. & Petty, R.E. (1982). The need for cognition. *Journal of Personality and Social Psychology*, **42**, 116–31.

Cacioppo, J.T., Petty, R.E. & Kao, C.F. (1984). The efficient assessment of need for cognition. *Journal of Personality Assessment*, **48**, 306–7.

Callahan, J. & Sashin, J.I. (1987). Models of affect–response and anorexia nervosa. *Annals of the New York Academy of Sciences*, **504**, 241–59.

Calvin, W.H. (1990). *The cerebral symphony*. New York: Bantam Books.

Camara, E.G. & Danao, T.C. (1989). The brain and the immune system: a psychosomatic network. *Psychosomatics*, **30**, 140–6.

Campos, J.J., Campos, R.G. & Barrett, K.C. (1989). Emergent themes in the study of emotional development and emotion regulation. *Developmental Psychology*, **25**, 394–402.

Camras, L.A., Holland, E.A. & Patterson, M.J. (1993). Facial expression. In M. Lewis & J.M. Haviland (Eds.), *Handbook of emotions*, pp. 199–208. New York: Guilford.

Cannon, W.B. (1927). The James–Lange theory of emotion: a critical examination and an alternative theory. *American Journal of Psychology*, **39**, 106–24.

Cannon, W.B. (1929). *Bodily changes in pain, hunger, fear and rage*, 2nd ed. New York: Appelton.

Cantwell, D.P., Sturzenberger, S., Burroughs, J., Salkin, B., & Green, J.K. (1977). Anorexia nervosa: an affective disorder? *Archives of General Psychiatry*, **34**, 1087–93.

Carlat, D.J. & Camargo, C.A. (1991). Review of bulimia nervosa in males. *American Journal of Psychiatry*, **148**, 831–43.

Carter, M.M., Hollon, S.D., Carson, R. & Shelton, R.C. (1995). Effects of safe person in induced distress following a biological challenge in panic disorder with agoraphobia. *Journal of Abnormal Psychology*, **104**, 156–63.

Cartwright, R.D. (1977). *Nightlife: explorations in dreaming*. New Jersey: Prentice-Hall.

Cartwright, R.D. (1993). Who needs their dreams? The usefulness of dreams in psychotherapy. *Journal of the American Academy of Psychoanalysis*, **21**, 539–47.

Cartwright, R.D., Tipton, L. & Wicklund, J. (1980). Focusing on dreams: a preparation program for psychotherapy. *Archives of General Psychiatry*, **37**, 275–7.

Carver, C.S. (1989). How should multifaceted personality constructs be tested? Issues illustrated by self-monitoring, attributional style, and hardiness. *Journal of Personality and Social Psychology*, **56**, 577–85.

Casper, R.C. (1983). Some provisional ideas concerning the psychologic structure in anorexia nervosa and bulimia. In P.L. Darby, P.E. Garfinkel, D.M. Garner & D.V. Coscina (Eds.), *Anorexia nervosa: recent developments in research*, pp. 387–92. New York: Alan R. Liss.

Casper, R.C. (1990). Personality features of women with good outcome from restricting anorexia nervosa. *Psychosomatic Medicine*, **52**, 156–70.

Casper, R.C., Eckert, E.D., Halmi, K.I., Goldberg, S.C. & Davis, J.M. (1980). Bulimia: its incidence and clinical importance in patients with anorexia nervosa. *Archives of General Psychiatry*, **37**, 1030–5.

Catchlove, R.F.H., Cohen, K.R., Braha, R.E.D. & Demers-Desrosiers, L.A. (1985). Incidence and implications of alexithymia in chronic pain patients. *Journal of Nervous and Mental Disease*, **173**, 246–8.

Cattell, R.B. & Burdsal, C.A. (1975). The radial parcel double factoring design: a solution to the item-vs-parcel controversy. *Multivariate Behavioral Research*, **10**, 165–79.

Cattell, R.B., Eber, H.W. & Tatsuoka, M.M. (1980). *Handbook for the Sixteen Personality Factor Questionnaire (16PF)*. Champaign, IL: Institute for Personality and Ability Testing.

Chambless, D.L., Cherney, J., Caputo, G.C. & Rheinstein, B.J.G. (1987). Anxiety disorders and alcoholism. *Journal of Anxiety Disorders*, **1**, 24–40.

Charman, D.K. (1979). Do different personalities have different hemispheric asymmetries? A brief communique of an initial experiment. *Cortex*, **15**, 655–7.

Charney, D.S., Deutch, A.Y., Krystal, J.H., Southwick, S.M. & Davis, M. (1993). Psychobiologic mechanisms of posttraumatic stress disorder. *Archives of General Psychiatry*, 50, 294–305.

Choy, T. & de Bosset, F. (1992). Post-traumatic stress disorder: an overview. *Canadian Journal of Psychiatry*, 37, 578–83.

Christensen, A.J. & Smith, T.W. (1993). Cynical hostility and cardiovascular reactivity during self-disclosure. *Psychosomatic Medicine*, 55, 193–202.

Christman, S.D. (1994). The many sides of the two sides of the brain. *Brain and Cognition*, 26, 91–8.

Christman, S.D. (1995). Independence versus integration of rights and left hemisphere processing: effects of handedness. In F.L. Kitterle (Ed.), *Hemispheric communication: mechanisms and models*, pp. 231–253. Hillsdale, NJ: Erlbaum.

Cicchetti, D., Ganiban, J. & Barnett, D. (1991). Contributions from the study of high-risk populations to understanding the development of emotion regulation. In J. Garber & K.A. Dodge (Eds.), *The development of emotion regulation and dysregulation*, pp. 15–48. Cambridge: Cambridge University Press.

Cicchetti, D. & Tucker, D. (1994). Development and self-regulatory structures of the mind. *Development and Psychopathology*, 6, 533–49.

Ciompi, L. (1991). Affects as central organising and integrating factors: a new psychosocial/biological model of the psyche. *British Journal of Psychiatry*, 159, 97–105.

Clark, D.M. (1986). A cognitive approach to panic. *Behaviour Research and Therapy*, 24, 461–70.

Clerici, M., Albonetti, S., Papa, R., Penati, G. & Invernizzi, G. (1992). Alexithymia and obesity. *Psychotherapy and Psychosomatics*, 57, 83–93.

Cloninger, C.R. (1987). Neurogenic adaptive mechanisms in alcoholism. *Science*, 236, 410–16.

Cloninger, C.R., Martin, R.L., Guze, S.B. & Clayton, P.J. (1986). A prospective follow-up and family study of somatization in men and women. *American Journal of Psychiatry*, 143, 873–8.

Cloninger, C.R., Svrakic, D.M. & Przybeck, T.R. (1993). A psychobiological model of temperament and character. *Archives of General Psychiatry*, 50, 975–90.

Cochrane, C.E., Brewerton, T.D., Wilson, D.B. & Hodges, E.L. (1993). Alexithymia in eating disorders. *International Journal of Eating Disorders*, 14, 219–22.

Cohen, B.M., Renshaw, P.F. & Yurgelun-Todd, D. (1995). Imaging the mind: magnetic resonance spectroscopy and functional brain imaging. *American Journal of Psychiatry*, 152, 655–8.

Cohen, J. (1993). Die zwei Arten der psychoanalytischen Rekonstruktion: warum Analysen beide benötigen. (The two classes of psychoanalytic reconstruction: why analyses require both.) *Jahrbuch der Psychoanalyse*, **30**, 65–100. (An English translation is available from the author.)

Cohen, J. & Kinston, W. (1984). Repression theory: a new look at the cornerstone. *International Journal of Psychoanalysis*, **65**, 411–22.

Cohen, K.R., Auld, F. & Brooker, H. (1994). Is alexithymia related to psychosomatic disorder and somatizing? *Journal of Psychosomatic Research*, **38**, 119–27.

Cohen, K.R., Auld, F., Demers, L.A. & Catchlove, R.F.H. (1985). Alexithymia: the development of a valid and reliable projective measure (the objectively scored archetypal 9 test). *Journal of Nervous and Mental Disease*, **173**, 621–7.

Cohen, K.R., Demers-Desrosiers, L.A. & Catchlove, R.F.H. (1983). The SAT$_9$: a quantitative scoring system for the AT$_9$ test as a measure of symbolic function central to alexithymic presentation. *Psychotherapy and Psychosomatics*, **39**, 77–88.

Cohen, M.E. & White, P.D. (1950). Life situations, emotions, and neurocirculatory asthenia (anxiety, neurasthenia, and effort syndrome). In H.G. Wolff (Ed.), *Life stress and bodily disease*, Nervous and Mental Disease, Research Publication No. 29. Baltimore, MD: Williams & Wilkins.

Cole, D.A. (1987). Utility of confirmatory factor analysis in test validation research. *Journal of Consulting and Clinical Psychology*, **55**, 584–94.

Cole, G. & Bakan, P. (1985). Alexithymia, hemisphericity, and conjugate lateral eye movements. *Psychotherapy and Psychosomatics*, **44**, 139–43.

Comrey, A.L. (1988). Factor-analytic methods of scale development in personality and clinical psychology. *Journal of Consulting and Clinical Psychology*, **56**, 754–61.

Conte, H.R., Buckley, P., Picard, S. & Karasu, T.B. (1995). Relationships between psychological mindedness and personality traits and ego functioning: validity studies. *Comprehensive Psychiatry*, **36**, 11–17.

Conte, H.R., Plutchik, R., Jung, B.B., Picard, S., Karasu, T.B. & Lotterman, A. (1990). Psychological mindedness as a predictor of psychotherapy outcome: a preliminary report. *Comprehensive Psychiatry*, **31**, 426–31.

Costa, P.T. & McCrae, R.R. (1980). Influence of extraversion and neuroticism on subjective well-being: happy and unhappy people. *Journal of Personality and Social Psychology*, **38**, 668–78.

Costa, P.T. & McCrae, R.R. (1985). *The NEO Personality Inventory manual*. Odessa, FL: Psychological Assessment Resources.

Costa, P.T. & McCrae, R.R. (1987a). Personality assessment in psychosomatic medicine. *Advances in Psychosomatic Medicine*, **17**, 71–82.

Costa, P.T. & McCrae, R.R. (1987*b*). Neuroticism, somatic complaints, and disease: is the bark worse than the bite? *Journal of Personality*, **55**, 299–316.

Costa, P.T. & McCrae, R.R. (1992). *Revised NEO Personality Inventory (NEO PI-R) and NEO Five-Factor Inventory (NEO-FFI) professional manual*. Odessa, FL: Psychological Assessment Resources.

Cox, B.J., Kuch, K., Parker, J.D.A., Shulman, I.D. & Evans, R.J. (1994). Alexithymia in somatoform disorder patients with chronic pain. *Journal of Psychosomatic Research*, **38**, 523–7.

Cox, B.J., Swinson, R.P., Shulman, I.D. & Bourdeau, D. (1995). Alexithymia in panic disorder and social phobia. *Comprehensive Psychiatry*, **36**, 195–8.

Craig, T.K.J., Boardman, A.P., Mills, K., Daly-Jones, O. & Drake, H. (1993). The South London somatisation study I: Longitudinal course and the influence of early life experiences. *British Journal of Psychiatry*, **163**, 579–88.

Crisp, A.H. (1968). Primary anorexia nervosa. *Gut*, **9**, 370–2.

Crisp, A.H. (1980). *Anorexia nervosa: let me be*. London: Academic Press.

Crisp, A.H., Palmer, R.L. & Kalucy, R.A. (1976). How common is anorexia nervosa? A prevalence study. *British Journal of Psychiatry*, **128**, 549–54.

Crittenden, P.M. (1994). Peering into the black box: an exploratory treatise on the development of self in young children. In D. Cicchetti & S.L. Toth (Eds.), *Rochester symposium on developmental psychopathology, Vol. 5. Disorders and dysfunctions of the self*, pp. 79–148. Rochester, NY: University of Rochester Press.

Cronbach, L.J. & Meehl, P.E. (1955). Construct validity in psychological tests. *Psychological Bulletin*, **52**, 281–302.

Crossman, D.L. & Polich, J.H.(1989). Hemispheric and personality differences between 'left-' and 'right-brain' individuals for tachistoscopic verbal and spatial tasks. *Personality and Individual Differences*, **10**, 747–55.

Crown, S. & Crisp, A.H. (1979). *Manual of the Crown-Crisp Experiential Index*. London: Hodder & Stoughton.

Crown, S., Crown, J.M. & Fleming, A. (1975). Aspects of the psychology and epidemiology of rheumatoid disease. *Psychological Medicine*, **5**, 291–9.

Cutting, J. (1992). The role of right hemisphere dysfunction in psychiatric disorders. *British Journal of Psychiatry*, **160**, 583–8.

DaCosta, J.M. (1871). On irritable heart: a clinical study of a form of functional cardiac disorder and its consequences. *American Journal of Medical Sciences*, **61**, 2–53.

Daruna, J.H. & Morgan, J.E. (1990). Psychosocial effects on immune function: neuroendocrine pathways. *Psychosomatics*, **31**, 4–12.

Darwin, C. (1872). *The expression of the emotions in man and animals.* Chicago: University of Chicago Press, 1965.

Davidson, R.J. (1993). The neuropsychology of emotion and affective style. In M. Lewis & J.M. Haviland (Eds.), *Handbook of emotions,* pp. 143–54. New York: Guilford Press.

Davidson, R. J. (1994). Complexities in the search for emotion-specific physiology. In P. Ekman & R.J. Davidson (Eds.), *The nature of emotion: fundamental questions,* pp. 237–42. New York: Oxford University Press.

Davidson, R.J. & Ekman, P. (1994). Afterword: what are the minimal cognitive prerequisites for emotion? In P. Ekman, & R.J. Davidson (Eds.), *The nature of emotion: fundamental questions,* pp. 232–4. New York: Oxford University Press.

Davidson, R.J., Ekman, P., Saron, C.D., Senulis, J.A. & Friesen, W.V. (1990). Approach–withdrawal and cerebral asymmetry: emotional expression and brain physiology I. *Journal of Personality and Social Psychology,* **58**, 330–41.

Davidson, R.J. & Fox, N.A. (1988). Cerebral asymmetry and emotion: developmental and individual differences. In D.L. Molfese & S.J. Segalowitz (Eds.), *Brain lateralization in children: developmental implications,* pp. 191–206. New York: Guilford Press.

Deary, I.J., Fowkes, F.G.R., Donnan, P.T. & Housley, E. (1994). Hostile personality and risks of peripheral arterial disease in the general population. *Psychosomatic Medicine,* **56**, 197–202.

Defourny, M., Hubin, P. & Luminet, D. (1976/77). Alexithymia, 'pensée opératoire', and predisposition to coronopathy. *Psychotherapy and Psychosomatics,* **27**, 106–14.

de Groot, J.M., Rodin, G. & Olmsted, M.P. (1995). Alexithymia, depression, and treatment outcome in bulimia nervosa. *Comprehensive Psychiatry,* **36**, 53–60.

DeJong, C.A.J., van den Brink, W., Harteveld, F.M. & van der Wielen, E.G.M. (1993). Personality disorders in alcoholics and drug addicts. *Comprehensive Psychiatry,* **34**, 87–94.

Delle Chiaie, R., Cianconi, P., Didonna, A., Saito, A., Regine, F. & Pancheri, P. (1994). *Alexithymia in opioid addicts. State dependent reaction or permanent trait?* Presented at the 20th European Conference on Psychosomatic Research, Gent, Belgium.

Dembroski, T.M. & Costa, P.T. (1987). Coronary prone behavior: components of the Type A pattern and hostility. *Journal of Personality,* **55**, 211–35.

Dembroski, T.M., MacDougall, J.M., Costa, P.T. & Grandits, G.A. (1989). Components of hostility as predictors of sudden death and myocardial infarction in the multiple risk factor intervention trial. *Psychosomatic Medicine,* **51**, 514–22.

Dembroski, T.M., MacDougall, J.M., Williams, R.B., Haney, T. & Blumenthal, J.A. (1985). Components of Type A, hostility and anger-in. Relationship to angiographic findings. *Psychosomatic Medicine*, **47**, 219–33.

Demers-Desrosiers, L.A. (1982). Influence of alexithymia on symbolic function. *Psychotherapy and Psychosomatics*, **38**, 103–20.

Demers-Desrosiers, L.A. (1985). Empirical journey into the measurement of symbolic function as a dimension of alexithymia. *Psychotherapy and Psychosomatics*, **44**, 65–71.

Demers-Desrosiers, L.A., Cohen, K.R., Catchlove, R.F.H. & Ramsay, R.A. (1983). The measure of symbolic function in alexithymic pain patients. *Psychotherapy and Psychosomatics*, **39**, 65–76.

Deri, S.K. (1984). *Symbolization and creativity*. New York: International Universities Press.

Derogatis, L.R. (1977). *SCL-90. Administration, scoring and procedures manual. Clinical psychometric research*. Baltimore, MD: Johns Hopkins University School of Medicine.

Derryberry, D. & Tucker, D.M. (1992). Neural mechanisms of emotion. *Journal of Consulting and Clinical Psychology*, **60**, 329–38.

Deter, H. & Herzog, W. (1994). Anorexia nervosa in a long-term perspective: results of the Heidelberg-Manneheim study. *Psychosomatic Medicine*, **56**, 20–7.

Deutsch, F. (1959). *On the mysterious leap from the mind to the body*. New York: International Universities Press.

Dewaraja, R. & Sasaki, Y. (1990). A right to left hemisphere callosal transfer deficit of nonlinguistic information in alexithymia. *Psychotherapy and Psychosomatics*, **54**, 201–7.

Digman, J.M. (1990). Personality structure: emergence of the five-factor model. *Annual Review of Psychology*, **41**, 417–40.

Dodes, L.M. (1990). Addiction, helplessness, and narcissistic rage. *Psychoanalytic Quarterly*, **59**, 398–419.

Dodge, K.A. & Garber, J. (1991). Domains of emotion regulation. In J. Garber & K.A. Dodge (Eds.), *The development of emotion regulation and dysregulation*, pp. 3–11. Cambridge: Cambridge University Press.

Donovan, J.M. (1986). An etiological model of alcoholism. *American Journal of Psychiatry*, **143**, 1–11.

Dorpat, T.L. (1985). *Denial and defense in the therapeutic situation*. Northvale, NJ: Aronson.

Drewnowski, A., Yee, D.K. & Krahn, D.D. (1988). Bulimia in college women: incidence and recovery rates. *American Journal of Psychiatry*, **145**, 753–5.

Drewnowski, A., Yee, D.K., Kurth, C.L. & Krahn, D.D. (1994). Eating pathology and DSM-III-R bulimia nervosa: a continuum of behavior. *American Journal of Psychiatry*, **151**, 1217–19.

Drossman, D.A., McKee, D.C., Sandler, R.S., Mitchell, C.M., Cramer, E.M., Lowman, B.C. & Burger, A.L. (1988). Psychosocial factors in the irritable bowel syndrome: a multivariate study of patients and non-patients with irritable bowel syndrome. *Gastroenterology*, **95**, 701–8.

Dubovsky, S.L. & Thomas, M. (1995*a*). Serotonergic mechanisms and current and future psychiatric practice. *Journal of Clinical Psychiatry*, **56** (suppl. 2), 38–48.

Dubovsky, S.L. & Thomas, M. (1995*b*). Beyond specifity: effects of serotonin and serotonergic treatments on psychobiological dysfunction. *Journal of Psychosomatic Research*, **39**, 429–44.

Dunbar, F. (1935). *Emotions and bodily changes: a survey of literature on psychosomatic interrelationships 1910–1933*. New York: Columbia University Press.

Dunn, B.R., Bartscher, J., Turaniczo, M. & Gram, P. (1989). Relationship between lateral eye movements, brain organization, and cognitive style. *Brain and Cognition*, **10**, 171–88.

Dunn, J. & Brown, J. (1991). Relationships, talk about feelings, and the development of affect regulation in early childhood. In J. Garber & K.A. Dodge (Eds.), *The development of emotion regulation and dysregulation*, pp. 89–108. Cambridge: Cambridge University Press.

Eagle, M.N. (1984). *Recent developments in psychoanalysis: a critical evaluation*. New York: McGraw-Hill.

Edgcumbe, R.M. (1984). Modes of communication: the differentiation of somatic and verbal expression. *Psychoanalytic Study of the Child*, **39**, 137–54.

Ehrlichman, H. & Weinberger, A. (1978). Lateral eye movements and hemispheric asymmetry: a critical review. *Psychological Bulletin*, **85**, 1080–101.

Ehrlichman, H. & Barrett, J. (1983). Right hemisphere specialization for mental imagery: a review of the evidence. *Brain and Cognition*, **2**, 55–76.

Ekman, P. (1993). Facial expression and emotion. *American Psychologist*, **48**, 384–92.

Ekman, P. & Davidson, R.J. (1994). *The nature of emotion: fundamental questions*. New York: Oxford University Press.

Emde, R.N. (1984). The affective self: continuities and transformations from infancy. In J.D. Call, E. Galenson, & R.L. Tyson (Eds.), *Frontiers of infant psychiatry*, vol. 2, pp. 38–54. New York: Basic Books.

Emde, R.N. (1988*a*). Development terminable and interminable. I. Innate and motivational factors from infancy. *International Journal of Psychoanalysis*, **69**, 23–42.

Emde, R.N. (1988b). Development terminable and interminable. II. Recent psychoanalytic theory and therapeutic considerations. *International Journal of Psychoanalysis*, **69**, 283–96.

Emde, R.N. (1991). Positive emotions for psychoanalytic theory: surprises from infancy research and new directions. *Journal of the American Psychoanalytic Association*, **39** (Suppl.), 5–44.

Endler, N.S. & Parker, J.D.A. (1995). Assessing a patient's ability to cope. In J.N. Butcher (Ed.), *Clinical personality assessment: Practical approaches*, pp. 329–352. New York: Oxford University Press.

Engel, G.L. (1955). Studies of ulcerative colitis: III. The nature of the psychologic processes. *American Journal of Medicine*, **19**, 231–56.

Engel, G.L. (1958). Studies of ulcerative colitis: V. Psychological aspects and their implications for treatment. *American Journal of Digestive Diseases*, **3**, 315–37.

Engel, G.L. (1959). 'Psychogenic' pain and the pain-prone patient. *American Journal of Medicine*, **26**, 899–918.

Engel, G.L. (1962). *Psychological development in health and disease*. Philadelphia: Saunders.

Engel, G.L. (1968). A life setting conducive to illness: the giving up-given up complex. *Annals of Internal Medicine*, **69**, 293–300.

Engel, G.L. (1971). Sudden and rapid death during psychological stress. *Annals of Internal Medicine*, **74**, 771–82.

Engel, G.L. (1977). The need for a new medical model: a challenge for biomedicine. *Science*, **196**, 129–36.

Engel, G.L. & Reichsman, F. (1956). Spontaneous and experimentally induced depressions in an infant with a gastric fistula. A contribution to the problem of depression. *Journal of the American Psychoanalytic Association*, **4**, 428–52.

Engel, G.L. & Schmale, A.H. (1967). Psychoanalytic theory of somatic disorder: conversion, specificity and the disease onset situation. *Journal of the American Psychoanalytic Association*, **15**, 344–65.

Engel, K. & Meier, I. (1988). Clinical process studies on anxiety and aggressiveness: affects in the inpatient therapy of anorexia nervosa. *Psychotherapy and Psychosomatics*, **50**, 125–33.

Erdelyi, M.H. (1990). Repression, reconstruction, and defense: history and integration of the psychoanalytic and experimental frameworks. In J.L. Singer (Ed.) *Repression and dissociation: implications for personality theory, psychopathology and health*, pp. 1–31. Chicago: University of Chicago Press.

Erikson, E.H. (1959). Identity and the Life Cycle. *Psychological Issues*. Volume 1. New York: International Universities Press.

Escobar, J.I. (1987). Cross-cultural aspects of the somatization trait. *Hospital and Community Psychiatry*, **38**, 174–80.

Escobar, J.I., Swartz, M., Rubio-Stipec, M. & Manu, P. (1991). Medically unexplained symptoms: distribution, risk factors, and comorbidity. In L.J. Kirmayer & J.M. Robbins (Eds.), *Current concepts of somatiziation: research and clinical perspectives*, pp. 63–78. Washington, DC: American Psychiatric Press.

Esler, M., Julius, S., Zweifler, A., Randall, O., Harburg, E., Gardiner, H. & De Quattro, V. (1977). Mild high renin essential hypertension: a neurogenic human hypertension? *New England Journal of Medicine*, **296**, 405–11.

Exner, J.E. (1986). *The Rorschach: a comprehensive system. Vol. 1. Basic foundations*, 2nd ed. New York: Wiley.

Eysenck, H.J. (1963). Emotion as a determinant of integrative learning: an experimental study. *Behavior Research and Therapy*, **1**, 197–211.

Eysenck, H.J. (1982). Development of a theory. In C.D. Spielberger (Ed.), *Personality, genetics and behavior*, pp. 1–38. New York: Praeger.

Eysenck, H.J. (1990). Biological dimensions of personality. In L.A. Pervin (Ed.), *Handbook of personality theory: theory, and research*. New York: Guilford.

Eysenck, H.J. (1991*a*). Dimensions of personality: 16, 5 or 3?–criteria for a taxonomic paradigm. *Personality and Individual Differences*, **12**, 773–90.

Eysenck, H.J. (1991*b*). Personality, stress and disease: an interactionist perspective. *Psychological Inquiry*, **2**, 221–32.

Eysenck, H.J. (1991*c*). Reply to criticisms of the Grossarth–Maticek studies. *Psychological Inquiry*, **2**, 297–323.

Eysenck, H.J. (1992). Psychosocial factors, cancer, and ischaemic heart disease. *British Medical Journal*, **305**, 457–9.

Eysenck, H.J. & Eysenck, M.W. (1985). *Personality and individual differences: a natural science approach*. New York: Plenum.

Eysenck, H.J. & Eysenck, S.B.G. (1968). *Manual of the Eysenck Personality Inventory*. San Diego, CA: Educational and Industrial Testing Service.

Eysenck, H.J. & Eysenck, S.B.G. (1975). *Manual of the Eysenck Personality Questionnaire*. San Diego, CA: Educational and Industrial Testing Service.

Fahy, T. & Eisler, I. (1993). Impulsivity and eating disorders. *British Journal of Psychiatry*, **162**, 193–7.

Fairbairn, W.R.D. (1952). *Psychoanalytic studies of the personality*. London: Tavistock. [Published in US as *An object relations theory of the personality*. New York: Basic Books, 1954.]

Fairburn, C.G. & Beglin, S.J. (1990). Studies of the epidemiology of bulimia nervosa. *American Journal of Psychiatry*, **147**, 401–8.

Fairburn, C.G. & Cooper, P.J. (1984*a*). The clinical features of bulimia nervosa. *British Journal of Psychiatry*, **144**, 238–46.

Fairburn, C.G. & Cooper, P.J. (1984b). Rumination in bulimia nervosa. *British Medical Journal*, **288**, 826–7.

Fairburn, C.G., Jones, R., Peveler. R.C., Hope, R.A. & O'Connor, M. (1993). Psychotherapy and bulimia nervosa: longer-term effects of interpersonal psychotherapy, behavior therapy, and cognitive behavior therapy. *Archives of General Psychiatry*, **50**, 419–28.

Fairburn, C.G., Norman, P.A., Welch, S.L., O'Connor, M.E., Doll, H.A. & Peveler, R.C. (1995). A prospective study of outcome in bulimia nervosa and the long-term effects of three psychological treatments. *Archives of General Psychiatry*, **52**, 304–12.

Falconer, W. (1796). *The influence of the passions upon disorders of the body.* London: C. Dilly & J. Phillips.

Farah, M.J. (1984). The neurological basis of mental imagery: a componential analysis. *Cognition*, **18**, 245–72.

Farah, M.J., Gazzaniga, M.S., Holtzman, J.D. & Kosslyn, S.M. (1985). A left hemisphere basis for visual mental imagery? *Neuropsychologia*, **23**, 115–18.

Faravelli, C. & Albanesi, G. (1987). Agoraphobia with panic attacks: 1-year prospective follow-up. *Comprehensive Psychiatry*, **28**, 481–7.

Faravelli, C. & Pallanti, S. (1989). Recent life events and panic disorder. *American Journal of Psychiatry*, **146**, 622–6.

Farthing, G.W., Venturino, M. & Brown, S.W. (1984). Suggestion and distraction in the control of pain: test of two hypotheses. *Journal of Abnormal Psychology*, **3**, 266–76.

Faryna, A., Rodenhauser, P. & Torem, M. (1986). Development of an Analog Alexithymia Scale: testing in a nonpatient population. *Psychotherapy and Psychosomatics*, **45**, 201–6.

Fava, G.A., Baldaro, B. & Osti, R.M.A. (1980). Towards a self-rating scale for alexithymia. *Psychotherapy and Psychosomatics*, **34**, 34–9.

Fava, M., Copeland, P.M., Schweiger, U. & Herzog, D.B. (1989). Neurochemical abnormalities of anorexia nervosa and bulimia nervosa. *American Journal of Psychiatry*, **146**, 963–71.

Federman, R. & Mohns, E. (1984). A validity study of the MMPI alexithymia subscale conducted on migraine headache outpatients. *Psychotherapy and Psychosomatics*, **41**, 29–32.

Felten, D.L., Felten, S.Y., Bellinger, D.L. & Madden, K.S. (1993). Fundamental aspects of neural-immune signalling. *Psychotherapy and Psychosomatics*, **60**, 46–56.

Fenichel, O. (1945). *The psychoanalytic theory of neurosis.* New York: Norton.

Ferenczi, S. (1951). *Final contributions.* New York: Basic Books.

Ferenczi, S. (1988). *The clinical diary of Sandor Ferenczi.* (Ed.) J. Dupont. Cambridge, MA: Harvard University Press.

Fernandez, A., Sriram, T.G., Rajkumar, S. & Chandrasekar, A.N. (1989). Alexithymic characteristics in rheumatoid arthritis: a controlled study. *Psychotherapy and Psychosomatics*, **51**, 45–50.

Field, T. (1985). Attachment as psychobiological attunement: being on the same wavelength. In M. Reite & T. Field (Eds.), *The psychobiology of attachment and separation*, pp.415–54. Orlando, FL: Academic Press.

Fink, P. (1993). Admission patterns of persistent somatization patients. *General Hospital Psychiatry*, **15**, 211–18.

Finn, P.R., Martin, J. & Pihl, R.O. (1987). Alexithymia in males at high risk for alcoholism. *Psychotherapy and Psychosomatics*, **47**, 18–21.

Fisch, R.Z. (1989). Alexithymia, masked depression and loss in a holocaust survivor. *British Journal of Psychiatry*, **154**, 708–10.

Flannery, J.G. (1977). Alexithymia I. The communication of physical symptoms. *Psychotherapy and Psychosomatics*, **28**, 133–40.

Flannery, J.G. (1978). Alexithymia II. The association with unexplained physical distress. *Psychotherapy and Psychosomatics*, **30**, 193–7.

Fonagy, P. (1991). Thinking about thinking: some clinical and theoretical considerations in the treatment of a borderline patient. *International Journal of Psychoanalysis*, **72**, 639–56.

Fonagy, P. & Moran, G. (1994). Psychoanalytic formulation and treatment: chronic metabolic disturbance in insulin-dependent diabetes mellitus. In A. Erskine & D. Judd (Eds.), *The imaginative body*, pp. 60–86. London: Whurr Publishers.

Foss, L. & Rothenberg, K. (1987). *The second medical revolution: from biomedicine to infomedicine*. Boston: New Science Library, Shambhala Publications.

Fox, N.A. & Davidson, R.J. (1984). Hemispheric substrates of affect: a developmental model. In N.A. Fox & R.J. Davidson (Eds.), *The psychobiology of affective development*, pp. 353–81. Hillsdale, NJ: Erlbaum.

Frankel, F.H., Apfel-Savitz, R., Nemiah, J.C. & Sifneos, P.E. (1977). The relationship between hypnotizability and alexithymia. *Psychotherapy and Psychosomatics*, **28**, 172–8.

Freeman, C.P.L. & Munro, J.K.M. (1988). Drug and group treatments for bulimia/bulimia nervosa. *Journal of Psychosomatic Research*, **32**, 647–60.

Freud, A. (1936). *The ego and the mechanisms of defense*. New York: International Universities Press, 1966.

Freud, S. (1895a). On the grounds for detaching a particular syndrome from neurasthenia under the description 'anxiety neurosis'. *Standard Edition*, **3**, 90–115, 1962.

Freud, S. (1895b). Obsessions and phobias. *Standard Edition*, **3**, 71–82. London: Hogarth Press, 1962.

Freud, S. (1896). The aetiology of hysteria. *Standard Edition*, **3**, 187–221. London: Hogarth Press, 1962.

Freud, S. (1898). Sexuality in the aetiology of the neuroses. *Standard Edition*, 3, 261–285. London: Hogarth Press, 1962.

Freud, S. (1905). Psychical (or mental) treatment. *Standard Edition*, 7, 283–302. London: Hogarth Press, 1953.

Freud, S. (1914). On narcissism: an introduction. *Standard Edition*, 14, 67–102. London: Hogarth Press, 1957.

Freud, S. (1915a). Repression. *Standard Edition*, 14, 143–158. London: Hogarth Press, 1957.

Freud, S. (1915b). Instincts and their vicissitudes. *Standard Edition*, 14; 117–40. London: Hogarth Press, 1957.

Freud, S. (1917). Introductory lectures on psychoanalysis. Part III: General theory of neurosis. *Standard Edition*, 16, 358–77. London: Hogarth Press, 1963.

Freud, S. (1918). From the history of an infantile neurosis. *Standard Edition*, 17, 13–122. London: Hogarth Press, 1955.

Freud, S. (1919). Introduction to 'psychoanalysis and the war neuroses'. *Standard Edition*, 17, 206–10. London: Hogarth Press, 1955.

Freud, S. (1920). Beyond the pleasure principle. *Standard Edition*, 18, 3–64. London: Hogarth Press, 1955.

Freud, S. (1923). The ego and the id. *Standard Edition*, 19, 3–59. London: Hogarth Press, 1961.

Freud, S. (1926). Inhibitions, symptoms, and anxiety. *Standard Edition*, 20, 77–175. London: Hogarth Press, 1959.

Freud, S. (1940). Splitting of the ego in the process of defense. *Standard Edition*, 23, 271–8. London: Hogarth Press, 1964.

Freyberger, H. (1977). Supportive psychotherapeutic techniques in primary and secondary alexithymia. *Psychotherapy and Psychosomatics*, 28, 337–42.

Freyberger, H., Kunsebeck, H.W., Lempa, W., Wellmann, W. & Avenarius, H.J. (1985). Psychotherapeutic interventions in alexithymic patients. With special regard to ulcerative colitis and Crohn patients. *Psychotherapy and Psychosomatics*, 44, 72–81.

Fricchione, G. & Howantiz, E. (1985). Aprosodia and alexithymia – a case report. *Psychotherapy and Psychosomatics*, 43, 156–60.

Friedman, H.S. & Booth-Kewley, S. (1987). The 'disease-prone personality'. A meta-analytic view of the construct. *American Psychologist*, 42, 539–55.

Friedman, M. & Rosenman, R.H. (1959). Association of specific overt behavior pattern with blood and cardiovascular findings. *Journal of the American Medical Association*, 169, 1286–96.

Friedman, M.J. (1988). Toward rational pharmacotherapy for post-traumatic stress disorder: an interim report. *American Journal of Psychiatry*, 145, 281–5.

Friedman, M., Thoresen, C.E., Gill, J.J., Ulmer, D., Powell, L.H., Price, V.A., Brown, B., Thompson, L., Rabin, D.D., Breall, W.S., Bourg, E., Levy, R. & Dixon, T. (1986). Alteration of type A behavior and its effect on cardiac recurrences in post myocardial infarction patients: summary results of the recurrent coronary prevention project. *American Heart Journal*, **112**, 653–63.

Frijda, N.H. (1986). *The emotions*. Cambridge: Cambridge University Press.

Frosch, A. (1995). The preconceptual organization of emotion. *Journal of the American Psychoanalytic Association*, **43**, 423–47.

Frosch, J. (1990). *Psychodynamic psychiatry: theory and practice, vol. 1*. Madison, CT: International Universities Press.

Frosch, W.A. (1970). Psychoanalytic evaluation of addiction and habituation. *Journal of the American Psychoanalytic Association* 18, 209–18.

Fukunishi, I. (1992). Psychosomatic problems surrounding kidney transplantation. *Psychotherapy and Psychosomatics*, **57**, 42–9.

Fukunishi, I., Chishima, Y. & Anze, M. (1994). Posttraumatic stress disorder and alexithymia in burn patients. *Psychological Reports*, **75**, 1371–6.

Fukunishi, I., Hattori, M., Nakamura, H. & Nakagawa, T. (1995a). Hostility is related to narcissism controlling for social desirability: studies of college students and patients with myocardial infarction. *Journal of Psychosomatic Research*, **39**, 215–20.

Fukunishi, I., Ichikawa, M., Ichikawa, T. & Matsuzawa, K. (1994). Effect of family group psychotherapy on alcoholic families. *Psychological Reports*, **74**, 568–70.

Fukunishi, I., Ichikawa, M., Ichikawa, T., Matsuzawa, K., Fujimura, K., Tabe, T., Iida, Y. & Saito, S. (1992a). Alexithymia and depression in families with alcoholics. *Psychopathology*, **25**, 326–30.

Fukunishi, I., Moroji, T. & Okabe, S. (1995b). Stress in middle-aged women: influence of Type A behaviour and narcissism. *Psychotherapy and Psychosomatics*, **63**, 159–64.

Fukunishi, I. & Rahe, R.H. (1995). Alexithymia and coping with stress in healthy persons: alexithymia as a personality trait is associated with low social support and poor responses to stress. *Psychological Reports*, **76**, 1299–304.

Fukunishi, I., Saito, S. & Ozaki, S. (1992b). The influence of defense mechanisms on secondary alexithymia in hemodialysis patients. *Psychotherapy and Psychosomatics*, **57**, 50–6.

Furman, E. (1992). On feeling and being felt with. *Psychoanalytic Study of the Child*, **47**, 67–84.

Gabel, S. (1988). The right hemisphere in imagery, hypnosis, rapid eye movement sleep and dreaming: empirical studies and tentative conclusions. *Journal of Nervous and Mental Disease*, **176**, 323–31.

Gaddini, R. (1978). Transitional object origins and the psychosomatic symptom. In A. Grolnick, L. Barkin & W. Muensterberger (Eds.), *Between reality and fantasy: transitional objects and phenomena*, pp. 111–31. New York: Aronson.

Gage, B.C. & Egan, K.J. (1984). The effect of alexithymia on morbidity in hypertensives. *Psychotherapy and Psychosomatics*, **41**, 136–44.

Gainotti, G., Caltagirone, C. & Zoccolotti, P. (1993). Left/right and cortical/subcortical dichotomies in the neuropsychological study of human emotions. *Cognition and Emotion*, **7**, 71–93.

Galenson, E. (1984). Influences on the development of the symbolic function. In J.D. Call, E. Galenson, & R.L. Tyson (Eds.), *Frontiers of infant psychiatry*, vol. 2, pp. 30–37. New York: Basic Books.

Galin, D. (1974). Implications for psychiatry of left and right cerebral specialization: a neurophysiological context for unconscious processes. *Archives of General Psychiatry*, **31**, 572–83.

Garber, J. & Dodge, K.A. (1991). *The development of emotion regulation and dysregulation*. Cambridge: Cambridge University Press.

Gardner, H., Brownell, H. H., Wapner, W. & Michelow, D. (1983). Missing the point: the role of the right hemisphere in the processing of complex linguistic materials. In E. Perecman (Ed.), *Cognitive processing in the right hemisphere*, pp. 169–91. New York: Academic Press.

Gardos, G., Schniebolk, S., Mirin, S.M., Wolk, P.C. & Rosenthal, K. (1984). Alexithymia: towards validation and measurement. *Comprehensive Psychiatry*, **25**, 278–82.

Garfinkel, P.E. & Garner, D.M. (1982). *Anorexia nervosa: a multidimensional perspective*. New York: Brunner/Mazel.

Garfinkel, P.E., Kaplan, A.S., Garner, D.M. & Darby, P.L. (1983). The differentiation of vomiting/weight loss as a conversion disorder from anorexia nervosa. *American Journal of Psychiatry*, **140**, 1019–22.

Garfinkel, P.E., Moldofsky, H. & Garner, D.M. (1980). The heterogeneity of anorexia nervosa. Bulimia as a distinct subgroup. *Archives of General Psychiatry*, **37**, 1036–40.

Garner, D.M. (1991). *Eating Disorder Inventory-2: professional manual*. Odessa, FL: Psychological Assessment Resources.

Garner, D.M., Olmsted, M.P. & Garfinkel, P.E. (1983*a*). Does anorexia nervosa occur on a continuum? *International Journal of Eating Disorders*, **2**, 11–20.

Garner, D.M., Olmsted, M.P. & Polivy, J. (1983*b*). Development and validation of a multidimensional eating disorder inventory for anorexia nervosa and bulimia. *International Journal of Eating Disorders*, **2**, 15–34.

Garner, D.M., Olmsted, M.P., Polivy, J. & Garfinkel, P.E. (1984). Comparison between weight-preoccupied women and anorexia nervosa. *Psychosomatic Medicine*, **46**, 255–66.

Gaskin, M.E., Greene, A.F., Robinson, M.E. & Geisser, M.E. (1992). Negative affect and the experience of chronic pain. *Journal of Psychosomatic Research*, **36**, 707–13.

Gediman, H.K. (1984). Actual neurosis and psychoneurosis. *International Journal of Psychoanalysis*, **65**, 191–202.

George, M.S., Ketter, T.A., Parekh, P.I., Horwitz, B., Herscovitch, P. & Post, R.M. (1995). Brain activity during transient sadness and happiness in healthy women. *American Journal of Psychiatry*, **152**, 341–51.

George, M.S., Ketter, T.A. & Post, R.M. (1994). Prefrontal cortex dysfunction in clinical depression. *Depression*, **2**, 59–72.

Gerstley, L.J., Alterman, A.I., McLellan, A.T. & Woody, G.E. (1990). Antisocial personality disorder in patients with substance abuse disorders: a problematic diagnosis. *American Journal of Psychiatry*, **147**, 173–8.

Gilbert, B.O., Johnson, S.B., Silverstein, J. & Malone, J. (1989). Psychological and physiological responses to acute laboratory stressors in insulin-dependent diabetes mellitus adolescents and nondiabetic controls. *Journal of Pediatric Psychology*, **14**, 577–91.

Glover, E. (1932). On the etiology of drug addiction. *International Journal of Psychoanalysis*, **13**, 298–328.

Glover, E. (1939). *Psychoanalysis*. London: Staples.

Goldberg, L.R. (1993). The structure of phenotypic personality traits. *American Psychologist*, **48**, 26–34.

Goldberg, S. (1991). Recent developments in attachment theory and research. *Canadian Journal of Psychiatry*, **36**, 393–400.

Goldberg, S., MacKay-Soroka, S. & Rochester, M. (1994). Affect, attachment and maternal responsiveness. *Infant Behavior and Development*, **17**, 335–9.

Goldbloom, D.S., Kennedy, S.H., Kaplan, A.S. & Woodside, D.B. (1989). Anorexia nervosa and bulimia nervosa. *Canadian Medical Association Journal*, **140**, 1149–54.

Golden, C.J., Sawicki, R.F. & Franzen, M.D. (1984). Test construction. In G. Goldstein & M. Hersen (Eds.), *Handbook of psychological assessment*, pp. 19–37. New York: Pergamon.

Goldenberg, D.L. (1989). Psychological symptoms and psychiatric diagnosis in patients with fibromyalgia. *Journal of Rheumatology*, **16** (suppl. 19), 127–30.

Goldstein, H.S., Edelberg, R., Meier, C.F. & Davis, L. (1988). Relationship of blood pressure and heart rate to experienced anger and expressed anger. *Psychosomatic Medicine*, **50**, 321–9.

Goldstein, L. (1984). A reconsideration of right hemispheric activity during visual imagery, REM sleep, and depression. *Research Communications in Psychology, Psychiatry, and Behaviour*, **9**, 139–48.

Goldstein, L., Stoltzfus, N.W. & Gardocki, J. F. (1972). Changes in inter-hemispheric amplitude relationships in EEG during sleep. *Physiology and Behavior*, **8**, 811–15.

Goleman, D. (1995). *Emotional intelligence*. New York: Bantam.

Goodman, A. (1993). The addictive process: a psychoanalytic understanding. *Journal of the American Academy of Psychoanalysis*, **21**, 89–105.

Goodsitt, A. (1983). Self-regulatory disturbances in eating disorders. *International Journal of Eating Disorders*, **2**, 51–60.

Goodsitt, A. (1985). Self psychology and the treatment of anorexia nervosa. In D.M. Garner & P.E. Garfinkel (Eds.), *Handbook of psychotherapy for anorexia nervosa and bulimia*, pp. 55–82. New York: Guilford Press.

Gorman, J.M., Liebowitz, M.R., Fyer, A.J. & Stein, J. (1989). A neuroanatomical hypothesis for panic disorder. *American Journal of Psychiatry*, **146**, 148–61.

Gottschalk, L.A. (1974). Quantification and psychological indicators of emotions: the content analysis of speech and other objective measures of psychological states. *International Journal of Psychiatric Medicine*, **5**, 587–610.

Gottschalk, L.A. & Gleser, G. (1969). *The measurement of psychological states through the analysis of verbal behavior*. Berkeley: University of California Press.

Gough, H.G. (1969). *Manual for the California Psychological Inventory* (rev. ed.). Palo Alto, CA: Consulting Psychologist Press.

Gough, H.G. (1987). *California Psychological Inventory* [Administrator's guide]. Palo Alto, CA: Consulting Psychologist Press.

Grace, J. & Malloy, P. (1992). Neuropsychiatric aspects of right hemisphere learning disability. *Neuropsychiatry, Neuropsychology, and Behavioral Neurology*, **5**, 194–204.

Graham, J.R. (1987). *The MMPI: a practical guide*. New York: Oxford Press.

Graham, J.R. & Strenger, V.E. (1988). MMPI characteristics of alcoholics: a review. *Journal of Consulting and Clinical Psychology*, **56**, 197–205.

Graves, P.L. & Thomas, C.B. (1981). Themes of interaction in medical students' Rorschach responses as predictors of midlife health or disease. *Psychosomatic Medicine*, **43**, 215–25.

Gray, J.A. (1994). Is there emotion-specific physiology. In P. Ekman & R.J. Davidson (Eds.), *The nature of emotion: fundamental questions*, pp. 243–7. New York: Oxford University Press.

Green, B.L., Grace, M.C., Lindy, J.D., Gleser, G.C. & Leonard, A. (1990). Risk factors for PTSD and other diagnoses in a general sample of Vietnam veterans. *American Journal of Psychiatry*, **147**, 729–33.

Greenberg, D.B. (1990). Chronic mononucleosis, chronic fatigue syndrome, and anxiety and depressive disorders. *Psychosomatics*, **31**, 129–37.

Greenberg, L.S. & Safran, J.D. (1989). Emotion in psychotherapy. *American Psychologist*, **44**, 19–29.

Greenberg, M.S. & Farah, M.J. (1986). The laterality of dreaming. *Brain and Cognition*, **5**, 307–21.

Greenberg, M.T., Kusche, C.A. & Speltz, M. (1990). Emotional regulation, self-control, and psychopathology: the role of relationships in early childhood. In J. Masling (Ed.), *Empirical studies of psychoanalytic theories*, vol. 3, pp. 21–55. Hillsdale, NJ: Analytic Press.

Greene, W.A., Goldstein, S. & Moss, A.J. (1972). Psychosocial aspects of sudden death. *Archives of Internal Medicine*, **129**, 725–31.

Greer, S. & Morris, T. (1975). Psychological attributes of women who develop breast cancer: a controlled study. *Journal of Psychosomatic Research*, **19**, 147–53.

Gross, J.J. & Muñoz, R.F. (1995). Emotion regulation and mental health. *Clinical Psychology: Science and Practice*, **2**, 151–64.

Grossarth-Maticek, R. (1991). Some comments on the Yugoslav and Heidelberg studies. *Psychological Inquiry*, **2**, 294–6.

Grossarth-Maticek, R. & Eysenck, H.J. (1995). Self-regulation and mortality from cancer, coronary heart disease, and other causes: a prospective study. *Personality and Individual Differences*, **19**, 781–95.

Grossarth-Maticek, R. & Eysenck, H.J. (1990). Personality, stress, and disease: description and validity of a new inventory. *Psychological Reports*, **66**, 355–73.

Grossarth-Maticek, R., Eysenck, H.J. & Vetter, H. (1988). Personality type, smoking habit and their interaction as predictors of cancer and coronary heart disease. *Personality and Individual Differences*, **9**, 479–95.

Grotstein, J.S. (1981). *Splitting and projective identification*. New York, Aronson.

Grotstein, J. S. (1983). Some perspectives on self psychology. In A. Goldberg (Ed.), *The future of psychoanalysis*. New York: International Universities Press.

Grotstein, J.S. (1986). The psychology of powerlessness: disorders of self-regulation and interactional regulation as a newer paradigm for psychopathology. *Psychoanalytic Inquiry*, **6**, 93–118.

Grotstein, J.S. (1987). The borderline as a disorder of self-regulation. In J.S. Grotstein, Solomon, M.F. & Lang, J.A. (Eds.), *The borderline patient: emerging concepts in diagnosis, psychodynamics, and treatment*, pp. 347–83. Hillsdale, NJ: Analytic Press.

Grotstein, J.S. (1990). Nothingness, meaningless, chaos, and the 'black hole' II: The 'black hole'. *Contemporary Psychoanalysis*, **26**, 377–407.

Grotstein, J.S. (1996). Bion's 'O', Kant's 'thing-in-itself', and Lacan's 'Real': Toward the conception of the 'Transcendent Position.' *Melanie Klein and Object Relations.* In press.

Group for the Advancement of Psychiatry Committee on Alcoholism and the Addictions (1991). Substance use disorders: a psychiatric priority. *American Journal of Psychiatry*, **148**, 1291–300.

Gull, W.W. (1874). Anorexia nervosa. Transcripts of the Clinical Society (London), **7**, 22–8. Reprinted in R.M. Kaufman & M. Heiman (Eds.), *Evolution of psychosomatic concepts. Anorexia nervosa: a paradigm.* New York: International Universities Press, 1964.

Gunderson, J.G. & Sabo, A.N. (1993). The phenomenological and conceptual interface between borderline personality disorder and PTSD. *American Journal of Psychiatry*, **150**, 19–27.

Gur, R.E. (1975). Conjugate lateral eye movements as an index of hemispheric activation. *Journal of Personality and Social Psychology*, **5**, 751–7.

Haan, N. (1963). Proposed model of ego functioning: coping and defense mechanisms in relationship to IQ change. *Psychological Monograph*, **77** (No. 8), 1–27.

Haddad, P.M. (1994). Depression: counting the costs. *Psychiatric Bulletin*, **18**, 25–8.

Hamilton, N.G. (1990). The containing function and the analyst's projective identification. *International Journal of Psychoanalysis*, **71**, 445–53.

Harburg, E., Gleiberman, L., Russell, M. & Cooper, M.L. (1991). Anger-coping styles and blood pressure in black and white males: Buffalo, New York. *Psychosomatic Medicine*, **53**, 153–4.

Hartmann, H. (1939). *Ego psychology and the problem of adaptation.* New York: International Universities Press.

Hatsukami, D., Eckert, E., Mitchell, J.E. & Pyle, R.L. (1984). Affective disorder and substance abuse in women with bulimia. *Psychological Medicine*, **14**, 701–4.

Haviland, M.G., Hendryx, M.S., Cummings, M.A., Shaw, D.G. & MacMurray, J.P. (1991). Multidimensionality and state dependency of alexithymia in recently sober alcoholics. *Journal of Nervous and Mental Disease*, **179**, 284–90.

Haviland, M.G., Hendryx, M.S., Shaw, D.G. & Henry, J.P. (1994). Alexithymia in women and men hospitalized for psychoactive substance dependence. *Comprehensive Psychiatry*, **35**, 124–8.

Haviland, M.G., MacMurray, J.P. & Cummings, M.A. (1988a). The relationship between alexithymia and depressive symptoms in a sample of newly abstinent alcoholic inpatients. *Psychotherapy and Psychosomatics*, **49**, 37–40.

Haviland, M.G., Shaw, D.G., Cummings, M.A. & MacMurray, J.P. (1988b). Alexithymia: Subscales and relationship to depression. *Psychotherapy and Psychosomatics*, **50**, 164–70.

Haviland, M.G., Shaw, D.G., MacMurray, J.P. & Cummings, M.A. (1988c). Validation of the Toronto Alexithymia Scale with substance abusers. *Psychotherapy and Psychosomatics*, **50**, 81–7.

Heiberg, A. (1980). Alexithymic characteristics and somatic illness. *Psychotherapy and Psychosomatics*, **34**, 261–6.

Heiberg, A. & Heiberg, A. (1977). Alexithymia – an inherited trait? A study of twins. *Psychotherapy and Psychosomatics*, **28**, 221–5.

Hellige, J. (1993). *Hemispheric asymmetry: what's right and what's left.* Cambridge: Harvard University Press.

Helz, J.W. & Templeton, B. (1990). Evidence of the role of psychosocial factors in diabetes mellitus: a review. *American Journal of Psychiatry*, **147**, 1275–82.

Henderson, M. & Freeman, C.P.L. (1987). A self-rating scale for bulimia: the 'BITE'. *British Journal of Psychiatry*, **150**, 18–24.

Hendryx, M.S., Haviland, M.G. & Shaw, D.G. (1991). Dimensions of alexithymia and their relationships to anxiety and depression. *Journal of Personality Assessment*, **56**, 227–37.

Henzel, H.A. (1984). Diagnosing alcoholism in patients with anorexia nervosa. *American Journal of Drug and Alcohol Abuse*, **10**, 461–6.

Herbert, T.B., Cohen, S., Marsland, A.L., Bachen, E.A., Rabin, B.S., Muldoon, M.F. & Manuck, S.B. (1994). Cardiovascular reactivity and the course of immune response to an acute psychological stressor. *Psychosomatic Medicine*, **56**, 37–44.

Herbert, T.B, & Cohen, S. (1993). Stress and immunity in humans: a meta-analytic review. *Psychosomatic Medicine*, **55**, 364–79.

Herman, J.L. & van der Kolk, B.A. (1987). Traumatic antecedents of borderline personality disorder. In B.A. van der Kolk (Ed.), *Psychological trauma*, pp. 111–26. Washington, DC: American Psychiatric Press.

Herzog, D.B. (1991). Recent advances in bulimia nervosa. Symposium presented at the 144th annual meeting of the American Psychiatric Association. New Orleans, May 11–16.

Herzog, D.B., Keller, M.B. & Lavori, P.W. (1988). Outcome in anorexia nervosa and bulimia nervosa–a review of the literature. *Journal of Nervous and Mental Disease*, **176**, 131–43.

Hesse, P. & Cicchetti, D. (1982). Perspectives on an integrated theory of emotional development. In D. Cicchetti & P. Hesse (Eds.), *New directions for child development: emotional development*, pp. 3–48. San Francisco: Jossey-Bass.

Hesselbrock, M.N., Meyer, R.E. & Keener, J.J. (1985). Psychopathology in hospitalized alcoholics. *Archives of General Psychiatry*, **42**, 1050–5.

Hickie, I., Lloyd, A., Wakefield, D. & Parker, G. (1990). The psychiatric status of patients with the chronic fatigue syndrome. *British Journal of Psychiatry*, **156**, 534–40.

Higuchi, S., Suzuki, K., Yamada, K., Parrish, K. & Kono, H. (1993). Alcoholics with eating disorders: prevalence and clinical course. A study from Japan. *British Journal of Psychiatry*, **162**, 403–6.

Hobson, J.A. & McCarley, R.W. (1977). The brain as a dream-state generator: an activation–synthesis hypothesis of the dream process. *American Journal of Psychiatry*, **134**, 1335–48.

Hobson, R.P. (1994). On developing a mind. *British Journal of Psychiatry*, **165**, 577–81.

Hofer, M.A. (1983). On the relationship between attachment and separation processes in infancy. In R. Plutchik (Ed.), *Emotion: Theory, research and experience: vol. II. Emotions in early development*, pp. 199–219. New York: Academic Press.

Hofer, M.A. (1984). Relationships as regulators: a psychobiologic perspective on bereavement. *Psychosomatic Medicine*, **46**, 183–97.

Hofer, M.A. (1987). Early social relationships: a psychobiologist's view. *Child Development*, **58**, 633–47.

Hoffman, L. (1992). On the clinical utility of the concept of depressive affect as signal affect. *Journal of the American Psychoanalytic Association*, **40**, 405–23.

Hofmann-Patsalides, B.M. (1994). *Paternal incest, somatization, and disturbances in affect symbolization (alexithymia): a Rorschach study*. Doctoral dissertation, California Institute of Integral Studies, California.

Hogan, C.C. (1995). *Psychosomatics, psychoanalysis, and inflammatory disease of the colon*. Madison, CT: International Universities Press.

Hogan, R. & Nicholson, R.A. (1988). The meaning of personality test scores. *American Psychologist*, **43**, 621–6.

Holderness, C.C., Brooks-Gunn, J. & Warren, M.P. (1994). Co-morbidity of eating disorders and substance abuse. Review of the literature. *International Journal of Eating Disorders*, **16**, 1–34.

Holroyd, K.A. & Coyne, J. (1987). Personality and health in the 1980s: psychosomatic medicine revisited? *Journal of Personality*, **55**, 359–75.

Hoppe, K.D. (1977). Split brains and psychoanalysis. *Psychoanalytic Quarterly*, **46**, 220–44.

Hoppe, K.D. (1988). Hemispheric specialization and creativity. *Psychiatric Clinics of North America*, **11**, 303–15.

Hoppe, K.D. & Bogen, J.E. (1977). Alexithymia in twelve commissurotomized patients. *Psychotherapy and Psychosomatics*, **28**, 148–55.

Horney, K. (1952). The paucity of inner experiences. *American Journal of Psychoanalysis*, **12**, 3–9.

Horton, P.C. (1981). *Solace: the missing dimension in psychiatry*. Chicago: University of Chicago Press.

Hsu, L.K.G. (1980). Outcome of anorexia nervosa – a review of the literature (1954–1978). *Archives of General Psychiatry*, **37**, 1041–6.

Hsu, L.K.G., Crisp, A.H. & Callender, J.S. (1992). Psychiatric diagnoses in recovered and unrecovered anorectics 22 years after onset of illness: a pilot study. *Comprehensive Psychiatry*, **33**, 123–7.

Huba, G.J., Singer, J.L., Anhensel, C.S. & Antrobus, J.S. (1982). *Short Imaginal Processes Inventory Manual*. Port Huron, MI: Research Psychologist Press.

Hudson, J.I., Laffer, P.S. & Pope, H.G., Jr. (1982). Bulimia related to affective disorder by family history and response to dexamethasone suppression test. *American Journal of Psychiatry*, **139**, 685–7.

Hudson, J.I. & Pope, H.G. (1989). Fibromyalgia and psychopathology: is fibromyalgia a form of 'affective spectrum disorder?' *Journal of Rheumatology*, **16** (suppl. 19), 15–22.

Hudson, J.I. & Pope, H.G. (1990). Affective spectrum disorder: does antidepressant response identify a family of disorders with a common pathophysiology? *American Journal of Psychiatry*, **147**, 552–64.

Humphrey, M.E. & Zangwill, O.L. (1951). Cessation of dreaming after brain injury. *Journal of Neurology, Neurosurgery, and Psychiatry*, **14**, 322–5.

Hyer, L., Woods, M.G., Summers, M.N., Boudewyns, P. & Harrison, W.R. (1990). Alexithymia among Vietnam veterans with posttraumatic stress disorder. *Journal of Clinical Psychiatry*, **51**, 243–7.

Iezzi, A., Stokes, G.S., Adams, H.E., Pilon, R.N. & Ault, L. (1994). Somatothymia in chronic pain patients. *Psychosomatics*, **35**, 460–8.

Isenstadt, L. (1980). From panic to signal anxiety: the acquisition of signal structure in a hyperactive boy. *International Review of Psychoanalysis*, **7**, 469–81.

Izard, C.E. (1971). *The face of emotion*. New York: Appleton-Century-Crofts.

Izard, C.E. (1977). *Human emotions*. New York: Plenum Press.

Izard, C.E. (1994). Cognition is one of four types of emotion-activating systems. In P. Ekman, & R.J. Davidson (Eds.), *The nature of emotion: fundamental questions*, pp. 203–7. New York: Oxford University Press.

Izard, C.E. & Buechler, S. (1980). Aspects of consciousness and personality in terms of differential emotions theory. In R. Plutchik, & H. Kellerman (Eds.), *Emotion: theory, research, and experience. Vol.1. Theories of emotion*, pp. 165–87. New York: Academic Press.

Izard, C.E. & Kobak, R.R. (1991). Emotions system functioning and emotion regulation. In J. Garber & K.A. Dodge (Eds.), *The development of emotion regulation and dysregulation*, pp. 303–21. Cambridge: Cambridge University Press.

Jackson, D.N. (1974). *Basic Personality Inventory*. London, Ontario: Research Psychologist Press.

Jacobson, J.G. (1994). Signal affects and our psychoanalytic confusion of tongues. *Journal of the American Psychoanalytic Association* **42**, 15–42.

James, F.R. & Large, R.G. (1991). Quantifying alexithymia and hypno-
tisability in pain clinic attenders and normal controls. In M.R. Bond,
J.E. Charlton & C.J. Woolf (Eds.), *Proceedings of the VIth World Congress on Pain*, pp. 247–50. New York: Elsevier Science.

James, L., Singer, A., Zurynski, Y., Gordon, E., Kraiuhin, C., Harris,
A., Howson, A. & Meares, R. (1987). Evoked response potentials
and regional cerebral blood flow in somatization disorder. *Psychotherapy and Psychosomatics*, **47**, 190–6.

James, W. (1884). What is an emotion? *Mind*, **9**, 199–205.

Jamner, L.D., Shapiro, D., Hui, K.K., Oakley, M.E. & Lovett, M.
(1993). Hostility and differences between clinic, self-determined and
ambulatory blood pressure. *Psychosomatic Medicine*, **55**, 203–11.

Janet, P. (1889). *L'automatisme psychologique*. Paris: Alcan.

Jimerson, D.C., Lesem, M.D., Kaye, W.H., Hegg, A.P. & Brewerton,
T.D. (1990). Eating disorders and depression: is there a serotonin
connection? *Biological Psychiatry*, **28**, 443–54.

Jimerson, D.C., Walton, B.E., Sifneos, P.E., Franko, D.L. & Covino,
N.A. (1991). Alexithymia and affect-deficit symptoms in bulimia. Pa-
per presented at the 144th annual meeting of the American Psychiatric
Association, New Orleans, May 11–16.

Jimerson, D.C., Wolfe, B.E., Franko, D.L., Covino, N.A. & Sifneos,
P.E. (1994). Alexithymia ratings in bulimia nervosa: clinical correlates. *Psychosomatic Medicine*, **56**, 90–3.

Johannessen, D.J., Cowley, D.S., Walker, R.D., Jensen, C.F. & Parker,
L. (1989). Prevalence, onset, and clinical recognition of panic states
in hospitalized male alcoholics. *American Journal of Psychiatry*, **146**,
1201–3.

Johnson, C. & Connors, M.E. (1987). *The etiology and treatment of bulimia
nervosa: a biopsychosocial perspective*. New York: Basic Books.

Johnson, C. & Larson, R. (1982). Bulimia: an analysis of moods and behaviour. *Psychosomatic Medicine*, **44**, 341–51.

Johnson-Sabine, E.C., Wood, K.H. & Wakeling, A. (1984). Mood
changes in bulimia nervosa. *British Journal of Psychiatry*, **145**, 512–16.

Johnston, L.D. & O'Malley, P.M. (1986). Why do the nation's students
use drugs and alcohol? Self-reported reasons from nine national surveys. *Journal of Drug Issues*, **16**, 29–66.

Jonas, J., Gold, M., Sweeny, D. & Potlash, A.L.C. (1987). Eating disorders and cocaine abuse: a survey of 259 cocaine abusers. *Journal of
Clinical Psychiatry*, **48**, 47–50.

Jones, A.D., Cheshire, N. & Moorhouse, H. (1985). Anorexia nervosa,
bulimia and alcoholism – association of eating disorder and alcohol.
*Journal of Psychiatric Research*, **19**, 377–80.

Jones, J.M. (1995). *Affects as process: an inquiry into the centrality of affect in
psychological life*. Hillsdale, NJ: Analytic Press.

Jordan, M.S. & Lumley, M.A. (1993). Alexithymia and rheumatoid arthritis. Poster presented at the annual meeting of the American Psychosomatic Society, Charleston, SC, March, 1993.

Julkunen, J., Hurri, H. & Kankainen, J. (1988). Psychological factors in the treatment of chronic low back pain. *Psychotherapy and Psychosomatics*, **50**, 173–81.

Julkunen, J., Salonen, R., Kaplan, G.A., Chesney, M.A. & Salonen, J. (1994). Hostility and the progression of carotid atherosclerosis. *Psychosomatic Medicine*, **56**, 519–25.

Kant, I. (1787). *Kritik der reimen Vernunft. (Critique of Pure Reason.)* In: Immanuel Kant's *Sämtliche Werke*, Vol. 2. Frankfurt: Insel, 1956.

Kaplan, C., Lipkin, M. & Gordon, G.H. (1988). Somatization in primary care: patients with unexplained and vexing medical complaints. *Journal of General Internal Medicine*, **3**, 177–89.

Kardiner, A. (1941). *The traumatic memories of war.* New York: Hoeber.

Karush, A. (1989). Instinct and affect. In A.M. Cooper, O.F. Kernberg & E.S. Person (Eds.), *Psychoanalysis: toward the second century*, pp. 76–90. New Haven. CT: Yale University Press.

Karush, A., Daniels, G.E., Flood, C. & O'Connor, J.F. & Stern, L.O. (1977). *Psychotherapy in ulcerative colitis.* Philadelphia: W.B. Saunders.

Katan, A. (1961). Some thoughts about the role of verbalization in early childhood. *Psychoanalytic Study of the Child*, **16**, 184–8.

Katon, W. (1984). Panic disorder and somatization. Review of 55 cases. *American Journal of Medicine*, **77**, 101–6.

Katon, W., Kleinman, A. & Rosen, G. (1982). Depression and somatization: a review. Part I. *American Journal of Medicine*, **72**, 127–35.

Katon, W., Lin, E., Von Korff, M., Russo, J., Lipscomb, P. & Bush, T. (1991). Somatization: a spectrum of severity. *American Journal of Psychiatry*, **148**, 34–40.

Katon, W., Vitaliano, P.P., Anderson, K., Jones, M. & Russo, J. (1987). Panic disorder: residual symptoms after the acute attacks abate. *Comprehensive Psychiatry*, **28**, 151–8.

Kauffman, S.A. (1993). *The origins of order: self-organization and selection in evolution.* New York and Oxford: Oxford University Press.

Kauffman, S.A. (1995). *At home in the universe.* New York and Oxford: Oxford University Press.

Kauhanen, J. (1993). *Dealing with emotions and health: a population study of alexithymia in middle-aged men.* Kuopio, Finland: Kuopio University Publications D. Medical Sciences 25.

Kauhanen, J., Julkunen, J. & Salonen, J.T. (1991). Alexithymia and perceived symptoms: criterion validity of the Toronto Alexithymia Scale. *Psychotherapy and Psychosomatics*, **56**, 247–52.

Kauhanen, J., Julkunen, J. & Salonen, J.T. (1992a). Validity and reliability of the Toronto Alexithymia Scale (TAS) in a population study. *Journal of Psychosomatic Research*, **36**, 687–94.

Kauhanen, J., Julkunen, J. & Salonen, J.T. (1992b). Coping with inner feelings and stress: heavy alcohol use in the context of alexithymia. *Behavioral Medicine*, **18**, 121–6.

Kauhanen, J., Kaplan, G.A., Cohen, R.D., Salonen, R. & Salonen, J.T. (1994). Alexithymia may influence the diagnosis of coronary heart disease. *Psychosomatic Medicine*, **56**, 237–44.

Kauhanen, J., Kaplan, G.A., Julkunen, J., Wilson, T.W. & Salonen, J.T. (1993). Social factors in alexithymia. *Comprehensive Psychiatry*, **34**, 1–5.

Kaye, W.H., Gwirtsman, H.E., George, D.T., Weiss, S.R. & Jimerson, D.C. (1986). Relationship of mood alterations to bingeing behaviour in bulimia. *British Journal of Psychiatry*, **149**, 479–85.

Keller, D.S., Carroll, K.M., Nich, C. & Rounsaville, B.J. (1995). Alexithymia in cocaine abusers: response to psychotherapy and pharmacotherapy. *American Journal on Addictions*, **4**, 234–44.

Kellner, R. (1975). Psychotherapy in psychosomatic disorders: a survey of controlled studies. *Archives of General Psychiatry*, **32**, 1021–8.

Kellner, R. (1985). Functional somatic symptoms and hypochondriasis: a survey of empirical studies. *Archives of General Psychiatry*, **42**, 821–33.

Kellner, R. (1986). *Hypochondriasis and somatization*. New York: Praeger.

Kellner, R. (1987). Hypochondriasis and somatization. *Journal of the American Medical Association*, **258**, 2718–22.

Kellner, R. (1990). Somatization: theories and research. *Journal of Nervous and Mental Disease*, **178**, 150–60.

Kellner, R. (1991). *Psychosomatic syndromes and somatic symptoms*. Washington, DC: American Psychiatric Press.

Kellner, R. (1994). Psychosomatic syndromes, somatization and somatoform disorders. *Psychotherapy and Psychosomatics*, **61**, 4–24.

Kelman, N. (1952). Clinical aspects of externalized living. *American Journal of Psychoanalysis*, **12**, 15–23.

Keltikangas-Järvinen, L. (1982). Alexithymia in violent offenders. *Journal of Personality Assessment*, **46**, 462–7.

Keltikangas-Järvinen, L. (1985). Concept of alexithymia I. The prevalence of alexithymia in psychosomatic patients. *Psychotherapy and Psychosomatics*, **44**, 132–8.

Keltikangas-Järvinen, L. (1987). Concept of alexithymia II. The consistency of alexithymia. *Psychotherapy and Psychosomatics*, **47**, 113–20.

Keltikangas-Järvinen, L. (1989). 'Psychosomatic personality' – a personality constellation or an illness-related reaction? *British Journal of Medical Psychology*, **62**, 325–31.

Keltikangas-Järvinen, L. (1990). Alexithymia and type A behaviour compared in psychodynamic terms of personality. *British Journal of Medical Psychology*, **63**, 131–5.

Keltikangas-Järvinen, L. & Jokinen, J. (1989). Type A behavior, coping mechanisms and emotions related to somatic risk factors of coronary heart disease in adolescents. *Journal of Psychosomatic Research*, **33**, 17–28.

Kenyon, L.W., Ketterer, M.W., Gheorghiade, M. & Goldstein, S. (1991). Psychological factors related to prehospital delay during acute myocardial infarction. *Circulation*, **84**, 1969–76.

Kernberg, O.K. (1984). *Severe personality disorders*. New Haven: Yale University Press.

Khantzian, E.J. (1978). The ego, the self and opiate addiction: theoretical and treatment considerations. *International Review of Psychoanalysis*, **5**, 189–8.

Khantzian, E.J. (1982). Psychological (structural) vulnerabilities and the specific appeal of narcotics. *Annals of the New York Academy of Sciences*, **398**, 24–32.

Khantzian, E.J. (1985). The self-medication hypothesis of addictive disorders: focus on heroin and cocaine dependence. *American Journal of Psychiatry*, **142**, 1259–64.

Khantzian, E.J. (1990). Self-regulation and self-medication factors in alcoholism and the addictions: similarities and differences. In M. Galanter (Ed.), *Recent developments in alcoholism*, vol. 8. New York: Plenum.

Khantzian, E.J. (1993). Affects and addictive suffering: a clinical perspective. In L. Ablon, D. Brown, E.J. Khantzian & J.E. Mack (Eds.), *Human feelings: explorations in affect development and meaning*, pp. 259–79. Hillsdale, NJ: Analytic Press.

Khantzian, E.J. & Treece, C. (1985). DSM-III psychiatric diagnosis of narcotic addicts. *Archives of General Psychiatry*, **42**, 1067–71.

Kiecolt-Glaser, J.K. & Glaser, R. (1995). Psychoneuroimmunology and health consequences: data and shared mechanisms. *Psychosomatic Medicine*, **57**, 269–74.

Killingmo, B. (1989). Conflict and deficit: implications for technique. *International Journal of Psychoanalysis*, **70**, 65–79.

Kinder, B.N. & Curtiss, G. (1990). Alexithymia among empirically derived subgroups of chronic back pain patients. *Journal of Personality Assessment*, **54**, 351–62.

King, L.A., Emmons, R.A. & Woodley, S. (1992). The structure of inhibition. *Journal of Research in Personality*, **26**, 85–102.

Kinston, W. & Cohen, J. (1986). Primal repression: clinical and theoretical aspects. *International Journal of Psychoanalysis*, **67**, 337–56.

Kinston, W. & Cohen, J. (1988). Primal repression and other states of mind. *Scandinavian Psychoanalytic Review*, **11**, 81–105.

Kirmayer, L.J. (1987). Languages of suffering and healing: alexithymia as a social and cultural process. *Transcultural Psychiatric Research Review*, **24**, 119–36.

Kirmayer, L.J. & Robbins, J.M. (1991a). Three forms of somatization in primary care: prevalence, co-occurrence, and sociodemographic characteristics. *Journal of Nervous and Mental Disease*, **179**, 647–55.

Kirmayer, L.J. & Robbins, J.M. (1991b). Functional somatic syndromes. In L.J. Kirmayer & J.M. Robbins (Eds.), *Current concepts of somatization: research and clinical perspectives*, pp. 79–106. Washington, DC: American Psychiatric Press.

Kirmayer, L.J. & Robbins, J.M. (1991c). Introduction: concepts of somatization. In L.J. Kirmayer & J.M. Robbins (Eds.), *Current concepts of somatization: research and clinical perspectives*, pp. 1–19. Washington, DC: American Psychiatric Press.

Kirmayer, L.J. & Robbins, J.M. (1993). Cognitive and social correlates of the Toronto Alexithymia Scale. *Psychosomatics*, **34**, 41–52.

Kirmayer, L.J., Robbins, J.M., Dworkin, M. & Yaffe, M.J. (1993). Somatization and the recognition of depression and anxiety in primary care. *American Journal of Psychiatry*, **150**, 734–41.

Kirmayer, L.J., Robbins, J.M. & Kapusta, M.A. (1988). Somatization and depression in fibromyalgia syndrome. *American Journal of Psychiatry*, **145**, 950–4.

Kirmayer, L.J., Robbins, J.M. & Paris, J. (1994). Somatoform disorders: personality and the social matrix of somatic distress. *Journal of Abnormal Psychology*, **103**, 125–36.

Kissen, D.M. & Eysenck, H.J. (1962). Personality and male lung cancer patients. *Journal of Psychosomatic Research*, **6**, 123–37.

Kissen, M. (1995). *Affect, object, and character structure*. Madison, CT: International Universities Press.

Kleiger, J.H. & Jones, N.F. (1980). Characteristics of alexithymic patients in a chronic respiratory illness population. *Psychotherapy and Psychosomatics*, **34**, 25–33.

Kleiger, J.H. & Kinsman, R.A. (1980). The development of an MMPI alexithymia scale. *Psychotherapy and Psychosomatics*, **34**, 17–24.

Klein, D.F. (1964). Delineation of two drug-responsive anxiety syndromes. *Psychopharmacology*, **5**, 397–408.

Klein, D.F. (1981). Anxiety reconceptualized. In D.F. Klein & J.G. Rabkin (Eds.), *Anxiety: new research and changing concepts*, pp. 235–63. New York: Raven Press.

Klein, D.F. (1994). Testing the suffocation false alarm theory of panic disorder. *Anxiety*, **1**, 1–7.

Klein, M. (1935). A contribution to the psychogenesis of manic-depressive states. *Contributions to psycho-analysis*. London: Hogarth Press.

Klein, M. (1940). Mourning and its relation to manic-depressive state. In: *Contributions to psycho-analysis, 1921–1945*. London: Hogarth Press and the Institute of Psychoanalysis, 1950, pp. 311–38.

Kleinman, A. (1986). *Social origins of distress and disease: depression, neurasthenia, and pain in modern China*. New Haven: Yale University Press.

Knapp, P.H. (1981). Core processes in the organization of emotions. *Journal of the American Psychoanalytic Association*, 9, 415–34.

Knapp, P.H. (1983). Emotions and bodily changes: a reassessment. In L. Temoshok, C. Van Dyke, & L.S. Zegans (Eds.), *Emotions in health and illness: theoretical and research foundations*, pp. 15–27. New York: Grune & Stratton.

Kneier, A.W. & Temoshok, L. (1984). Repressive coping reactions in patients with malignant melanoma as compared to cardiovascular disease patients. *Journal of Psychosomatic Research*, 28, 145–55.

Kobak, R.R. & Sceery, A. (1988). Attachment in late adolescence: working models, affect regulation, and representations of self and others. *Child Development*, 59, 135–46.

Kohut, H. (1971). *The analysis of the self: a systematic approach to the psychoanalytic treatment of narcissistic personality disorders*. New York: International Universities Press.

Kohut, H. (1977). *The restoration of the self*. New York: International Universities Press.

Kohut, H. (1984). *How does analysis cure?* Chicago: University of Chicago Press.

Kohut, H. & Wolf, E. (1978). The disorders of the self and their treatment: an outline. *International Journal of Psychoanalysis*, 60, 3–27.

Kolb, L.C. (1987). A neuropsychological hypothesis explaining post-traumatic stress disorders. *American Journal of Psychiatry*, 144, 989–95.

Kondas, O. & Kordacova, J. (1990). Prehledove studie: alexitymia a jej metodicke zachytenie. *Ceskoslovenska Psychologie*, 34, 411–25.

Kopp, C.B. (1989). Regulation of distress and negative emotions: a developmental view. *Developmental Psychology*, 25, 343–54.

Kosslyn, S.M. (1987). Seeing and imagining in the cerebral hemispheres: a computational approach. *Psychological Review*, 94, 148–75.

Kosten, T.R., Krystal, J.H., Giller, E.L., Jr. & Dan, E. (1992). Alexithymia as a predictor of treatment response in post-traumatic stress disorder. *Journal of Traumatic Stress*, 5, 41–50.

Kraepelin, E. (1909–1915). *Psychiatrie: ein Lehrbuch fuer Studierende und Arzte*, 8th ed. (4 vols. publ. between 1909–1915). Leipzig: Barth.

Kring, A.M., Kerr, S.L., Smith, D.A. & Neale, J.M. (1993). Flat affect in schizophrenia does not reflect diminished subjective experience of emotion. *Journal of Abnormal Psychology*, 102, 507–17.

Kroeber, T.C. (1963). The coping functions of the ego mechanisms. In R.W. White (Ed.), *The study of lives: essays on personality in honor of Henry A. Murray*, pp. 178–189. New York: Atherton Press.

Krystal, H. (1962). The opiate withdrawal syndrome as a state of stress. *Psychiatric Quarterly*, **36** (suppl.), 53–65.

Krystal, H. (1968). *Massive psychic trauma*. New York: International Universities Press.

Krystal, H. (1974). The genetic development of affects and affect regression. *Annual of Psychoanalysis*, **2**, 98–126.

Krystal, H. (1975). Affect tolerance. *Annual of Psychoanalysis*, **3**, 179–219.

Krystal, H. (1978a). Self-representation and the capacity for self care. *Annual of Psychoanalysis*, **6**, 209–46.

Krystal, H. (1978b). Trauma and affects. *The Psychoanalytic Study of the Child*, **33**, 81–115.

Krystal, H. (1979). Alexithymia and psychotherapy. *American Journal of Psychotherapy*, **33**, 17–31.

Krystal, H. (1981). The aging survivor of the holocaust: integration and self-healing in posttraumatic states. *Journal of Geriatric Psychiatry*, **14**, 165–89.

Krystal, H. (1982). Adolescence and the tendencies to develop substance dependence. *Psychoanalytic Inquiry*, **2**, 581–617.

Krystal, H. (1982/83). Alexithymia and the effectiveness of psychoanalytic treatment. *International Journal of Psychoanalytic Psychotherapy*, **9**, 353–88.

Krystal, H. (1988). *Integration and self-healing: affect, trauma, alexithymia*. Hillsdale, NJ: Analytic Press.

Krystal, H. (1990). An information processing view of object-relations. *Psychoanalytic Inquiry*, **10**, 221–51.

Krystal, H. (1992). Psychoanalysis as a 'normal' science. *Journal of the American Academy of Psychoanalysis*, **20**, 395–412.

Krystal, H. (1997). Desomatization and the consequences of infantile psychic trauma. *Psychoanalytic Inquiry*, **17**, 136–50.

Krystal, J.H., Giller, E.L. & Cicchetti, D.V. (1986). Assessment of alexithymia in posttraumatic stress disorder and somatic illness: introduction of a reliable measure. *Psychosomatic Medicine*, **48**, 84–94.

Krystal, H. & Raskin, H. (1970). *Drug dependence*. Detroit: Wayne State University Press.

Kuchenhoff, J. (1993). Defense mechanisms and defense organizations: their role in the adaptation to the acute stage of Crohn's disease. In U. Hentschel, G.J.W. Smith, W. Ehlers & J.G. Draguns (Eds.), *The concept of defense mechanisms in contemporary psychology: theoretical, research, and clinical perspectives*, pp. 412–23. New York: Springer-Verlag.

Kushner, M.G. & Sher, K.J. (1993). Comorbidity of alcohol and anxiety disorders among college students: effects of gender and family history of alcoholism. *Addictive Behaviors*, **18**, 543–52.

Kushner, M.G., Sher, K.J. & Beitman, B.D. (1990). The relation between alcohol problems and the anxiety disorders. *American Journal of Psychiatry*, **147**, 685–95.

Lacan, J. (1966). *Écrits*. Paris: Seuil. [Re-published: *Écrits: 1949–1960*. (Trans.) A. Sheridan. New York: W.W. Norton, 1977.]

Lacey, J.H. (1993). Self-damaging and addictive behaviour in bulimia nervosa: a catchment area study. *British Journal of Psychiatry*, **163**, 190–4.

Lacey, J.H. & Evans, C.D.H. (1986). The impulsivist: a multi-impulsive personality disorder. *British Journal of Addiction*, **81**, 715–23.

Laessle, R., Schweiger, U. & Pirke, K.M. (1988). Depression as a correlate of starvation in patients with eating disorders. *Biological Psychiatry*, **23**, 719–25.

Lake, B. (1985). Concept of ego strength in psychotherapy. *British Journal of Psychiatry*, **147**, 471–8.

Lane, R.D., Quinlan, D.M., Schwartz, G.E., Walker, P.A. & Zeitlin, S.B. (1990). The levels of emotional awareness scale: a cognitive-developmental measure of emotion. *Journal of Personality Assessment*, **55**, 124–34.

Lane, R.D. & Schwartz, G.E. (1987). Levels of emotional awareness: a cognitive–developmental theory and its application to psychopathology. *American Journal of Psychiatry*, **144**, 133–43.

Lane, R., Sechrest, L., Reidel, R., Brown, V., Kaszniak, A. & Schwartz, G. (1995). Alexithymia and nonverbal emotion processing deficits. (Abstract). *Psychosomatic Medicine*, **57**, 84.

Lange, C.G. (1885). *Om sindsbevoegelser: et psyko-fysiologiske studie. (The emotions.* Baltimore: Williams and Wilkins, 1922.)

Langs, R.J. (1978/79). Some communicative properties of the bipersonal field. *International Journal of Psychoanalytic Psychotherapy*, **7**, 87–135.

Laquatra, T.A. & Clopton, J.R. (1994). Characteristics of alexithymia and eating disorders in college women. *Addictive Behaviors*, **19**, 373–80.

Latimer, P.R. (1981) Irritable bowel syndrome: a behavioral model. *Behavioral Research Therapy*, **19**, 475–83.

Lazare, A., Klerman, G.L. & Armor, D.J. (1970). Oral, obsessive and hysterical personality patterns: replication of factor analysis in an independent sample. *Journal of Psychiatric Research*, **7**, 275–9.

Lazarus, R.S. (1991). *Emotion and adaptation*. New York: Oxford University Press.

LeDoux, J.E. (1992). Emotion and the amygdala. In J.P. Aggleton (Ed.), *The amygdala: neurobiological aspects of emotion, memory, and mental dysfunction*, pp. 339–51. New York: Wiley-Liss.

LeDoux, J.E. (1994). Cognitive–emotional interactions in the brain. In P. Ekman & R.J. Davidson (Eds.), *The nature of emotion: fundamental questions*, pp. 216–23. New York: Oxford University Press.

Lee, K.A., Vaillant, G.E., Torrey, W.C. & Elder, G.H. (1995). A 50-year prospective study of the psychological sequelae of world war II combat. *American Journal of Psychiatry*, **152**, 516–22.

Lee, Y-H., Rim, H-D. & Lee, J-Y. (1996). Development and validation of a Korean version of the 20-item Toronto Alexithymia Scale (TAS-20K). *Journal of the Korean Neuropsychiatric Association*, **35**, 888–99.

Leff, J. (1973). Culture and the differentiation of emotional states. *British Journal of Psychiatry*, **123**, 299–306.

Leff, J. (1977). The cross-cultural study of emotions. *Culture, Medicine and Psychiatry*, **1**, 317–50.

Leighton, A., Lambo, T., Hughes, C., Leighton, D., Murphy, J. & Macklin, D. (1963). *Psychiatric disorder among the Yoruba*. New York: Cornell University Press.

Leon, A.C., Portera, L. & Weissman, M.M. (1995). The social costs of anxiety disorders. *British Journal of Psychiatry*, **166** (suppl. 27), 19–22.

Leon, G.R., Carroll, K., Chernyk, B. & Finn, S. (1985). Binge eating and associated habit patterns within college student and identified bulimic populations. *International Journal of Eating Disorders*, **4**, 43–57.

Lesse, S. (1983). The masked depression syndrome – results of a seventeen-year clinical study. *American Journal of Psychotherapy*, **37**, 456–75.

Lesser, I.M. (1981). A review of the alexithymia concept. *Psychosomatic Medicine*, **43**, 531–43.

Lesser, I.M. (1985). Current concepts in psychiatry: alexithymia. *New England Journal of Medicine*, **312**, 690–2.

Lesser, I.M., Ford, C.V. & Friedmann, C.T.H. (1979). Alexithymia in somatizing patients. *General Hospital Psychiatry*, **1**, 256–61.

Lesser, I.M. & Lesser, B.Z. (1983). Alexithymia: examining the development of a psychological concept. *American Journal of Psychiatry*, **140**, 1305–8.

Levin, J.D. (1987). *Treatment of alcoholism and other addictions: a self psychology approach*. Northvale, NJ: Aronson.

Levitan, H. (1981). The implications of certain dreams reported by patients with the anorexia–bulimia nervosa syndrome. *Canadian Journal of Psychiatry*, **30**, 137–49.

Levitan, H. (1989). Failure of the defensive functions of the ego in psychosomatic patients. In S. Cheren (Ed.), *Psychosomatic medicine: theory, physiology, and practice*, vol. 1, pp. 135–57. Madison, CT: International Universities Press.

Levy, A.B., Dixon, K.N. & Stern, S.L. (1989). How are depression and bulimia related? *American Journal of Psychiatry*, **146**, 162–9.

Ley, R.G. (1979) Cerebral asymmetries, emotional experience, and imagery: implications for psychotherapy. In A.A. Sheikh & J.T. Shaffer (Eds.), *The potential of fantasy and imagination*, pp. 41–65. New York: Brandon House.

Ley, R.G. & Bryden, M.P. (1979). Hemispheric differences in processing emotions and faces. *Brain and Language*, **7**, 127–38.

Lichtenberg, J.D. (1983). *Psychoanalysis and infant research*. Analytic Press: Hillsdale, NJ.

Lichtenberg, J.D. (1989). *Psychoanalysis and Motivation*. Hillsdale, NJ: Analytic Press.

Linden, W., Wen, F. & Paulhaus, D.L. (1994). Measuring alexithymia: reliability, validity, and prevalence. In J. Butcher & C. Spielberger (Eds.), *Advances in personality assessment*, pp. 125–43. Hillsdale, NJ: Lawrence Erlbaum.

Liotti, G. (1992). Disorganized/disoriented attachment in the etiology of the dissociative disorders. *Dissociation*, **5**, 196–204.

Lipowski, Z.J. (1977) Psychosomatic medicine in the seventies: an overview. *American Journal of Psychiatry*, **134**, 233–44.

Lipowski, Z.J. (1987). Somatization: medicine's unsolved problem. *Psychosomatics*, **28**, 294–7.

Lipowski, Z.J. (1988). Somatization: the concept and its clinical application. *American Journal of Psychiatry*, **145**, 1358–68.

Lipowski, Z.J. (1990). Somatization and depression. *Psychosomatics*, **31**, 13–21.

Liskow, B. et al. (1986). Is Briquet's syndrome a heterogeneous disorder? *American Journal of Psychiatry*, **143**, 626–9.

Littman, A.B. (1993). Review of psychosomatic aspects of cardiovascular disease. *Psychotherapy and Psychosomatics*, **60**, 148–67.

Littman, A. et al. (1993). The use of buspirone in the treatment of stress, hostility, and type A behavior in cardiac patients. *Psychotherapy and Psychosomatics*, **59**, 107-10.

Loas, G. et al. (1993). L'alexithymie chez le sujet sain: validation de l'echelle d'alexithymie de Toronto (TAS) dans une population 'tout venant' de 144 sujets, application au calcul de la prevalence. *Annual Medicine Psychologie*, **151**, 660-3.

Lodhi, P.H. & Thakur, S. (1993). Personality of drug addicts: Eysenckian analysis. *Personality and Individual Differences*, **15**, 121–8.

Loewenstein, R.J. (1990). Somatoform disorders in victims of incest and child abuse. In R.P. Kluft (Ed.), *Incest-related syndromes of adult psychopatholgy*, pp.75–111. Washington, DC: American Psychiatric Press.

Loiselle, C.G. & Dawson, C. (1988). Toronto Alexithymia Scale: relationships with measures of patient self-disclosure and private self-consciousness. *Psychotherapy and Psychosomatics*, **50**, 109–16.

Lolas, F., de la Parra, G., Aronsohn, S. & Collin, C. (1980). On the measurement of alexithymic behavior. *Psychotherapy and Psychosomatics*, **33**, 139–46.

Lolas, F., von Rad, M. & Scheibler, D. (1981). Situational influences on verbal affective expression of psychosomatic and psychoneurotic patients. *Journal of Nervous and Mental Disease*, **169**, 619–23.

Lopez Ibor, J.J. (1972). Masked depressions. *British Journal of Psychiatry*, **120**, 245–58.

Luby, E.D., Marrazzi, M. & Sperti, S. (1987). Anorexia nervosa: a syndrome of starvation dependence. *Comprehensive Therapy*, **13**, 16–21.

Lucas, A.R., Beard, C.M., O'Fallon, W.M. & Kurland, L.T. (1991). 50-year trends in the incidence of anorexia nervosa in Rochester, Minn.: a population-based study. *American Journal of Psychiatry*, **148**, 917–22.

Lumley, M.A., Downey, K., Stettner, L., Wehmer, F. & Pomerleau, O.F. (1994). Alexithymia and negative affect: relationship to cigarette smoking, nicotine dependence, and smoking cessation. *Psychotherapy and Psychosomatics*, **61**, 156–62.

Lydiard, R.B. (1992). Anxiety and the irritable bowel syndrome. *Psychiatric Annals*, **22**, 612–18.

Lynch, J.L. (1993). Editorial comment. *Integrative Physiological and Behavioral Science*, **28**, 368.

Lynch, J.J., Lynch, K.E. & Friedman, E. (1992). A cry unheard: sudden reductions in blood pressure while talking about feelings of hopelessness and helplessness. *Integrative Physiological and Behavioral Science*, **27**, 151–69.

Lynn, S.J. & Rhue, J.W. (1988). Fantasy proneness: hypnosis, developmental antecedents, and psychopathology. *American Psychologist*, **43**, 35–44.

MacAlpine, I. (1952). Psychosomatic symptom formation. *The Lancet*, **i**, 278–82.

MacLean, P.D. (1949). Psychosomatic disease and the 'visceral brain': recent developments bearing on the Papez theory of emotion. *Psychosomatic Medicine*, **11**, 338–53.

MacLean, P.D. (1990). *The triune brain in evolution: role in paleocerebral functions*. New York: Oxford University Press.

MacLean, P.D. (1993). Cerebral evolution of emotions. In M. Lewis & J.M. Haviland (Eds.), *Handbook of emotions*, pp. 67–83. New York: Guilford.

Magai, C. & Hunziker, J. (1993). Tolstoy and the riddle of developmental transformation: a lifespan analysis of the role of emotions in personality development. In M. Lewis & J.M. Haviland (Eds.), *Handbook of emotions*, pp. 247–59. New York: Guilford Press.

Magai, C. & McFadden, S.H. (1995). *The role of emotions in social and personality development*, New York: Plenum Press.

Magni, G., Di Mario, F., Rizzardo, R., Pulin, S. & Naccarato, R. (1986). Personality profiles of patients with duodenal ulcer. *American Journal of Psychiatry*, **143**, 1297–300.

Maier, S.F., Watkins, L.R. & Fleshner, M. (1994). Psychoneuroimmunology: the interface between behavior, brain and immunity. *American Psychologist*, **49**, 1004–17.

Main, M. (1991). Metacognitive knowledge, metacognitive monitoring, and singular (coherent) vs. multiple (incoherent) models of attachment: findings and directions for future research. In C.M. Parkes, P. Marris & J. Stevenson-Hinde (Eds.), *Attachment across the life cycle*, pp. 127–59. New York: Routledge.

Main, M., Kaplan, N. & Cassidy, J. (1985). Security in infancy, childhood and adulthood: a move to the level of representation. In I. Bretherton & E. Waters (Eds.), *Growing points in attachment theory and research: monographs of the Society for Social Research in Child Development*, **50**, 1–2, Serial No. 299, 66–104.

Malatesta, C.Z. (1990). The role of emotions in the development and organization of personality. In R.A. Thompson (Ed.), *Nebraska symposium on motivation (vol. 36): socioemotional development*, pp. 1–56. Lincoln: University of Nebraska Press.

Manassis, K., Bradley, S., Goldberg, S., Hood, J. & Swinson, R.P. (1994). Attachment in mothers with anxiety disorders and their children. *Journal of the American Academy of Child and Adolescent Psychiatry*, **33**, 1106–13.

Mandal, M.K. & Singh, S.K. (1990). Lateral asymmetry in identification and expression of facial emotions. *Cognition and Emotion*, **4**, 61–70.

Mann, L.S., Wise, T.N., Trinidad, A. & Kohanski, R. (1994). Alexithymia, affect recognition, and the five-factor model of personality in normal subjects. *Psychological Reports*, **74**, 563–7.

Manu, P., Lane, T.J. & Matthews, D.A. (1992). Chronic fatigue syndromes in clinical practice. *Psychotherapy and Psychosomatics*, **58**, 60–8.

Marcus, M.D. & Wing, R.R. (1987). Binge eating among the obese. *Annals of Behavioral Medicine*, **9**, 23–7.

Margraf, J., Ehlers, A. & Roth, W.T. (1986). Biological models of panic disorder and agoraphobia – a review. *Behaviour, Research and Therapy*, **24**, 553–67.

Margulies, A. (1993). Empathy, virtuality, and the birth of complex emotional states: do we find or do we create feelings in the other? In S.L. Ablon, D. Brown, E.J. Khantzian & J.E. Mack (Eds.), *Human feelings: explorations in affect development and meaning*, pp. 181–202. Hillsdale, NJ: Analytic Press.

Marks, I.M. (1987). Behavioral aspects of panic disorder. *American Journal of Psychiatry*, **144**, 1160–5.

Marshall, G.N., Wortman, C.B., Vickers, R.R., Kusulas, J.W. & Hervig, L.K. (1994). The five-factor model of personality as a framework for personality-health research. *Journal of Personality and Social Psychology*, **67**, 278–86.

Martin, E.D. & Sher, K.J. (1994). Family history of alcoholism, alcohol use disorders and the five-factor model of personality. *Journal of Studies in Alcoholism*, **55**, 81–90.

Martin, J.B. & Pihl, R.O. (1986). Influence of alexithymic characteristics on physiological and subjective stress responses in normal individuals. *Psychotherapy and Psychosomatics*, **45**, 66–77.

Martin, J.B., Pihl, R.O. & Dobkin, P. (1984). Schalling-Sifneos Personality Scale: findings and recommendations. *Psychotherapy and Psychosomatics*, **41**, 145–152.

Marty, P. & DeBray, R. (1989). Current concepts of character disturbance. In S. Cheren (Ed.), *Psychosomatic medicine: theory, physiology, and practice*, vol. 1, pp. 159–84. Madison, CT: International Universities Press.

Marty, P. & de M'Uzan, M. (1963). La 'pensée opératoire'. *Revue Francaise de Psychanalyse*, **27** (suppl.), 1345–56.

Marzi, C.A., Bisiacchi, P. & Nicoletti, R. (1991). Is interhemispheric transfer of visuomotor information asymmetric? Evidence from a meta-analysis. *Neuropsychologia*, **29**, 1163–77.

Masterson, J.F. (1977). Primary anorexia nervosa in the borderline adolescent: an object relations view. In P. Hartocollis (Ed.), *Borderline personality disorders*, pp. 475–94. New York: International Universities Press.

Mastrovito, R.C., Deguire, K.S., Clarkin, J., Thaler, T., Lewis, J.L. & Cooper, E. (1979). Personality characteristics of women with gynecological cancer. *Cancer Detection and Prevention*, **2**, 281–7.

Matte-Blanco, I. (1988). *Thinking, feeling, and being: clinical reflections on the fundamental antinomy of human beings and world*. London and New York: Routledge.

Matthews, K.A., Glass, D.C., Rosinman, R.H. & Bortner, R.W. (1977). Competitive drive, pattern A, and coronary heart disease: a further analysis of some data from the Western Collaborative Group Study. *Journal of Chronic Diseases*, **30**, 489–98.

Mavissakalian, M. (1990). The relationship between panic disorder/agoraphobia and personality disorders. *Psychiatric Clinics of North America*, **13**, 661–84.

Mayer, J.D., DiPaolo, M. & Salovey, P. (1990). Perceiving affective content in ambiguous visual stimuli: a component of emotional intelligence. *Journal of Personality Assessment*, **54**, 772–81.

Mayes, L.C. & Cohen, D.J. (1992). The development of a capacity for imagination in early childhood. *Psychoanalytic Study of the Child*, **47**, 23–47.

Mayou, R. (1993). Somatization. *Psychotherapy and Psychosomatics*, **59**, 69–83.

McAdams, D.P. (1992). The five-factor model of personality: a critical appraisal. *Journal of Personality*, **60**, 329–61.

McCrae, R.R. (1982). Consensual validation of personality traits: evidence from self-reports and ratings. *Journal of Personality and Social Psychology*, **43**, 293–303.

McCrae, R.R. (1987). Creativity, divergent thinking, and openness to experience. *Journal of Personality and Social Psychology*, **52**, 1258–65.

McCrae, R.R. (1991). The five-factor model and its assessment in clinical settings. *Journal of Personality Assessment*, **57**, 399–414.

McCrae, R.R. & Costa, P.T. (1985). Openness to experience. In R. Hogan & W.H. Jones (Eds.), *Perspectives in psychology: theory, measurement and interpersonal dynamics*, vol. 1, pp. 145–72. Greenwich: JAI Press.

McCrae, R.R. & Costa, P.T. (1987). Validation of a five-factor model of personality across instruments and observers. *Journal of Personality and Social Psychology*, **52**, 81–90.

McCrae, R.R. & Costa, P.T. (1991). Adding *Liebe und arbeit*: the full five-factor model and well-being. *Personality and Social Psychology Bulletin*, **17**, 227–32.

McCrae, R.R. & Costa, P.T. (1997). Conceptions and correlates of openness to experience. In R. Hogan, J. Johnson & S.R. Briggs (Eds.), *Handbook of personality psychology*, pp. 825–47. San Diego: Academic Press.

McCrae, R.R. & John, O.P. (1992). An introduction to the five-factor model and its applications. *Journal of Personality*, **60**, 175–215.

McDonald, P.W. & Prkachin, K.M. (1987). The Schalling-Sifneos Personality Scale: reliability and descriptive data from a large non-clinical sample. *Canadian Psychology*, **28a**, 390.

McDonald, P.W. & Prkachin, K.W. (1990). The expression and perception of facial emotion in alexithymia: a pilot study. *Psychosomatic Medicine*, **52**, 199–210.

McDougall, J. (1972). The anti-analysand in analysis. In S. Lebovici & D. Widlocher (Eds.), *Ten years of psychoanalysis in France*, pp. 333–54. New York: International Universities Press, 1980.

McDougall, J. (1974). The psychosoma and the psychoanalytic process. *International Review of Psychoanalysis*, **1**, 437–59.

McDougall, J. (1978). Primitive communications and the use of the countertransference. *Contemporary Psychoanalysis*, **16**, 417–59.

McDougall, J. (1980a) *Plea for a measure of abnormality*. New York: International Universities Press.

McDougall, J. (1980b). A child is being eaten. *Contemporary Psychoanalysis*, **16**, 417–59.

McDougall, J. (1982a). Alexithymia: a psychoanalytic viewpoint. *Psychotherapy and Psychosomatics*, **38**, 81–90.

McDougall, J. (1982b). Alexithymia, psychosomatosis, and psychosis. *International Journal of Psychoanalytic Psychotherapy*, **9**, 379–88.

McDougall, J. (1985). *Theaters of the mind: illusion and truth on the psycho-analytic stage.* New York: Basic Books.

McFarlane, A.C. (1988). The aetiology of post-traumatic stress disorders following a natural disaster. *British Journal of Psychiatry,* **152**, 110–21.

McGlone, J. (1978). Sex differences in functional brain asymmetry. *Cortex,* **14**, 122–8.

McNair, D.M., Lorr, M. & Droppleman, L.F. (1971/1981). *Manual for Profile of Moods States.* San Diego, CA: EDITS.

McNaughton, N. (1989). *Biology and emotion.* Cambridge: Cambridge University Press.

Meehl, P.E. (1945). The 'dynamics' of structured personality tests. *Journal of Clinical Psychology,* **1**, 296–303.

Melamed, S. (1987). Emotional reactivity and elevated blood pressure. *Psychosomatic Medicine,* **49**, 217–25.

Mendelson, G. (1982). Alexithymia and chronic pain: prevalence, correlates and treatment results. *Psychotherapy and Psychosomatics,* **37**, 154–64.

Merskey, H.A. (1982). Comments on 'chronic pain as a variant of depressive disease: the pain-prone disorder'. *Journal of Nervous and Mental Disease,* **170**, 409–11.

Mesquita, B. & Frijda, N.H. (1992). Cultural variations in emotions: a review. *Psychological Bulletin,* **112**, 179–204.

Meyer, G.J. & Shack, J.R. (1989). The structural convergence of mood and personality: Evidence for old and new directions. *Journal of Personality and Social Psychology,* **57**, 691–706.

Michels, R., Frances, A. & Shear, M.K. (1985). Psychodynamic models of anxiety. In A.H. Tuma & J.M. Maser (Eds.), *Anxiety and the anxiety disorders,* pp. 595–618. Hillsdale, NJ: Erlbaum.

Mikulincer, M. & Orbach, I. (1995). Attachment styles and repressive defensiveness: the accessibility and architecture of affective memories. *Journal of Personality and Social Psychology,* **68**, 917–25.

Milkman, H. & Frosch, W.A. (1973). On the preferential abuse of heroin and amphetamine. *Journal of Nervous and Mental Disease,* **156**, 242–8.

Millard, R.W. & Kinsler, B.L. (1992). Evaluation of constricted affect in chronic pain: an attempt using the Toronto Alexithymia Scale. *Pain,* **50**, 287–92.

Miller, T.R. (1991). The psychotherapeutic utility of the five-factor model of personality: a clinician's experience. *Journal of Personality Assessment,* **57**, 415–33.

Minuchin, S., Rosman, B.L. & Baker, L. (1978). *Psychosomatic families: anorexia nervosa in context.* Cambridge, MA: Harvard University Press.

Mirin, S.M., Weiss, R.D., Griffin, M.L. & Michael, J.L. (1991). Psychopathology in drug abusers and their families. *Comprehensive Psychiatry*, **32**, 36–51.

Mitchell, J.E., Raymond, N. & Specker, S. (1993). A review of the controlled trials of pharmacotherapy and psychotherapy in the treatment of bulimia nervosa. *International Journal of Eating Disorders*, **14**, 229–47.

Mitrani, J.L. (1995). Toward an understanding of unmentalized experience. *Psychoanalytic Quarterly*, **64**, 68–112.

Miyaoka, H. (1992). Clinical significance of alexithymia. *Japanese Journal of Psychosomatic Medicine* (suppl.), **32**, 24.

Moldofsky, H. (1989). Nonrestorative sleep and symptoms after a febrile illness in patients with fibrositis and chronic fatigue syndromes. *Journal of Rheumatology*, **16** (suppl. 19), 150–3.

Moldofsky, H. (1993). Sleep and chronic fatigue syndrome. In D.M. Dawson & T.D. Sabin (Eds.), *Chronic fatigue syndrome*, pp. 141–152. Little Brown.

Monrad-Krohn, G. H. (1947). Dysprosody or altered 'melody of language'. *Brain*, **70**, 405–15.

Mora, G. (1967). History of psychiatry. In A.M. Freedman & H.I. Kaplan (Eds.), *Comprehensive textbook of psychiatry*, pp. 2–34. Baltimore, MD: Williams and Wilkins.

Morris, T. & Greer, S. (1980). A type C for cancer? *Cancer Detection and Prevention*, **3**, abstract no. 102.

Morrison, J. (1989). Childhood sexual histories of women with somatization disorder. *American Journal of Psychiatry*, **146**, 239–241.

Morton, R. (1694). *Phthisiologica: or a treatise of consumptions*. London: S. Smith and B. Walford.

Mueller, J. (1983). Neuroanatomic correlates of emotion. In L. Temoshok, C. Van Dyke & L.S. Zegans (Eds.), *Emotions in health and illness: theoretical and research foundations*, pp. 95–121. New York: Grune & Stratton.

Musaph, H. (1974). The role of aggression in somatic symptom formation. *International Journal of Psychiatry and Medicine*, **5**, 449–60.

Mushatt, C. (1982/83). Anorexia nervosa: a psychoanalytic commentary. *International Journal of Psychoanalysis and Psychotherapy*, **9**, 257–65.

Mutén, E. (1991). Self-reports, spouse ratings, and psychophysiological assessment in a behavioral medicine program: an application of the five-factor model. *Journal of Personality Assessment*, **57**, 449–64.

Myers, L.B. (1995). Alexithymia and repression: the role of defensiveness and trait anxiety. *Personality and Individual Differences*, **19**, 489–92.

Nasser, M. (1988). Culture and weight consciousness. *Journal of Psychosomatic Research*, **32**, 573–7.

Nathan, P.E. (1988). The addictive personality is the behavior of the addict. *Journal of Consulting and Clinical Psychology*, **56**, 183–8.

Nathanson, D.L. (1992). *Shame and pride: affect, sex, and the birth of the self*. New York: Norton.

Nemiah, J.C. (1977). Alexithymia. Theoretical considerations. *Psychotherapy and Psychosomatics*, **28**, 199–206.

Nemiah, J.C. (1982). A reconsideration of psychological specificity in psychosomatic disorders. *Psychotherapy and Psychosomatics*, **38**, 39–45.

Nemiah, J.C. (1984). The psychodynamic view of anxiety. In R.O. Pasnau (Ed.), *Diagnosis and treatment of anxiety disorders*, pp. 117–37. Washington, DC: American Psychiatric Press.

Nemiah, J.C. (1988). The psychodynamic view of anxiety: an historical approach. In M. Roth, R. Noyes Jr. & G.D. Burrows (Eds.), *Handbook of anxiety, vol. 1. Biological, clinical, and cultural perspectives*, pp. 277–303. Elsevier: Amsterdam.

Nemiah, J.C. (1989). Janet redivivus: the centenary of *L'automatisme psychologique*. *American Journal of Psychiatry*, **146**, 1527–9.

Nemiah, J.C. (1991). Dissociation, conversion, and somatization. In A. Tasman & S.M. Goldfinger (Eds.), *American psychiatric press review of psychiatry*, vol. 10, pp. 248–60. Washington, DC: American Psychiatric Press.

Nemiah, J.C., Freyberger, H. & Sifneos, P.E. (1976). Alexithymia: a view of the psychosomatic process. In O.W. Hill (Ed.), *Modern trends in psychosomatic medicine*, vol. 3, pp. 430–9. London: Butterworths.

Nemiah, J.C. & Sifneos, P.E. (1970). Affect and fantasy in patients with psychosomatic disorders. In O.W. Hill (Ed.), *Modern trends in psychosomatic medicine*, vol. 2, pp. 26–34. London: Butterworths.

Newton, T.L. & Contrada, R.J. (1994). Alexithymia and repression: contrasting emotion-focused coping styles. *Psychosomatic Medicine*, **56**, 457–62.

Newton, J.R., Freeman, C.P. & Munro, J. (1993). Impulsivity and dyscontrol in bulimia nervosa: is impulsivity an independent phenomenon or a marker of severity? *Acta Psychiatrica Scandinavica*, **87**, 389–94.

Nielson, A.C. & Williams, T.A. (1980). Depression in ambulatory medical patients. *Archives of General Psychiatry*, **37**, 999–1004.

Norring, C., Sohlberg, S., Rosmark, B., Humble, K., Holmgren, S. & Nordqvist, C. (1989). Ego functioning in eating disorders: description and relation to diagnostic classification. *International Journal of Eating Disorders*, **8**, 607–21.

Norton, N.C. (1989). Three scales of alexithymia: do they measure the same thing? *Journal of Personality Assessment*, **53**, 621–37.

Notarius, C.I. & Levenson, R.W. (1979). Expressive tendencies and physiological response to stress. *Journal of Personality and Social Psychology*, **37**, 1204–10.

Noyes, R., Clancy, J., Woodman, C., Holt, C., Suelzer, M., Christian-sen, J. & Anderson, D.J. (1993). Environmental factors related to the outcome of panic disorder: a seven-year follow-up study. *Journal of Nervous and Mental Disease*, **181**, 529–38.

Nunnally, J.C. (1978). *Psychometric theory*, 2nd ed. New York: McGraw-Hill.

Ogden, T.H. (1989). *The primitive edge of experience*, Northvale, NJ: Aronson.

Olivardia, R., Pope, H.G., Mangweth, B. & Hudson, J.I. (1995). Eating disorders in college men. *American Journal of Psychiatry*, **152**, 1279–85.

Oppenheim, B.S. (1918). Report on neurocirculatory asthenia and its management. *Military Surgeon*, **42**, 711–44.

Orth-Gomér, K. & Undén, A. (1990). Type A behavior, social support, and coronary risk: interaction and significance for mortality in cardiac patients. *Psychosomatic Medicine*, **52**, 59–72.

Ortony, A., Clore, G.L. & Collins, A. (1988). *The cognitive structure of emotions*. Cambridge: Cambridge University Press.

Osofsky, J.D. (1992). Affective development and early relationships: clinical implications. In J.W. Barron, M.N. Eagle & D.L. Wolitzky (Eds.), *Interface of psychoanalysis and psychology*, pp. 233–44. Washington, DC: American Psychological Association.

Osofsky, J.D. & Eberhart-Wright, A. (1988). Affective exchanges between high risk mothers and infants. *International Journal of Psychoanalysis*, **69**, 221–31.

Osti, R.M.A., Trombini, G. & Magnani, B. (1980). Stress and distress in essential hypertension. *Psychotherapy and Psychosomatics*, **33**, 193–7.

Ouellet, L., Nielson, T., Cartier, A. & Montplaiser, J. (1994). EEG coherence and dream content differences in alexithymic subjects. *Journal of Sleep Research*, **3** (suppl. 1), 180.

Oxman, T.E., Rosenberg, S.D., Schnurr, P.P. & Tucker, G.J. (1985). Linguistic dimensions of affect and thought in somatization disorder. *American Journal of Psychiatry*, **142**, 1150–5.

Oyebode, F. & Oyebode, J. (1990). Letter to the editor: differentiation of the emotions. *Psychiatric Bulletin*, **14**, 425–31.

Paez, D., Basabe, N., Valdoseda, M. & Iraurgi, I. (1995). Confrontation – inhibition, alexithymia and health. In J.W. Pennebaker (Ed.), *Emotions, disclosure, and health*. Washington, DC: American Psychological Association.

Pandey, R., Mandal, M.K., Taylor, G.J. & Parker, J.D.A. (1996). Cross-cultural alexithymia: development and validation of a Hindi translation of the Twenty-Item Toronto Alexithymia Scale. *Journal of Clinical Psychology*, **52**, 173–6.

Papciak, A.S., Feuerstein, M., Belar, C.D. & Pistone, L. (1986–87). Alexithymia and pain in an outpatient behavioral medicine clinic. *International Journal of Psychiatry in Medicine*, **16**, 347–57.

Papciak, A.S., Feuerstein, M. & Spiegel, J.A. (1985). Stress reactivity in alexithymia: decoupling of physiological and cognitive responses. *Journal of Human Stress*, **11**, 135–42.

Papez, J.W. (1937). A proposed mechanism of emotion. *Archives of Neurology and Psychiatry*, **38**, 725–43.

Paris, J. (1995). Memories of abuse in borderline patients: true or false? *Harvard Review of Psychiatry*, **3**, 10–17.

Parker, J.D.A., Bagby, R.M. & Taylor, G.J. (1989a). Toronto Alexithymia Scale, EPQ and self-report measures of somatic complaints. *Personality and Individual Differences*, **10**, 599–604.

Parker, J.D.A., Bagby, R.M. & Taylor, G.J. (1991a). Alexithymia and depression: distinct or overlapping constructs? *Comprehensive Psychiatry*, **32**, 387–94.

Parker, J.D.A., Bagby, R.M., Taylor, G.J., Endler, N.S. & Schmitz, P. (1993a). Factorial validity of the 20-item Toronto Alexithymia Scale. *European Journal of Personality*, **7**, 221–32.

Parker, J.D.A., Taylor, G.J. & Bagby, R.M. (1989b). The alexithymia construct: relationship with sociodemographic variables and intelligence. *Comprehensive Psychiatry*, **30**, 434–41.

Parker, J.D.A., Taylor, G.J. & Bagby, R.M. (1992). Relationship between conjugate lateral eye movements and alexithymia. *Psychotherapy and Psychosomatics*, **57**, 94–101.

Parker, J.D.A., Taylor, G.J. & Bagby, R.M. (1993b). Alexithymia and the processing of emotional stimuli: an experimental study. *New Trends in Experimental and Clinical Psychiatry*, **9**, 9–14.

Parker, J.D.A., Taylor, G.J. & Bagby, R.M. (1993c). Alexithymia and the recognition of facial expressions of emotion. *Psychotherapy and Psychosomatics*, **59**, 197–202.

Parker, J.D.A., Taylor, G.J., Bagby, R.M. & Acklin, M.W. (1993d). Alexithymia in panic disorder and simple phobia: a comparative study. *American Journal of Psychiatry*, **150**, 1105–7.

Parker, J.D.A., Taylor, G.J., Bagby, R.M. & Thomas, S.(1991b). Problems with measuring alexithymia. *Psychosomatics*, **32**, 196–202.

Parry-Jones, B. (1994). Merycism or rumination disorder. A historical investigation and current assessment. *British Journal of Psychiatry*, **165**, 303–14.

Pasini, A., Delle Chiaie, R., Seripa, S. & Ciani, N. (1992). Alexithymia as related to sex, age, and educational level: results of the Toronto Alexithymia Scale in 417 normal subjects. *Comprehensive Psychiatry*, **33**, 42–6.

Pauli, P., Schwenzer, M., Brody, S., Rau, H. & Birbaumer, N. (1993). Hypochondriacal attitudes, pain sensitivity, and attentional bias. *Journal of Psychosomatic Research*, **37**, 745–52.

Paulson, J.E. (1985). State of the art of alexithymia measurement. *Psychotherapy and Psychosomatics*, **44**, 57–64.

Pelosi, A.J. & Appelby, L. (1992). Psychological influences on cancer and ischaemic heart disease. *British Medical Journal*, **304**, 1295–8.

Pennebaker, J.W. (1985). Traumatic experience and psychosomatic disease: exploring the roles of behavioural inhibition, obsession, and confiding. *Canadian Psychology*, **26**, 82–95.

Pennebaker, J.W. & Susman, J.R. (1988). Disclosure of traumas and psychosomatic processes. *Social Science and Medicine*, **26**, 327–32.

Pennebaker, J.W. & Watson, D. (1991). The psychology of somatic symptoms. In L.J. Kirmayer & J.M. Robbins (Eds.), *Current concepts of somatization: research and clinical perspectives*, pp. 21–35. Washington, DC: American Psychiatric Press.

Perini, C., Rauchfleisch, U. & Bühler, F.R. (1985). Personality characteristics and renin in essential hypertension. *Psychotherapy and Psychosomatics*, **43**, 44–8.

Perlman, L.V., Ferguson, S., Bergum, K., Isenberg, E.L. & Hammarsten, J.F. (1971). Precipitation of CHF: social and emotional factors. *Annals of Internal Medicine*, **75**, 1–7.

Perry, J.C. & Cooper, S.H. (1989). What do cross-sectional measures of defense mechanisms predict? In G.E. Vaillant (Ed.), *Empirical studies of ego mechanisms of defense*, pp. 47–59. Washington, DC: American Psychiatric Press.

Pert, C.B., Ruff, M.R., Weber, R.J. & Herkenham, M. (1985). Neuropeptides and their receptors: a psychosomatic network. *Journal of Immunology*, **135**, 820s–6s.

Pervin, L.A. (1988). Affect and addiction. *Addictive Behaviors*, **13**, 83–6.

Peyrot, M. & McMurray, J.F., Jr. (1985). Psychosocial factors in diabetes control: adjustment of insulin-treated adults. *Psychosomatic Medicine*, **47**, 542–57.

Philippot, P. (1993). Inducing and assessing differentiated emotion-feeling states in the laboratory. *Cognition and Emotion*, **7**, 171–93.

Piaget, J. (1962). *Play, dreams, and imitation in childhood*. New York: Norton.

Piaget, J. (1967). *Six psychological studies*. New York: Random House.

Piaget, J. (1981). *Intelligence and affectivity*. Palo Alto, CA: Annual Reviews, Inc.

Pierce, M.J., Faryna, A., Davidson, A., Markart, R. & Krystal, J.H. (1989). A comparison of interview and self-report alexithymia measures (abstract). *Psychosomatic Medicine*, **51**, 244.

Pierloot, R.A., Houben, M.E. & Acke, G. (1988). Are anorexia nervosa patients alexithymic? *Acta Psychiatrica Belgica*, **88**, 222–32.

Pierloot, R. & Vinck, J. (1977). A pragmatic approach to the concept of alexithymia. *Psychotherapy and Psychosomatics*, **28**, 156–66.

Pilgrim, J.A. (1994). Psychological aspects of high and low blood pressure. *Psychological Medicine*, **24**, 9–14.

Pinard, G. (1987). Masked depression: a semantic or diagnostic dilemma. *Annals of the Royal College of Physicians and Surgeons of Canada*, **20**, 17–19.

Pinard, L., Negrete, J.C., Annable, L. & Audet, N. (1996). Alexithymia in substance abusers: persistence and correlates of variance. *American Journal on Addictions*, **5**, 32–9.

Pipp, S. & Harmon, R.J. (1987). Attachment as regulation. *Child Development*, **58**, 648–52.

Plutchik, R. (1980). A general psychoevolutionary theory of emotion. In R. Plutchik & H. Kellerman (Eds.), *Emotion: theory, research, and experience. Vol. 1. Theories of emotion*, pp. 3–33. New York: Academic Press.

Plutchik, R. (1993). Emotions and their vicissitudes: emotions and psychopathology. In M. Lewis & J.M. Haviland (Eds.), *Handbook of emotions*, pp. 53–66. New York: Guilford Press.

Pope, H.G., Hudson, J.I., Jonas, J.M. & Yurgelum-Todd, D. (1983). Bulimia treated with imipramine: a placebo controlled, double-blind study. *American Journal of Psychiatry*, **140**, 554–8.

Porcelli, P., Leoci, C., Guerra, V., Taylor, G.J. & Bagby, R.M. (1996). A longitudinal study of alexithymia and psychological distress in inflammatory bowel disease. *Journal of Psychosomatic Research*, **41**, 569–73.

Porcelli, P. Zaka, S., Leoci, C., Centonze, S. & Taylor, G.J. (1995). Alexithymia in inflammatory bowel disease. A case-control study. *Psychotherapy and Psychosomatics*, **64**, 49–53.

Porges, S.W. (1991). Vagal tone: an autonomic mediator of affect. In J. Garber & K.A. Dodge (Eds.), *The development of emotion regulation and dysregulation*, pp. 111–28. Cambridge: Cambridge University Press.

Postone, N. (1986). Alexithymia in chronic pain patients. *General Hospital Psychiatry*, **8**, 163–7.

Pribor, E.F. & Dinwiddie, S.H. (1992). Psychiatric correlates of incest in childhood. *American Journal of Psychiatry*, **149**, 52–6.

Pribor, E.F., Yutzy, S.H., Dean, J.T. & Wetzel, R.D. (1993). Briquet's syndrome, dissociation, and abuse. *American Journal of Psychiatry*, **150**, 1507–11.

Priel, B. & Shamai, D. (1995). Attachment style and perceived social support: effects on affect regulation. *Personality and Individual Differences*, **19**, 235–41.

Prince, J.D. & Berenbaum, H. (1993). Alexithymia and hedonic capacity. *Journal of Research in Personality*, **27**, 15–22.

Prince, R. (1987). Alexithymia and verbal psychotherapies in cultural context. *Transcultural Psychiatric Research Review*, **24**, 107–18.

Quitkin, F.M., Rifkin, A., Kaplan, J., Klein, D.F. & Oaks, G. (1972). Phobic anxiety syndrome complicated by drug dependence and addiction. *Archives of General Psychiatry*, **27**, 159–62.

Rabavilas, A.D. (1987). Electrodermal activity in low and high alexithymia neurotic patients. *Psychotherapy and Psychosomatics*, **47**, 101–4.

Rachman, S. (1980). Emotional processing. *Behaviour Research and Therapy*, **18**, 51–60.

Rachman, S. (1984). Agoraphobia: a safety-signal perspective. *Behaviour Research and Therapy*, **22**, 59–70.

Racle, G.L. (1980). Civilizations of the left cerebral hemisphere? *Journal of the Society for Accelerative Learning and Teaching*, **5**, 267–74.

Racle, G.L. (1986). Book review: the Japanese brain, uniqueness and universality, by Tadanobu Tsunoda. *Journal of the Society for Accelerative Learning and Teaching*, **11**, 57–9.

Radke-Yarrow, M., Cummings, E.M., Kuczynski, L. & Chapman, M. (1985). Patterns of attachment in two- and three-year olds in normal families and families with parental depression. *Child Development*, **56**, 884–93.

Rado, S. (1933). The psychoanalysis of pharmacothymia. *Psychoanalytic Quarterly*, **2**, 1–23.

Rangell, L. (1968). A further attempt to resolve the 'Problem of Anxiety'. *Journal of the American Psychoanalytic Association*, **16**, 371–404.

Rangell, L. (1984). Structure, somatic and psychic: the biopsychological base of infancy. In J.D. Call, E. Galenson & R. Tyson (Eds.), *Frontiers of infant psychiatry*, vol. 2, pp. 70–81. New York: Basic Books.

Rapaport, D. (1953). On the psychoanalytic theory of affects. In M. Gill (Ed.), *The collected papers of David Rapaport*, pp. 476–512. New York: Basic Books, 1967.

Rather, L.J. (1965). *Mind and body in eighteenth century medicine*. London: Wellcome Historical Medical Library.

Regier, D.A., Farmer, M., Rae, D., Locke, B., Keith, S., Judd, L. & Goodwin, F.K. (1990). Comorbidity of mental disorders with alcohol and other drug abuse. *Journal of the American Medical Association*, **264**, 2511–18.

Reich, J., Noyes, R. & Troughton, E. (1987). Dependent personality disorder associated with phobic avoidance in patients with panic disorder. *American Journal of Psychiatry*, **144**, 323–6.

Reiser, M. (1978). Psychoanalysis in patients with psychosomatic disorders. In T.B. Karasu & R.I. Steinmuller (Eds.), *Psychotherapeutics in medicine*. New York: Grune and Stratton.

Reiss, S., Peterson, R.A., Gursky, M. & McNally R.J. (1986). Anxiety sensitivity, anxiety frequency, and the prediction of fearfulness. *Behaviour Research and Therapy*, **24**, 1–8.

Reite, M. & Field, T. (Eds.) (1985). *The psychobiology of attachment and separation*. Orlando, FL: Academic Press.

Rice, D.P. & Miller, L.S. (1995). The economic burden of affective disorders. *British Journal of Psychiatry*, **166** (suppl. 27), 34–42.

Rimé, B., Ucros, C.G., Bestgen, Y. & Jeanjean, M. (1989). Type A
behavior pattern: specific coronary risk factor or general disease-
prone condition? *British Journal of Medical Psychology*, **62**, 229–40.

Rimon, R. (1969). A psychosomatic approach to rheumatoid arthritis: a
clinical study of 100 female patients. *Acta Rheumatica Scandinavica*,
suppl. 13, 1–154.

Rimon, R. & Laakso, R. L. (1985). Life stress and rheumatoid arthritis.
*Psychotherapy and Psychosomatics*, **43**, 38–43.

Rinsley, D.B. (1988). The dipsas revisited: comments on addiction and
personality. *Journal of Substance Abuse Treatment*, **5**, 1–7.

Robbins, J.M. & Kirmayer, L.J. (1991). Cognitive and social factors in
somatization. In L.J. Kirmayer & J.M. Robbins (Eds.), *Current concepts of somatization: research and clinical perspectives*, pp. 107–141.
Washington, DC: American Psychiatric Press.

Robbins, M. (1989). Primitive personality organization as an interper-
sonally adaptive modification of cognition and affect. *International
Journal of Psychoanalysis*, **70**, 443–59.

Rock, M.H. & Goldberger, L. (1978). Relationship between
agoraphobia and field dependence. *Journal of Nervous and Mental
Disease*, **166**, 781–6.

Rodin, G., Craven, J., Littlefield, C., Murray, M. & Daneman, D.
(1991). Eating disorders and intentional insulin undertreatment in adolescent females with diabetes. *Psychosomatics*, **32**, 171–6.

Rodrigo, G. & Lusiardo, M. (1992). Factor structure of the Spanish
version of the Toronto Alexithymia Scale. *Psychotherapy and Psychosomatics*, **58**, 197–201.

Rodrigo, G., Lusiardo, M. & Normey, L. (1989). Alexithymia: reliability and validity of the Spanish version of the Toronto Alexithymia
Scale. *Psychotherapy and Psychosomatics*, **51**, 162–8.

Rosenbaum, J.F., Biederman, J., Gersten, M., Hirshfeld, D.R.,
Meminger, S.R., Herman, J.B., Kagan, J., Reznick, J.S. & Snidman,
N. (1988). Behavioral inhibition in children of parents with panic dis-
order and agoraphobia. *Archives of General Psychiatry*, **45**, 463–70.

Rosenbaum, J.F., Pollock, R.A., Otto, M.W. & Pollack, M.H. (1995).
Integrated treatment of panic disorder. *Bulletin of the Menninger Clinic*,
**59** (suppl. A), 4–26.

Rosenman, R.H., Brand R.J., Jenkins, C.D., Friedman, M., Straus, R.
& Wurm, M. (1975). Coronary heart disease in the Western Collaborative Group Study: final follow-up experience of 8.5 years. *Journal
of the American Medical Association*, **233**, 872–7.

Rosenman, R.H. & Chesney, M.A. (1982). Stress, Type A behavior,
and coronary disease. In L. Goldberger & S. Breznitz (Eds.), *Handbook of stress: theoretical and clinical aspects*, pp. 547–65. New York:
Free Press.

Ross, C.A., Heber, S., Norton, G.R. & Anderson, G. (1989). Somatic symptoms in multiple personality disorder. *Psychosomatics*, **30**, 154–60.

Ross, E.D. (1981). The aprosodias: functional–anatomic organization of the affective components of language in the right hemisphere. *Archives of Neurology*, **38**, 561–9.

Ross, E.D. (1985). Modulation of affect and nonverbal communication by the right hemisphere. In M.M. Mesulam (Ed.), *Principles of behavioral neurology*, pp. 239–57. Philadelphia: F.A. Davis Company.

Ross, E.D., Homan, R.W. & Buck, R. (1994). Differential hemispheric lateralization of primary and social emotions: implications for developing a comprehensive neurology for emotions, repression, and the subconscious. *Neuropsychiatry, Neuropsychology, and Behavioral Neurology*, **7**, 1–19.

Roth, M. (1987). Some recent developments in relation to agoraphobia and related disorders and their bearing upon theories of their causation. *Psychiatric Journal of the University of Ottawa*, **12**, 150–5.

Rothbart, M.K. & Ahadi, S.A. (1994). Temperament and the development of personality. *Journal of Abnormal Psychology*, **103**, 55–66.

Rourke, B., Young, G. & Leenaars, A.A. (1989). A childhood learning disability that predisposes those afflicted to adolescent and adult depression and suicide risk. *Journal of Learning Disabilities*, **22**, 169–75.

Roy, R., Thomas, M. & Matas, M. (1984). Chronic pain and depression: a review. *Comprehensive Psychiatry*, **25**, 96–105.

Roy-Byrne, P.P., Geraci, M. & Uhde, T.W. (1986). Life events and the onset of panic disorder. *American Journal of Psychiatry*, **143**, 1424–27.

Roy-Byrne, P.P. & Cowley, D.S. (1994/1995). Course and outcome in panic disorder: a review of recent follow-up studies. *Anxiety*, **1**, 151–60.

Rubino, I.A., Grasso, S., Sonnino, A. & Pezzarossa, B. (1991). Is alexithymia a non-neurotic personality dimension? *British Journal of Medical Psychology*, **64**, 385–91.

Ruesch, J. (1948). The infantile personality. *Psychosomatic Medicine*, **10**, 134–44.

Ruesch, J. (1957). *Disturbed communication: the clinical assessment of normal and pathological communicative behavior*. New York: Norton.

Russell, G.F.M. (1985). Bulimia revisited. *International Journal of Eating Disorders*, **4**, 681–92.

Rybakowski, J. & Ziółkowski, M. (1990). Clinical and biochemical heterogeneity of alcoholism: the role of family history and alexithymia. *Drug and Alcohol Dependence*, **27**, 73–7.

Rybakowski, J., Ziółkowski, M., Zasadzka, T. & Brzezinski, R. (1988). High prevalence of alexithymia in male patients with alcohol dependence. *Drug and Alcohol Dependence*, **21**, 133–6.

Rybash, J.M. & Hoyer, G.W. (1992). Hemispheric specialization for categories and coordinate learning disabilities: social, academic, and adaptive functioning in adults and children. *Psychological Bulletin*, **107**, 196–209.

Safar, M.E., Kamiemiecka, H.A., Levenson, J.A., Dimitriu, V.M., & Pauleau, N.F. (1978). Hemodynamic factors and Rorschach testing in borderline and sustained hypertension. *Psychosomatic Medicine*, **40**, 620–30.

Salminen, J.K., Saarijärvi, S. & Äärelä, E. (1995). Two decades of alexithymia. *Journal of Psychosomatic Research*, **39**, 803–7.

Salminen, J.K., Saarijärvi, S., Äärelä, E. & Tamminen, T. (1994). Alexithymia -State or trait? One-year follow-up study of general hospital psychiatric consultation out-patients. *Journal of Psychosomatic Research*, **38**, 681–5.

Salovey, P., Hsee, C.K. & Mayer, J.D. (1993). Emotional intelligence and the self-regulation of affect. In D.M. Wegner & J.W. Pennebaker (Eds.), *Handbook of mental control*, pp. 258–77. Englewood Cliffs, NJ: Prentice Hall.

Salovey, P. & Mayer, J.D. (1989/90). Emotional intelligence. *Imagination, Cognition, and Personality*, **9**, 185–211.

Sanders, B. & Giolas, M.H. (1991). Dissociation and childhood trauma in psychologically disturbed adolescents. *American Journal of Psychiatry*, **148**, 50–4.

Sandin, B., Chorot, P., Miguel, A.S. & Jimenez, M.P. (1993). Stress behavior types, personality, alexithymia coping and state-trait anger expression. Presented at the 23rd European congress of behavior and cognitive therapies. London, September 22–5.

Sandler, J. (1972). The role of affects in psychoanalytic theory. In *Ciba foundation symposium 8: physiology, emotion and psychosomatic illness*, (pp. 31–56). Amsterdam: Elsevier.

Sandler, J. & Joffe, W.G. (1965). Notes on childhood depression. *International Journal of Psychoanalysis*, **46**, 88–96.

Sansone, R.A., Fine, M.A., Seuferer, S. & Bovenzi, J. (1989). The prevalence of borderline personality symptomatology among women with eating disorders. *Journal of Clinical Psychology*, **45**, 603–10.

Sashin, J.I. (1985). Affect tolerance: a model of affect-response using catastrophe theory. *Journal of Social and Biological Structure*, **8**, 175–202.

Saxe, G.N., Chinman, G., Berkowitz, R., Hall, K., Lieberg, G., Schwartz, J. & van der Kolk, B.A. (1994). Somatization in patients with dissociative disorders. *American Journal of Psychiatry*, **151**, 1329–34.

Schachter, S. (1964). The interactions of cognitive and physiological determinants of emotional state. In L. Berkowitz (Ed.), *Advances in experimental social psychology*, vol. 1., pp. 49–80. New York: Academic Press.

Schachter, S. & Singer, J. E. (1962). Cognitive, social and physiological determinants of emotional state. *Psychological Review*, **69**, 379–99.

Schafer, R. (1964). The clinical analysis of affects. *Journal of the American Psychoanalytic Association*, **12**, 275–99.

Schaffer, C.E. (1993). The role of adult attachment in the experience and regulation of affect. Doctoral dissertation, Yale University.

Scheier, M.F. & Bridges, M.W. (1995). Person variables and health: personality predispositions and acute psychological states as shared determinants for disease. *Psychosomatic Medicine*, **57**, 255–68.

Scherwitz, L.W., Perkins, L.L., Chesney, M.A., Hughes, G.H., Sidney, S. & Manolio, T.A. (1992). Hostility and health behaviours in young adults: the CARDIA study. *American Journal of Epidemiology*, **136**, 136–45.

Schiraldi, G. R. & Beck, K. H. (1988). Personality correlates of the Jenkins Activity Survey. *Social Behavior and Personality*, **16**, 109–15.

Schmale, A.H. (1958). Relationship of separation and depression to disease. *Psychosomatic Medicine*, **20**, 259–77.

Schmale, A.H. (1972). Giving up as a final common pathway to changes in health. *Advances in Psychosomatic Medicine*, **28**, 714–21.

Schmale, A.H. & Iker, H.P. (1966). The affect of hopelessness and the development of cancer. *Psychosomatic Medicine*, **28**, 714–21.

Schmidt, A.J.M., Wolfs-Takens, D.J., Oosterlaan, J. & van den Hout, M.A. (1994). Psychological mechanisms in hypochondriasis: attention-induced physical symptoms without sensory stimulation. *Psychotherapy and Psychosomatics*, **61**, 117–20.

Schmidt, U., Jiwany, A. & Treasure, J. (1993). A controlled study of alexithymia in eating disorders. *Comprehensive Psychiatry*, **34**, 54–8.

Schmitz, P.G. (1992). Personality, stress-reactions and disease. *Personality and Individual Differences*, **13**, 683–91.

Schneider, P.B. (1977). The observer, the psychosomatic phenomenon and the setting of the observation. *Psychotherapy and Psychosomatics*, **28**, 36–46.

Schneier, F.R., Johnson, J., Hornig, C.D., Liebowitz, M.R. & Weissman, M.M. (1992). Social phobia: comorbidity and morbidity in an epidemiologic sample. *Archives of General Psychiatry*, **49**, 282–8.

Schore, A.N. (1994). *Affect regulation and the origin of the self: the neurobiology of emotional development*. Hillsdale, NJ: Lawrence Erlbaum.

Schork, E.J., Eckert, E.D. & Halmi, K.A. (1994). The relationship between psychopathology, eating disorder diagnosis, and clinical outcome at 10-year follow-up in anorexia nervosa. *Comprehensive Psychiatry*, **35**, 113–23.

Schraa, J.C. & Dicks, J.F. (1981). Hypnotic treatment of the alexithymic patient: a case report. *American Journal of Clinical Hypnotherapy*, **23**, 207–10.

Schuckit, M.A. (1986). Genetic and clinical implications of alcoholism and affective disorder. *American Journal of Psychiatry*, **143**, 140–7.

Schuckit, M.A. (1994). Low level of response to alcohol as a predictor of future alcoholism. *American Journal of Psychiatry*, **151**, 184–9.

Schuckit, M.A. & Hesselbrock, V. (1994). Alcohol dependence and anxiety disorders: what is the relationship? *American Journal of Psychiatry*, **151**, 1723–34.

Schuckit, M.A., Klein, J., Twitchell, G. & Smith, T. (1994). Personality test scores as predictors of alcoholism almost a decade later. *American Journal of Psychiatry*, **151**, 1038–42.

Schuckit, M.A. & Monteiro, M.G. (1988). Alcoholism, anxiety and depression. *British Journal of Addiction*, **83**, 1373–80.

Schupak-Neuberg, E. & Nemeroff, C.J. (1993). Disturbances in identity and self-regulation in bulimia nervosa: implications for a metaphorical perspective of 'body as self'. *International Journal of Eating Disorders*, **13**, 335–47.

Schur, M. (1955). Comments on the metapsychology of somatization. *Psychoanalytic Study of the Child*, **10**, 110–64.

Schwartz, A. (1987). Drives, affects, behavior–and learning: approaches to a psychobiology of emotion and to an integration of psychoanalytic and neurobiologic thought. *Journal of the American Psychoanalytic Association*, **35**, 467–506.

Schwartz, A. (1992). Not art but science: applications of neurobiology, experimental psychology, and ethology to psychoanalytic technique. I: Neuroscientifically guided approaches to interpretive 'what's' and 'when's'. *Psychoanalytic Inquiry*, **12**, 445–74.

Schwartz, G.E. (1979). The brain as a health care system. In G.C. Stone, F. Cohen & N.E. Adler (Eds.), *Health psychology: a handbook*, pp. 549–71. San Francisco: Jossey-Bass.

Schwartz, G.E. (1983). Disregulation theory and disease: applications to the repression/cerebral disconnection/cardiovascular disorder hypothesis. *International Review of Applied Psychology*, **32**, 95–118.

Schwartz, G.E. (1989). Disregulation theory and disease: toward a general model for psychosomatic medicine. In S. Cheren (Ed.), *Psychosomatic medicine: theory, physiology, and practice*, vol. 1, pp. 91–117. Madison, CT: International Universities Press.

Schwartz, G.E. (1990). Psychobiology of repression and health: a systems approach. In J.L. Singer (Ed.), *Repression and dissociation: implications for personality theory, psychopathology, and health*, pp. 405–34. Chicago: University of Chicago Press.

Schwartz, H.J. (1985). Bulimia: psychoanalytic perspectives. *Journal of the American Psychoanalytic Association*, **34**, 439–62.

Segal, H. (1957). Notes on symbol formation. *International Journal of Psychoanalysis*, **38**, 391–7.

Segal, H. (1964). *Introduction to the work of Melanie Klein*. New York: Basic Books.

Segal, H. (1981). The function of dreams. In J.S. Grotstein (Ed.), *Do I dare disturb the universe?* pp. 580–7. Beverley Hills: Caesura Press.

Seligman, M. & Binik, Y. (1977). The safety signal hypothesis. In H. Davis & H. Huwitz (Eds.), *Pavlovian-operant interactions*, pp. 165–87. Hillsdale, NJ: Erlbaum.

Selvini Palazzoli, M. (1971). Anorexia nervosa. In S. Arieti (Ed.), *The world biennial of psychiatry and psychotherapy*, vol. 1, pp. 197–218. New York: Basic Books.

Selvini Palazzoli, M. (1974). *Self-starvation*. London: Chaucer.

Sensky, T. (1994). Somatization: syndromes or processes? *Psychotherapy and Psychosomatics*, **61**, 1–3.

Shands, H.C. (1975). How are 'psychosomatic' patients different from 'psychoneurotic' patients. *Psychotherapy and Psychosomatics*, **26**, 270–85.

Shanks, M.F. & Ho-Yen, D.O. (1995). A clinical study of chronic fatigue syndrome. *British Journal of Psychiatry*, **166**, 798–801.

Sharpe, M. & Bass, C. (1992). Pathophysiological mechanisms in somatization. *International Review of Psychiatry*, **4**, 81–97.

Shaver, P.R. & Brennan, K.A. (1992). Attachment styles and the 'big five' personality traits: their connections with each other and with romantic relationship outcomes. *Personality and Social Psychology Bulletin*, **18**, 536–45.

Shaw, J. & Creed, F. (1991). The cost of somatization. *Journal of Psychosomatic Research*, **35**, 307–12.

Shear, M.K., Cooper, A.M., Klerman, G.L., Busch, F.N. & Shapiro, T. (1993). A psychodynamic model of panic disorder. *American Journal of Psychiatry*, **150**, 859–66.

Sheehan, D.V. (1982). Medical intelligence: current concepts in psychiatry – Panic attacks and phobias. *New England Journal of Medicine*, **307**, 156–8.

Shekelle, R.B., Gale, M., Ostfeld, A.M. & Paul, O. (1983). Hostility, risk of coronary heart disease, and mortality. *Psychosomatic Medicine*, **45**, 109–14.

Shekelle, R.B., Hulley, S.B., Neston, J.D., Billings, J.H., Borboni, N.O., Gerace, T.A., Jacobs, D.R., Lasser, N.L., Mittlemark, M.B. & Stamler, J. (1985). The MRFIT behavior pattern study: type A behavior and incidence of coronary heart disease. *American Journal of Epidemiology*, **122**, 559–70.

Shekelle, R.B., Schoenberger, J.A. & Stamler, J. (1976). Correlates of the JAS Type A behavior pattern score. *Journal of Chronic Diseases*, **29**, 381–94.

Sher, K.J. & Trull, T.J. (1994). Personality and disinhibitory psycho-pathology: alcoholism and antisocial personality disorder. *Journal of Abnormal Psychology*, **103**, 92–102.

Shields, A.M., Cicchetti, D. & Ryan, R.M. (1994). The development of emotional and behavioral self-regulation and social competence among maltreated school-age children. *Development and Psychopathology*, **6**, 57–75.

Shipko, S. (1982). Alexithymia and somatization. *Psychotherapy and Psychosomatics*, **37**, 193–201.

Shipko, S., Alvarez, W.A. & Noviello, N. (1983). Towards a teleological model of alexithymia: alexithymia and post-traumatic stress disorder. *Psychotherapy and Psychosomatics*, **39**, 122–6.

Shipko, S. & Noviello, N. (1984). Psychometric properties of self-report scales of alexithymia. *Psychotherapy and Psychosomatics*, **41**, 85–90.

Shoenfeld, Y. & Schwartz, R.S. (1984). Immunologic and genetic factors in autoimmune diseases. *New England Journal of Medicine*, **311**, 1019–29.

Shorter, E. (1992). *From paralysis to fatigue: a history of psychosomatic illness in the modern era*. New York: The Free Press.

Shulman, L.E. & Bunim, J.J. (1962). Disorders of the joints. In T.R. Harrison, R.D. Adams, I.L. Bennett, W.H. Resnik, G.W. Thorn & M.M. Wintrobe (Eds.), *Principles of internal medicine*, pp. 1902–23. New York: McGraw-Hill.

Siever, L.J. & Davis, K.L. (1985). Overview: toward a dysregulation hypothesis of depression. *American Journal of Psychiatry*, **142**, 1017–31.

Siever, L.J. & Davis, K.L. (1991). A psychobiological perspective on the personality disorders. *American Journal of Psychiatry*, **148**, 1647–58.

Sifneos, P.E. (1967). Clinical observations on some patients suffering from a variety of psychosomatic diseases. *Acta Medicina Psychosomatica*, **7**, 1–10.

Sifneos, P.E. (1972/73). Is dynamic psychotherapy contraindicated for a large number of patients with psychosomatic disease? *Psychotherapy and Psychosomatics*, **21**, 133–6.

Sifneos, P.E. (1973). The prevalence of 'alexithymic' characteristics in psychosomatic patients. *Psychotherapy and Psychosomatics*, **22**, 255–62.

Sifneos, P.E. (1974). A reconsideration of psychodynamic mechanisms in psychosomatic symptom formation in view of recent clinical observations. *Psychotherapy and Psychosomatics*, **24**, 151–5.

Sifneos, P.E. (1975). Problems of psychotherapy of patients with alexithymic characteristics and physical disease. *Psychotherapy and Psychosomatics*, **26**, 65–70.

Sifneos, P.E. (1986). The Schalling–Sifneos Personality Scale-Revised. *Psychotherapy and Psychosomatics*, **45**, 161–5.

Sifneos, P.E. (1987). Anhedonia and alexithymia: a potential correlation. In D.C. Clark & J. Fawcett (Eds.), *Anhedonia and affect deficit states*, pp. 119–27. New York: PMA Publishing Corporation.

Sifneos, P.E. (1988). Alexithymia and its relationship to hemispheric specialization, affect and creativity. *Psychiatric Clinics of North America*, **11**, 287–92.

Sifneos, P.E. (1994). Affect deficit and alexithymia. *New Trends in Experimental and Clinical Psychiatry*, **10**, 193–5.

Sifneos, P.E., Apfel-Savitz, R. & Frankel, F.H. (1977). The phenomenon of 'alexithymia': observations in neurotic and psychosomatic patients. *Psychotherapy and Psychosomatics*, **28**, 47–57.

Silberman, E. K. & Weingartner, H. (1986). Hemispheric lateralization of functions related to emotion. *Brain and Cognition*, **5**, 322–53.

Silver, D., Glassman, E.J. & Cardish, R.J. (1988). The assessment of the capacity to be soothed: clinical and methodological issues. In Horton, P.C., Gewirtz, H. & Kreutter, K. (Eds.), *The solace paradigm: an eclectic search for psychological immunity*, pp. 91–119. Madison, CT: International Universities Press.

Simon, G.E. & VonKorff, M. (1991). Somatization and psychiatric disorder in the NIMH epidemiological catchment area study. *American Journal of Psychiatry*, **148**, 1494–500.

Singer, J.L. (1966). *Daydreaming: an introduction to the experimental study of inner experience.* New York: Random House.

Singer, M.T. (1977). Psychological dimensions in psychosomatic patients. *Psychotherapy and Psychosomatics*, **28**, 13–27.

Singer, J.L. (1979). Affect and imagination in play and fantasy. In C.E. Izard (Ed.), *Emotions in personality and psychopathology*, pp. 13–34. New York: Plenum Press.

Skodol, A.E., Oldham, J.M., Hyler, S.E., Kellman, H.D., Doidge, N. & Davies, M. (1993). Comorbidity of DSM-III-R eating disorders and personality disorders. *International Journal of Eating Disorders*, **14**, 403–16.

Slade, A. & Aber, J.L. (1992). Attachments, drives, and development: conflicts and convergences in theory. In J.W. Barron, M.N. Eagle & D.L. Wolitzky (Eds.), *Interface of psychoanalysis and psychology*, pp. 154–85. Washington, DC: American Psychological Association.

Smith, E.M. & Blalock, J.E. (1986). A complete regulatory loop between the immune and neuroendocrine systems operates through common signal molecules (hormones) and receptors. In N.P. Plotnikoff, R.E. Faith, A.J. Murgo & R.A. Good (Eds.), *Enkephalins and endorphins: stress and the immune system*, pp. 119–27. New York: Plenum.

Smith, G.R., Monson, R.A. & Ray, D.C. (1986). Patients with multiple unexplained symptoms. Their characteristics, functional health, and health care utilization. *Archives of Internal Medicine*, **146**, 69–72.

Smith, R.C., Greenbaum, D.S., Vancouver, J.B., Henry, R.C., Reinhart, M.A., Greenbaum, R.B., Dean, H.A. & Mayle, J.E. (1990). Psychosocial factors are associated with health care seeking rather than diagnosis in irritable bowel syndrome. *Gastroenterology*, **98**, 293–301.

Smith, T.W. (1992). Hostility and health: current status of a psychosomatic hypothesis. *Health Psychology*, **11**, 139–50.

Smith, T.W. & Frohm, F.D. (1985). What's so unhealthy about hostility? Construct validity and psychosocial correlates of the Cook and Medley Ho scale. *Health Psychology*, **4**, 503–20.

Smith, T.W. & Williams, P.G. (1992). Personality and health: advantages and limitations of the five-factor model. *Journal of Personality*, **60**, 395–423.

Smokler, I.A. & Shevrin, H. (1979). Cerebral lateralization and personality style. *Archives of General Psychiatry*, **36**, 949–54.

Smyth, K., Call, J., Hansell, S., Sparacino, J. & Strodtbeck, F. L. (1978). Type A behavior pattern and hypertension among inner-city black women. *Nursing Research*, **27**, 30–5.

Sohlberg, S. (1991). Impulsive regulation in anorexia nervosa and bulimia nervosa: some formulations. *Behavioural Neurology*, **4**, 189–202.

Solms, M. (1995). New findings on the neurological organization of dreaming: implications for psychoanalysis. *Psychoanalytic Quarterly*, **64**, 43–67.

Soloff, P.H. (1994). Is there any drug treatment of choice for the borderline patient? *Acta Psychiatrica Scandinavica*, **89** (suppl. 379), 50–5.

Sonne, S.C., Brady, K.T. & Morton, W.A. (1994). Substance abuse and bipolar affective disorder. *Journal of Nervous and Mental Disease*, **182**, 349–52.

Sours, J.A. (1980). *Starving to death in a sea of objects*. New York: Aronson.

Southwick, S.M., Krystal, J.H., Morgan, C.A., Johnson, D., Nagy, L.M., Nicolaou, A., Heninger, G.R. & Charney, D.S. (1993). Abnormal noradrenergic function in posttraumatic stress disorder. *Achieves of General Psychiatry*, **50**, 266–74.

Specker, S., de Zwaan, M., Raymond, N. & Mitchell, J. (1994). Psychopathology in subgroups of obese women with and without binge eating disorder. *Comprehensive Psychiatry*, **35**, 185–90.

Sperling, M. (1978). *Psychosomatic disorders in childhood*. New York: Aronson.

Spezzano, C. (1993). *Affect in psychoanalysis*. Hillsdale, NJ: Analytic Press.

Spielberger, C.D., Johnson, E.H., Russell, S.F., Crane, R.J., Jacobs, G.A. & Worden, T.J. (1985). The experience and expression of anger: construction and validation of an Anger Expression Scale. In M.A. Chesney & R.H. Rosenman (Eds.), *Anger and hostility in cardiovascular and behavioral disorders*, pp. 5–30. New York: McGraw-Hill.

Spoont, M.R. (1992). Modulatory role of serotonin in neural information processing: implications for human psychopathology. *Psychological Bulletin*, **112**, 330–50.

Spruiell, V. (1993). Deterministic chaos and the sciences of complexity: psychoanalysis in the midst of a general scientific revolution. *Journal of the American Psychoanalytic Association*, **41**, 3–43.

Sriram, T.G., Chaturvedi, S.K., Gopinath, P.S. & Shanmugam, V. (1987a). Controlled study of alexithymic characteristics in patients with psychogenic pain disorder. *Psychotherapy and Psychosomatics*, **47**, 11–17.

Sriram, T.G., Chaturvedi, S.K., Gopinath, P.S. & Subbakrishna, D.K. (1987b). Assessment of alexithymia: psychometric properties of the Toronto Alexithymia Scale (TAS) – a preliminary report. *Indian Journal of Psychiatry*, **29**, 133–8.

Sriram, T.G., Pratap, L. & Shanmugham, V. (1988). Towards enhancing the utility of Beth Israel Hospital Psychosomatic Questionnaire. *Psychotherapy and Psychosomatics*, **49**, 205–11.

Stabler, B., Surwit, R.S., Lane, J.D., Morris, M.A., Litton, J. & Feinglos M.N. (1987). Type A behavior pattern and blood glucose control in diabetic children. *Psychosomatic Medicine*, **49**, 313–16.

Stanghellini, G. & Ricca, V. (1995). Alexithymia and schizophrenias. *Psychopathology*, **28**, 263–72.

Stein, R. (1990). A new look at the theory of Melanie Klein. *International Journal of Psychoanalysis*, **71**, 499–511.

Steiner, J. (1979). The border between the paranoid–schizoid and the depressive positions in the borderline patient. *British Journal of Medical Psychology*, **52**, 385–91.

Stekel, W. (1925). *Peculiarities of behaviour, Volume I–II*. London: Williams & Norgate.

Stephanos, S., Biebl, W. & Plaum, F.G. (1976). Ambulatory analytical psychotherapy of psychosomatic patients: a report on the method of 'relaxation analytique'. *British Journal of Medical Psychology*, **49**, 305–13.

Steptoe, A. (1986). Contemporary psychosomatic theories of essential hypertension. In J.H. Lacey & D.A. Sturgeon (Eds.), *Proceedings of the 15th European conference on psychosomatic research*, pp. 189–92. London: Libbey.

Stern, A. (1938). Psychoanalytic investigation and therapy in the borderline group of neuroses. *Psychoanalytic Quarterly*, **7**, 467–89.

Stern, D.N. (1984). Affect attunement. In J.D. Call, E. Galenson & R.L. Tyson (Eds.), *Frontiers in infant psychiatry*, vol. 2, pp. 3–14. New York: Basic Books.

Stern, D.N. (1985). *The interpersonal world of the infant*. New York: Basic Books.

Stevens, J.H., Turner, C.W., Rhodewalt, F. & Talbot, S. (1984). The Type A behavior pattern and carotid artery atherosclerosis. *Psychosomatic Medicine*, **46**, 105–14.

Stewart, D.E. (1990). The changing faces of somatization. *Psychosomatics*, **31**, 153–8.

Stone, M.H. (1988). Theory of borderline personality disorder: is irritability the red thread that runs through borderline conditions? *Dissociation*, **1**, 2–15.

Stone, M.H. (1993). *Abnormalities of personality*. New York: Norton.

Striegel-Moore, R.H., Silberstein, L.R. & Rodin, J. (1986). Toward an understanding of risk factors for bulimia. *American Psychologist*, **41**, 246–63.

Strober, M. & Katz, J.L. (1987). Do eating disorders and affective disorders share a common etiology? *International Journal of Eating Disorders*, **6**, 171–80.

Strober, M., Salkin, B., Burroughs, J. & Morrell, W. (1982). Validity of the bulimia-restricter distinction in anorexia nervosa: parental personality characteristics and family psychiatric morbidity. *Journal of Nervous and Mental Disease*, **170**, 345–51.

Stroop, J.R. (1935). Studies in interference in serial verbal reactions. *Journal of Experimental Psychology*, **18**, 643–61.

Suarez, E.C. & Williams, R.B., Jr. (1989). Situational determinants of cardiovascular and emotional reactivity in high and low hostile men. *Psychosomatic Medicine*, **51**, 404–18.

Subbotsky, E.V. (1993). *Foundations of the mind*. Cambridge, MA: Harvard University Press.

Sugarman, A. & Kurash, C. (1982). The body as a transitional object in bulimia. *International Journal of Eating Disorders*, **1**, 57–67.

Sullivan, H.S. (1953). *The interpersonal theory of psychiatry*. New York: Norton.

Sulloway, F.J. (1979). *Freud, biologist of the mind*. New York: Basic Books.

Surwit, R.S. & Schneider, M.S. (1993). Role of stress in the etiology and treatment of diabetes mellitus. *Psychosomatic Medicine*, **55**, 380–93.

Sutker, P.B., Winstead, D.K., Galina, Z.H. & Allain, A.N. (1991). Cognitive deficits and psychopathology among former prisoners of war and combat veterans of the Korean conflict. *American Journal of Psychiatry*, **148**, 67–72.

Suzuki, K., Higuchi, S., Yamada, K., Mizutani, Y. & Kono, H. (1993). Young female alcoholics with and without eating disorders: a comparative study in Japan. *American Journal of Psychiatry*, **150**, 1053–8.

Swanson, D.W. (1984). Chronic pain as a third pathologic emotion. *American Journal of Psychiatry*, **141**, 210–14.

Swartz, M., Landerman, R., Blazer, D. & George, L. (1989). Somatization symptoms in the community: a rural/urban comparison. *Psychosomatics*, **30**, 44–53.

Swartz, M., Landerman, R., George, L.K., Blazer, D. & Escobar, J. (1991). Somatization disorder. In Robins, L.N, & Regier, D.A. (Eds.), *Psychiatric disorders in America*, pp. 220–57. New York: Free Press.

Swift, W., Andrews, D. & Barklage, N.E. (1986). The relationship between affective disorder and eating disorders: a review of the literature. *American Journal of Psychiatry*, **143**, 290–9.

Swift, W.J. & Letven, R. (1984). Bulimia and the basic fault: a psychoanalytic interpretation of the binging-vomiting syndrome. *Journal of the American Academy of Child Psychiatry*, **23**, 489–97.

Swiller, H.I. (1988). Alexithymia: treatment utilizing combined individual and group psychotherapy. *International Journal of Group Psychotherapy*, **38**, 47–61.

Szmukler, G.I. & Tantam, D. (1984). Anorexia nervosa: starvation dependence. *British Journal of Medical Psychology*, **57**, 303–10.

Tarter, R.E. (1988). Are there inherited behavioral traits that predispose to substance abuse? *Journal of Clinical and Consulting Psychology*, **56**, 189–96.

Tarter, R.E., Hegedus, A.M., Goldstein, G., Shelly, C. & Alterman, A.I. (1984). Adolescent sons of alcoholics: neuropsychological and personality characteristics. *Alcoholism: Clinical and Experimental Research*, **8**, 216–22.

Taylor, G.J. (1977). Alexithymia and the counter-transference. *Psychotherapy and Psychosomatics*, **28**, 141–7.

Taylor, G.J. (1984a). Alexithymia: concept, measurement, and implications for treatment. *American Journal of Psychiatry*, **141**, 725–32.

Taylor, G.J. (1984b). Psychotherapy with the boring patient. *Canadian Journal of Psychiatry*, **29**, 217–22.

Taylor, G.J. (1987a). *Psychosomatic medicine and contemporary psychoanalysis*. Madison, CT: International Universities Press.

Taylor, G.J. (1987b). Alexithymia: history and validation of the concept. *Transcultural Psychiatric Research Review*, **24**, 85–95.

Taylor, G.J. (1989). An integrated psychobiological model of panic disorder. Paper presented at the summer meeting of the Michigan Psychiatric Society, Toronto, July 28–30.

Taylor, G.J. (1992a). Psychoanalysis and psychosomatics: a new synthesis. *Journal of the American Academy of Psychoanalysis*, **20**, 251–75.

Taylor, G.J. (1992b). Psychosomatics and self-regulation. In J.W. Barron, M.N. Eagle & D.L. Wolitzky (Eds.), *Interface of psychoanalysis and psychology*, pp. 464–88. Washington, DC: American Psychological Association.

Taylor, G.J. (1993a). Book review. From paralysis to fatigue: a history of psychosomatic illness in the modern era. *Psychosomatic Medicine*, **55**, 88–9.

Taylor, G.J. (1993b). Clinical application of a dysregulation model of illness and disease: a case of spasmodic torticollis. *International Journal of Psychoanalysis*, **74**, 581–95.

Taylor, G.J. (1994). The alexithymia construct: conceptualization, validation, and relationship with basic dimensions of personality. *New Trends in Experimental and Clinical Psychiatry*, **10**, 61–74.

Taylor, G.J. (1995). Psychoanalysis and empirical research: the example of patients who lack psychological mindedness. *Journal of the American Academy of Psychoanalysis*, **23**, 263–81.

Taylor, G.J. & Bagby, R.M. (1988). Measurement of alexithymia. *Psychiatric Clinics of North America*, **11**, 351–66.

Taylor, G.J., Bagby, R.M. & Parker, J.D.A. (1991). The alexithymia construct: a potential paradigm for psychosomatic medicine. *Psychosomatics*, **32**, 153–64.

Taylor, G.J., Bagby, R.M. & Parker, J.D.A. (1992a). The Revised Toronto Alexithymia Scale: some reliability, validity, and normative data. *Psychotherapy and Psychosomatics*, **57**, 34–41.

Taylor, G.J., Bagby, R.M. & Parker, J.D.A. (1993). Is alexithymia a non-neurotic personality dimension? A response to Rubino, Grasso, Sonnino & Pezzarossa. *British Journal of Medical Psychology*, **66**, 281–7.

Taylor, G.J., Bagby, R.M., Ryan, D.P. & Parker, J.D.A. (1990a). Validation of the alexithymia construct: a measurement-based approach. *Canadian Journal of Psychiatry*, **35**, 290–7.

Taylor, G.J., Bagby, R.M., Ryan, D., Parker, J.D.A., Doody, K. & Keefe, P. (1988). Criterion validity of the Toronto Alexithymia Scale. *Psychosomatic Medicine*, **50**, 500–9.

Taylor, G.J. & Doody, K. (1985). Verbal measures of alexithymia: what do they measure. *Psychotherapy and Psychosomatics*, **43**, 32–7.

Taylor, G.J., Doody, K. & Newman, A. (1981). Alexithymic characteristics in patients with inflammatory bowel disease. *Canadian Journal of Psychiatry*, **26**, 470–4.

Taylor, G.J., Parker, J.D.A. & Bagby, R.M. (1990b). A preliminary investigation of alexithymia in men with psychoactive substance dependence. *American Journal of Psychiatry*, **147**, 1228–30.

Taylor, G.J., Parker, J.D.A., Bagby, R.M. & Acklin, M.W. (1992b). Alexithymia and somatic complaints in psychiatric out-patients. *Journal of Psychosomatic Research*, **36**, 417–24.

Taylor, G.J., Ryan, D. & Bagby, R.M. (1985). Toward the development of a new self-report alexithymia scale. *Psychotherapy and Psychosomatics*, **44**, 191–9.

Taylor, G.J. & Taylor, H.L. (1997). Alexithymia. In M. McCallum & W. Piper (Eds.), *Psychological mindedness*, pp. 77–104. Hillsdale, NJ: Erlbaum.

Taylor, S. (1995). Anxiety sensitivity: theoretical perspectives and recent findings. *Behaviour Research and Therapy*, **33**, 243–58.

Tellegen, A. (1985). Structures of mood and personality and their relevance to assessing anxiety, with an emphasis on self-report. In A. H. Tuma & J. D. Maser (Eds.), *Anxiety and the anxiety disorders*, pp. 681–706. Hillsdale, NJ: Erlbaum.

Tellegen, A. & Atkinson, G. (1974). Openness to absorbing and self-rating experiences ('absorption'), a trait related to hypnotic susceptibility. *Journal of Abnormal Psychology*, **83**, 268–77.

Temoshok, L. (1987). Personality, coping style, emotion and cancer: towards an integrative model. *Cancer Surveys*, **6**, 545–67.

Temoshok, L., Heller, B.W., Sagebiel, R.W., Blois, M.S., Sweet, D.M., DiClemente, R.J. & Gold, M.L. (1985). The relationship of psychosocial factors to prognostic indicators in cutaneous malignant melanomas. *Journal of Psychosomatic Research*, **29**, 139–53.

TenHouten, W.D., Hoppe, K.D., Bogen, J.E. & Walter, D.O. (1986). Alexithymia: an experimental study of cerebral commissurotomy patients and normal control subjects. *American Journal of Psychiatry*, **143**, 312–16.

Thailer, S.A., Friedman, R., Harshfield, G.A. & Pickering, T.G. (1985). Psychologic differences between high-, normal- and low-renin hypertensives. *Psychosomatic Medicine*, **47**, 294–7.

Thomas, A. & Chess, S. (1977). *Temperament and development*. New York: Brunner/Mazel.

Thomas, C.B., Duszynski, K.R. & Shaffer, J.W. (1979). Family attitudes reported in youth as potential predictors of cancer. *Psychosomatic Medicine*, **41**, 287–302.

Thompson, A.E. (1986). An object-relational theory to affect maturity: applications to the thematic apperception test. In M. Kissen (Ed.), *Assessing object relations phenomena*, pp. 207–24. Madison, CT: International Universities Press.

Thoreson, C.E. & Powell, L.H. (1992). Type A behavior pattern: new perspectives on theory, assessment, and intervention. *Journal of Consulting and Clinical Psychology*, **60**, 595–604.

Todarello, O., Casamassima, A., Daniele, S., Marinaccio, M., Fanciullo, F., Valentino, L., Tedesco, N. Wiesel, S., Simone, G. & Marinaccio, L. (1997). Alexithymia, immunity, and cervical intraepithelial neoplasia: replication. *Psychotherapy and Psychosomatics*, **66**, 208–13.

Todarello, O., Casamassima, A., Marinaccio, M., La Pesa, M.W., Caradonna, L., Valentino, L. & Marinaccio L. (1994). Alexithymia, immunity and cervical intraepithelial neoplasia: a pilot study. *Psychotherapy and Psychosomatics*, **61**, 199–204.

Todarello, O., La Pesa, M.W., Zaka, S., Martino, V. & Lattanzio, E. (1989). Alexithymia and breast cancer. *Psychotherapy and Psychosomatics*, **51**, 51–5.

Todarello, O., Taylor, G.J., Parker, J.D.A. & Fanelli, M. (1995). Alexithymia in essential hypertensive and psychiatric outpatients: a comparative study. *Journal of Psychosomatic Research*, **39**, 987–94.

Tomb, D.A. (1994). The phenomenology of post-traumatic stress disorder. *Psychiatric Clinics of North America*, **17**, 237–50.

Tomkins, S.S. (1962). *Affect/imagery/consciousness. Vol. 1: The positive affects*. New York: Springer.

Tomkins, S.S. (1963). *Affect/imagery/consciousness. Vol. 2: The negative affects*. New York: Springer.

Tomkins, S.S. (1981). The quest for primary motives: biography and autobiography of an idea. *Journal of Personality and Social Psychology*, **41**, 306–29.

Tomkins, S.S. (1984). Affect theory. In K.R. Scherer & P. Ekman (Eds.), *Approaches to emotion*, pp. 163–95. Hillsdale, NJ: Erlbaum.

Toner, B.B., Garfinkel, P.E. Garner, D.M. (1986). Long-term follow-up of anorexia nervosa. *Psychosomatic Medicine*, **48**, 520–9.

Traue, H.C., Gottwald, A., Henderson, P.R. & Bakal, D.A. (1985). Nonverbal expressiveness and EMG activity in tension headache sufferers and controls. *Journal of Psychosomatic Research*, **29**, 375–81.

Treece, C. (1984). Assessment of ego functioning in studies of narcotic addiction. In L. Bellak & L.A. Goldsmith (Eds). *The broad scope of ego function assessment*, pp. 268–90. New York: Wiley.

Triffleman, E.G., Marmar, C.R., Delucchi, K.L. & Ronfeldt, H. (1995). Childhood trauma and posttraumatic stress disorder in substance abuse inpatients. *Journal of Nervous and Mental Disease*, **183**, 172–6.

Turk, D.C. & Salovey, P. (1984). 'Chronic pain as a variant of depressive disease': a critical reappraisal. *Journal of Nervous and Mental Disease*, **172**, 398–404.

Tustin, F. (1981). *Autistic states in children*. London: Routledge & Kegan Paul.

Tustin, F. (1988). Psychotherapy with children who cannot play. *International Review of Psychoanalysis*, **15**, 93–106.

Tyrer, P. (1973). Relevance of bodily feelings in emotion. *The Lancet*, **i**, 915–16.

Tyrer, P., Fowler-Dixon, R., Ferguson, B. & Kelemen, A. (1990). A plea for the diagnosis of hypochondriacal personality disorder. *Journal of Psychosomatic Research*, **34**, 637–42.

Vaillant, G.E. (1971). Theoretical hierarchy of adaptive ego mechanisms. *Archives of General Psychiatry*, **24**, 107–18.

Vaillant, G.E. (1977). *Adaptation to life*. Boston, MA: Little, Brown.

Vaillant, G.E. (1983). *Natural history of alcoholism*. Cambridge, MA: Harvard University Press.

Vaillant, G.E. (1986). *Empirical studies of ego mechanisms of defense*. Washington, DC: American Psychiatric Press.

Vaillant, G.E. (1992). *Ego mechanisms of defense*. Washington, DC: American Psychiatric Press.

Vaillant, G.E. (1993). Is alcoholism more often the cause or the result of depression? *Harvard Review of Psychiatry*, 1, 94–9.

Vaillant, G.E. (1994). Ego mechanisms of defense and personality psychopathology. *Journal of Abnormal Psychology*, 103, 44–50.

van der Kolk, B.A. (1987). The separation cry and the trauma response: developmental issues in the psychobiology of attachment and separation. In B.A. van der Kolk (Ed.), *Psychological trauma*. Washington, DC: American Psychiatric Press.

van der Kolk, B.A. (1993). Biological considerations about emotions, trauma, memory, and the brain. In S.L. Ablon, D. Brown, E.J. Khantzian & J.E. Mack (Eds.), *Human feelings: explorations in affect development and meaning*, pp. 221–40. Hillsdale, NJ: Analytic Press.

van der Kolk, B.A. (1994). The body keeps the score: memory and the evolving psychobiology of posttraumatic stress. *Harvard Review of Psychiatry*, 1, 253–65.

van der Kolk, B.A., Blitz, R., Burr, W., Sherry, S. & Hartmann, E. (1984). Nightmares and trauma: a comparison of nightmares after combat with lifelong nightmares in veterans. *American Journal of Psychiatry*, 141, 187–90.

van der Kolk, B.A. & Greenberg, M.S. (1987). The psychobiology of the trauma response: hyperarousal, constriction, and addiction to traumatic re-exposure. In B.A. van der Kolk (Ed.), *Psychological trauma*, pp. 63–87. Washington, DC: American Psychiatric Press.

van der Kolk, B.A., Hostetler, A., Herron, N. & Fisler, R.E. (1994). Trauma and the development of borderline personality disorder. *Psychiatric Clinics of North America*, 17, 715–30.

van der Kolk, B.A. & van der Hart, O. (1989). Pierre Janet and the breakdown of adaptation in psychological trauma. *American Journal of Psychiatry*, 146, 1530–40.

Vassend, O. (1987). Personality, imaginative involvement, and self-reported somatic complaints: relevance to the concept of alexithymia. *Psychotherapy and Psychosomatics*, 47, 74–81.

Virchow, R. (1858). *Cellular pathology* (Trans. F. Chance). New York: De Witt.

Voeller, K.S. (1986). Right-hemisphere deficit syndrome in children. *American Journal of Psychiatry*, 143, 1004–9.

Voeller, K.S., Hanson, J.A. & Wendt, R.N. (1988). Facial affect recognition in children: a comparison of the performance of children with right and left hemisphere lesions. *Neurology*, 38, 1744–8.

Vogt, R., Burckstummer, G., Ernst, L., Meyer, K. & von Rad, M. (1977). Differences in phantasy life of psychosomatic and psychoneurotic patients. *Psychotherapy and Psychosomatics*, 28, 98–105.

Vollhardt, B.R., Ackerman, S.H., Grayzel, A.I. & Barland, P. (1982). Psychologically distinguishable groups of rheumatoid arthritis patients: a controlled, single blind study. *Psychosomatic Medicine*, **44**, 353–62.

Vollhardt, B.R., Ackerman, S.H. & Shindledecker, R.D. (1986). Verbal expression of affect in rheumatoid arthritis patients: a blind, controlled test for alexithymia. *Acta Psychiatrica Scandinavica*, **74**, 73–9.

von Rad, M., Lalucat, L. & Lolas, F. (1977). Differences of verbal behaviour in psychosomatic and psychoneurotic patients. *Psychotherapy and Psychosomatics*, **28**, 83–97.

Waelder, R. (1967). Inhibitions, symptoms and anxiety: forty years later. *Psychoanalytic Quarterly*, **36**, 1–36.

Walker, E., Katon, W., Harrop-Griffiths, J., Holm, L., Russo, J. & Hickok, L.R. (1988). Relationship of chronic pelvic pain to psychiatric diagnoses and childhood sexual abuse. *American Journal of Psychiatry*, **145**, 75–80.

Walker, E., Katon, W., Neraas, K., Jemelka, R.P. & Massoth, D. (1992). Dissociation in women with chronic pelvic pain. *American Journal of Psychiatry*, **149**, 534–7.

Walker, E.A., Roy-Byrne, P.P. & Katon, W.J. (1990). Irritable bowel syndrome and psychiatric illness. *American Journal of Psychiatry*, **147**, 565–72.

Wallace, E.R. (1988a). Mind–body. Monistic dual aspect interactionism. *Journal of Nervous and Mental Disease*, **176**, 4–21.

Wallace, E.R. (1988b). What is 'truth'? Some philosophical contributions to psychiatric issues. *American Journal of Psychiatry*, **145**, 137–47.

Wallach, J.D. & Lowenkopf, E.L. (1984). Five bulimic women. *International Journal of Eating Disorders*, **3**, 53–66.

Waller, J.V., Kauffman, R.M. & Deutsch, F. (1940). Anorexia nervosa: a psychosomatic entity. *Psychosomatic Medicine*, **2**, 3–16.

Walsh, B.T. (1991). Fluoxetine treatment of bulimia nervosa. *Journal of Psychosomatic Research*, **35** (Suppl. 1), 33–40.

Walsh, B.T., Steward, J.W., Wright, L., Harrison, W., Roose, S.P. & Glassman, A.H. (1982). Treatment of bulimia with monoamine oxidase inhibitors. *American Journal of Psychiatry*, **139**, 1629–30.

Warnes, H. (1985). Alexithymia and the grieving process. *Psychiatric Journal of the University of Ottawa*, **10**, 41–4.

Watson, D. (1991). Theoretical and psychometric issues in the study of somatic amplification. Unpublished manuscript, Department of Psychology, The University of Iowa, Iowa City, Iowa.

Watson, D. & Clark, L.A. (1984). Negative affectivity: the disposition to experience aversive emotional states. *Psychological Bulletin*, **96**, 465–90.

Watson, D. & Clark, L.A. (1991). *The PANAS-X: preliminary manual for the Positive and Negative Affect Schedule – Expanded Form*. Dallas, TX: Southern Methodist University.

Watson, D. & Clark, L.A. (1992). On traits and temperament: general and specific factors of emotional experience and their relation to the five-factor model. *Journal of Personality*, **60**, 441–76.

Watson, D. & Clark, L.A. (1993). Behavioral disinhibition versus constraint: a dispositional perspective. In D.M. Wegner & J.W. Pennebaker (Eds.), *Handbook of mental control*, pp. 506–27. New York: Prentice-Hall.

Watson, D. & Clark, L.A. (1994). Emotions, moods, traits, and temperaments: conceptual distinctions and empirical findings. In P. Ekman, & R.J. Davidson (Eds.), *The nature of emotion: fundamental questions*, pp. 89–96. New York: Oxford University Press.

Watson, D., Clark, L.A. & Carey, G. (1988). Positive and negative affectivity and their relation to anxiety and depressive disorders. *Journal of Abnormal Psychology*, **97**, 346–53.

Watson, D., Clark, L.A. & Harkness, A.R. (1994). Structures of personality and their relevance to psychopathology. *Journal of Abnormal Psychology*, **103**, 18–31.

Watson, D., Clark, L.A. & Tellegen, A. (1988). Development and validation of brief measures of positive and negative affect: the PANAS scales. *Journal of Personality and Social Psychology*, **54**, 1063–70.

Watson, D. & Tellegen, A. (1985). Toward a consensual structure of mood. *Psychological Bulletin*, **98**, 219–35.

Weich, M.J. (1978). Transitional language. In S.A. Grolnick, L. Barkin & W. Muensterberger (Eds.), *Between reality and fantasy: transitional objects and phenomena*, pp. 411–23. New York: Aronson.

Weidner, G., Friend, R., Ficarrotto, T.J. & Mendell, N.R. (1989). Hostility and cardiovascular reactivity to stress in women and men. *Psychosomatic Medicine*, **51**, 36–45.

Weidner, G., Sexton, G., McLennarn, R., Connor, S.L. & Matarazzo, J.D. (1987). The role of Type A behavior and hostility in an elevation of plasma lipids in adult women and men. *Psychosomatic Medicine*, **49**, 136–45.

Weiner, H. (1977). *Psychobiology and human disease*. New York: Elsevier.

Weiner, H. (1982). The prospects for psychosomatic medicine: selected topics. *Psychosomatic Medicine*, **44**, 491–517.

Weiner, H. (1984). What the future holds for psychosomatic medicine. *Psychotherapy and Psychosomatics*, **42**, 15–25.

Weiner, H. (1987). Some unexplored regions of psychosomatic medicine. *Psychotherapy and Psychosomatis*, **47**, 153–9.

Weiner, H. (1989). The dynamics of the organism: implications of recent biological thought for psychosomatic theory and research. *Psychosomatic Medicine*, **51**, 608–35.

Weiner, H. (1992). Specificity and specification: two continuing problems in psychosomatic research. *Psychosomatic Medicine*, **54**, 567–87.

Weiner, H. (in press). Psychosomatic medicine and the mind–body problem in psychiatry. In E.R. Wallace IV & J. Gach (Eds.), *The handbook of the history of psychiatry*. New Haven: Yale University Press.

Weiner, H. & Fawzy, F. (1989). An integrative model of health, disease, and illness. In S. Cheren (Ed.), *Psychosomatic medicine: theory, physiology and practice*, vol. 1, pp. 9–44. Madison, CT: International Universities Press.

Weiner, H., Thaler, M., Reiser, M.F. & Mirsky, I.A. (1957). Etiology of duodenal ulcer: I. Relation of specific psychological characteristics to rate of gastric secretion (serum pepsinogen). *Psychosomatic Medicine*, **19**, 1–10.

Weintraub, S. & Mesulam, M.M. (1983). Developmental learning disabilities of the right hemisphere. *Archives of Neurology*, **40**, 463–8.

Weintraub, S., Mesulam, M.M. & Kramer, L. (1981). Disturbances in prosody: a right-hemisphere contribution to language. *Archives of Neurology*, **38**, 742–4.

Weiss, K.J. & Rosenberg, D.J. (1985). Prevalence of anxiety disorder among alcoholics. *Journal of Clinical Psychiatry*, **46**, 3–5.

Weissman, M.M., Klerman, G.L., Markowitz, J. & Pihl, R.O.M. (1989). Suicidal ideation and suicide attempts in panic disorder and attacks. *New England Journal of Medicine*, **321**, 1209–14.

Welch, G., Hall, A. & Norring, C. (1990). The factor structure of the eating disorder inventory in a patient setting. *International Journal of Eating Disorders*, **9**, 79–85.

Werner, H. & Kaplan, B. (1963). *Symbol formation: an organismic-developmental approach to language and the expression of thought*. New York: Wiley.

West, M.L. & Sheldon-Keller, A.E. (1994). *Patterns of relating: an adult attachment perspective*. New York: Guilford.

White, R.W. (1974). Strategies of adaptation: an attempt at systematic description. In G.V. Coelho, D.A. Hamburg, & J.E. Adams (Eds.), *Coping and adaptation*, pp. 47–68. New York: Basic Books.

Wickramasekera, I. (1986). A model of people at high risk to develop chronic stress-related somatic symptoms: some predictions. *Professional Psychology: Research and Practice*, **17**, 437–47.

Wickramasekera, I. (1989). Somatizers, the health care system, and collapsing the psychological distance that the somatizer has to travel for help. *Professional Psychology: Research and Practice*, **20**, 105–11.

Wickramasekera, I. (1995). Somatization: concepts, data, and predictions from the high risk model of threat perception. *Journal of Nervous and Mental Disease*, **183**, 15–23.

Wieder, H. & Kaplan, E.H. (1969). Drug use in adolescents: psychodynamic meaning among alcoholics. *Psychoanalytic Study of the Child*, **24**, 399–431.

Wiggins, J.S. (1973). *Personality and prediction: principles of personality assessment*. Reading, MA: Addison-Wesley.

Williams, R.B. (1994). Neurobiology, cellular and molecular biology, and psychosomatic medicine. *Psychosomatic Medicine*, **56**, 308-15.

Williams, R.B., Jr., Haney, T.L., Lee, K.L., Kong, Y., Blumenthal, J. & Whalen, R. (1980). Type A behavior, hostility, and coronary atherosclerosis. *Psychosomatic Medicine*, **42**, 539-49.

Williams, R.B., Jr., Suarez, E. C., Kuhn, C. M., Zimmerman, E. A. & Schanberg, S. M. (1991). Biobehavioral basis of coronary-prone behavior in middle-aged men. Part I: Evidence for chronic SNS activation in Type As. *Psychosomatic Medicine*, **53**, 517-27.

Wilson, A., Passik, S.D. & Faude, J.P. (1990). Self-regulation and its failures. In J. Masling (Ed.), *Empirical studies of psychoanalytic theories*, vol. 3, pp. 149-213. Hillsdale, NJ: Analytic Press.

Wilson, A., Passik, S.D., Faude, J., Abrams, J. & Gordon, E. (1989). A hierarchical model of opiate addiction. Failures of self-regulation as a central aspect of substance abuse. *Journal of Nervous and Mental Disease*, **177**, 390-9.

Wilson, C.P., Hogan, C.C. & Mintz, I.L. (Eds.) (1985). *Fear of being fat: the treatment of anorexia nervosa and bulimia* (rev. ed.). Northvale, NJ: Aronson.

Wilson, C.P. & Mintz, I.L. (Eds.) (1989). *Psychosomatic symptoms: psychodynamic treatment of the underlying personality disorder*. Northvale, NJ: Aronson.

Winnicott, D.W. (1935). The manic defense. In *Collected papers: through paediatrics to psychoanalysis*, pp. 194-203. New York: Basic Books, 1958.

Winnicott, D.W. (1952). Psychoses and child care. In: *Collected papers: through paediatrics to psychoanalysis*, pp. 219-28. New York: Basic Books, 1958.

Winnicott, D.W. (1953). Transitional objects and transitional phenomena. *International Journal of Psychoanalysis*, **34**, 89-97.

Wise, T.N. & Mann, L.S. (1994). The relationship between somatosensory amplification, alexithymia, and neuroticism. *Journal of Psychosomatic Research*, **38**, 515-21.

Wise, T.N., Mann, L.S. & Epstein, S. (1991). Ego defense styles and alexithymia: a discriminant validation study. *Psychotherapy and Psychosomatics*, **56**, 141-5.

Wise, T.N., Mann, L.S. & Shay, L. (1992). Alexithymia and the five-factor model of personality. *Comprehensive Psychiatry*, **33**, 147-51.

Witelson, S.F. (1995). Neuroanatomical bases of hemispheric functional specialization in the human brain: possible developmental factors. In F.L. Kitterle (Ed.), *Hemispheric communication: mechanisms and models*, pp. 61-84. Hillsdale, NJ: Erlbaum.

Wolff, H.H. (1977). The contribution of the interview situation to the restriction of phantasy life and emotional experience in psychosomatic patients. *Psychotherapy and Psychosomatics*, **28**, 58–67.

Wonderlich, S.A., Fullerton, D., Swift, W.J. & Klein, M.H. (1994). Five-year outcome from eating disorders: relevance of personality disorders. *International Journal of Eating Disorders*, **15**, 133–243.

Woods, S.W. (1992). Regional cerebral blood flow imaging with SPECT in psychiatric disease: focus on schizophrenia, anxiety disorders, and substance abuse. *Journal of Clinical Psychiatry*, **53**, 20–5.

World Health Organization (1992). *International classification of diseases* (10th rev.).

Wright, T. (1601). *The passions of the minde in generalle*. London: Burre.

Wurmser, L. (1974). Psychoanalytic considerations of the etiology of compulsive drug use. *Journal of the American Psychoanalytic Association*, **22**, 820–41.

Wurmser, L. (1978). *The hidden dimension*. New York: Aronson.

Wurmser, L. (1984). More respect for the neurotic process: comments on the problem of narcissism in severe psychopathology, especially the addictions. *Journal of Substance Abuse Treatment*, **1**, 37–45.

Yates, A., Leehey, K. & Shisslak, C.M. (1983). Running – an analogue of anorexia? *New England Journal of Medicine*, **308**, 251–5.

Yehuda, R., Kahana, B., Binder-Brynes, K., Southwick, S.M., Mason, J.W. & Giller, E.L. (1995). Low urinary cortisol excretion in Holocaust survivors with posttraumatic stress disorder. *American Journal of Psychiatry*, **152**, 982–6.

Yelsma, P. (1992). Affective orientations associated with couples' verbal abusiveness. Paper presented at the 6th International Conference on Personal Relationships, Orono, Maine.

Yelsma, P. (1996). Affective orientations of perpetrators, victims, and functional spouses. *Journal of Interpersonal Violence*, **11**, 141–61.

Yeragani, V.K., Meiri, P.C., Balon, R., Patel, H. & Pohl, R. (1989). History of separation anxiety in patients with panic disorder and depression and normal controls. *Acta Psychiatrica Scandinavica*, **79**, 550–6.

Young, A.W. (1986). Subject characteristics in lateral differences for face processing by normals: age. In R. Bruyer (Ed.), *The neuropsychology of face perception and facial expression*, pp. 167–200. Hillsdale, NJ: Erlbaum.

Zajonc, R.B. (1984). On the primacy of affect. *American Psychologist*, **39**, 117–23.

Zalidis, S. (1994). Handling hyperventilation in general practice. *Journal of the Balint Society*, **22**, 1–14. London: Haverstock.

Zayfert, C., McCracken, L.M. & Gross, R.T. (1992). Alexithymia, disability, and emotional distress in chronic non-malignant pain. Paper presented at the 50th Anniversary Meeting of the American Psychosomatic Society, New York, April 1992.

Zeitlin, S.B., Lane, R.D., O'Leary, D.S. & Schrift, M.J. (1989). Interhemispheric transfer deficit and alexithymia. *American Journal of Psychiatry*, **146**, 1434–39.

Zeitlin, S.B. & McNally, R.J. (1993). Alexithymia and anxiety sensitivity in panic disorder and obsessive–compulsive disorder. *American Journal of Psychiatry*, **150**, 658–60.

Zeitlin, S.B., McNally, R.J. & Cassiday, K.L. (1993). Alexithymia in victims of sexual assault: an effect of repeated traumatization? *American Journal of Psychiatry*, **150**, 661–3.

Zerbe, K.J. (1992). Eating disorders in the 1990's: clinical challenges and treatment implications. *Bulletin of the Menninger Clinic*, **56**, 167–87.

Zerbe, K.J. (1993). Whose body is it anyway? Understanding and treating psychosomatic aspects of eating disorders. *Bulletin of the Menninger Clinic*, **57**, 161–77.

Ziółkowski, M., Gruss, T. & Rybakowski, J.K. (1995). Does alexithymia in male alcoholics constitute a negative factor for maintaining abstinence? *Psychotherapy and Psychosomatics*, **63**, 169–73.

Zuckerman, M. (1991). *Psychobiology of personality*. New York: Cambridge University Press.

Zuckerman, M. (1992). What is a basic factor and which factors are basic? Turtles all the way down. *Personality and Individual Differences*, **13**, 675–81.

Zuckerman, M., Kuhlman, D.M. & Camac, C. (1988). What lies beyond E and N? Factor analyses of scales believed to measure basic dimensions of personality. *Journal of Personality and Social Psychology*, **54**, 96–107.

# Index

Printed in the United States
70959LV00003B/70-81